The

Paleovation

Workbook

For Kelsey —
Cheers to happiness
& good health! All the
best in your career
— Kelly

A Daily Workbook to Reclaim Health and Vitality

Kelly C. Andrews, DC   ◆   Rachel D. Carlson, BS, RYT

ISBN-10: 1542822289

ISBN-13: 978-1542822282

The information presented as well as ideas, concepts and opinions expressed in this book are intended to be used for educational purposes only. This book is intended to supplement, not replace, the advice of a trained health professional. The reader should always consult his or her healthcare provider to determine the appropriateness of the information for their own situation or if they have any questions regarding a medical condition or treatment plan. The authors and publisher of this instructional book specifically disclaim any liability, loss, or risk, personal or otherwise, that is incurred or alleged to be incurred as a consequence, directly or indirectly, of the use, application or interpretation of any of the contents of this book. Reading the information in this book does not create a physician-patient relationship.

The authors are not responsible for websites, books, podcasts or videos (or their content) that are not of their ownership.

Several websites and authors are cited repeatedly. However, there are many quality websites not referenced and were not neglected due to content. The choice of website recommendations was based on the likelihood that the information would be available online long-term.

Book cover design by Anna Goebel, FreestyleGraphicDesign.com
Illustrations by Zak Jones, ZakMonster@hotmail.com
Back cover photo by Tony Packard
Front cover photos courtesy of Flickr creative commons

Published by:

Paleovation, LLC
Paleovation.com

Quantity discounts available for educational and promotional purposes. Email: BulkOrder@Paleovation.com

FOR YOU, OUR READER

The Paleovation Workbook is dedicated to those who are ready to
receive the gift of good health, whether this book is a gift to yourself
or you received it as a gift from another.

Is the Paleo Diet perfect for everyone?
Think of it this way – it's the perfect place to start on the path to better health.

TABLE OF CONTENTS

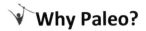 Why Paleo?

Our ancestors evolved and thrived on a "hunter-gatherer" diet which, in today's lingo, is commonly referred to as the Paleo Diet. But Paleo is more than just a diet, it's an entire lifestyle. Here are the basic principles:

Paleo Components	
Anti-Inflammatory Diet	**Healthy Lifestyle Factors**
✓ Eat a wide variety of minimally-processed, whole foods ✓ Avoid foods that cause inflammation ✓ Identify foods that are personally well-tolerated	✓ Exercise Sensibly ✓ Prioritize Sleep ✓ Minimize Stress

Perhaps you've already heard good things about Paleo or perhaps the Paleo concept is new to you. Regardless, even a brief examination of the Paleo Lifestyle reveals the amazing health benefits and improvements it offers:

- Quality sleep
- Weight regulation
- Joint fluidity
- Exercise recovery
- Enhanced focus
- Stronger bones
- Muscle flexibility
- Lower body fat
- Higher energy levels
- Clearer skin
- Reduced allergies
- Pacified old injury
- Improved digestion
- Better moods
- Normalized lipid panels
- Fewer aches and pains

It's also quickly apparent that there's no lack of Paleo information – books, websites, testimonials, cookbooks, podcasts and videos abound. In fact, there are so many Paleo resources that it can overwhelm or delay getting started! Where can I find easy-to-read information? What is the bottom line? Where do I begin? What about the naysayers? How will I implement Paleo long-term? Is there a simple way to stay on track?

Questions like these inspired *The Paleovation Workbook*. Our goal is to educate and assist people during the Paleo transition. This book will guide you through your first month, one day at a time, detailing the *how's* for effective implementation and explaining the *why's* (or *wise*) to support educated choices for long-term success. At the end of the month, we teach you to carefully reintroduce the eliminated foods to test personal tolerance.

Modern Health Decline

The prevalent processed and manufactured foods of recent generations are simply incompatible with our digestive systems. Because we are eating genetically-incompatible foods, modern dietary rules don't work: the 'mainstream' lifestyle suggestions below have not improved the growing rates of chronic disease and obesity.

- ✓ Increased exercise and consumption of fresh vegetables
- ✓ Reduced intake of salt, red meats and animal fats
- ✓ Consuming foods labeled *gluten-free, whole grain, low-fat, low-cholesterol, enriched, fortified* or *high fiber*

Modern health decline has transpired over several generations. Unfortunately, this means that marginal health has gradually been accepted as "normal" and is often blamed on external, uncontrollable factors:

- ☐ Aging
- ☐ Genetics
- ☐ Weather
- ☐ Germs
- ☐ Personal susceptibility
- ☐ Bad luck

Moreover, we are taught that pills are the solution to managing health problems, not what we eat. The reality is that food eaten in modern cultures has significantly deviated from the natural human diet. The following dietary practices have produced an inflamed, achy, fatigued, undernourished, overweight, disease-prone population:

- Manufactured pseudo-foods never found in nature such as high fructose corn syrup, canola oil or trans fat
- Chemical-laden foods containing preservatives, colorings, flavor enhancers or herbicide/pesticide residues
- Products from sick, confined animals fed antibiotics and hormones
- Preference for convenient products, fast food restaurants, meals from a box or meal replacement shakes
- Easy access to food, especially sweets and starches

> **Key Point:** Poor health is a result of nutritional problems. Our bodies are literally rejecting contemporary foods. No one should have to play victim to a diet that makes them unhealthy, fat and depressed. Paleo is a *solution*. Paleo is not just a diet – it's a *way of living* that promotes optimal health using human ancestry as a guideline.

⋎ **How to Use this Book**

This book is *your* guidebook – use it in ways most beneficial for you (starting now!). Circle your favorite ideas:

- Dog-ear pages
- Use sticky notes / flags
- Fill out relevant quizzes
- Tear out resource pages

- Write in the margins
- Go back and review
- Add additional journal pages
- Collaborate with a friend

- Highlight the reading
- Color code your notes
- Skip ahead to another topic
- Just skim and reflect

Each guided day includes a succinct reading section to boost your Paleo knowledge as well as daily goals, implementation strategies, activities, recipe suggestions and upcoming preparation. The text is designed to be easily scanned with topic headers, short paragraphs, bullet points, charts, graphics and key ideas in boxes. Expect each day to take between 30-45 minutes to read and complete.

Paleo-Wise Reading Sections

Quite literally, these are the Paleo *Whys*. To explain the basics of why the Paleo Diet and Lifestyle maximize health, we have selected the most significant points from the most pertinent topics. These are presented in daily snippets and often contain references to other Paleo resources for supplemental reading.

To provide the groundwork and basic understanding of the Paleo Diet, the beginning of the program requires a higher concentration of Paleo-Wise information. These sections taper down through the workbook.

Cooking Assistance

To expand your culinary repertoire, five Cooking Assignments are detailed during the program, roughly once per week. These Paleo staple recipes are in addition to regular meal preparation and provide home-made versions of *basic* foods that are either difficult to find or expensive to purchase. For those who can't or simply don't want to participate in those, other options are provided.

A *few* Paleo foundation recipes are located in the Resource Section. Due to individual variations in taste preferences and food tolerances, all other recipes will be your responsibility. Do not worry, a handful of recipes is enough to start the program and multiple suggestions are interspersed throughout the daily pages. Successful implementation of the Paleo Diet requires being flexible and self-sufficient...we'll point you in the right direction so you can build a personalized collection of favorite recipes and resources.

Further Reading / Viewing References (all available as direct links from **www.Paleovation.com**)

- ⌐ᵻ **Websites:** Online articles are designated with a mouse icon ⌐ᵻ, lighter text and underlined website. For example: ⌐ᵻ BalancedBites Fresh Blueberry Crumble. To locate the direct link, type: "balancedbites fresh blueberry crumble" (without the quotes) in your favorite search engine.
- 📖 **Books:** Designated with a book icon 📖 and italicized title.
- ⊛ **Videos or Movies:** Designated with a movie reel icon ⊛ and title.

Preparation Section

The preparation period is split into seven segments, A - G, to create a "week" of groundwork. However, this is a hypothetical timeframe. Actual prep time is variable with some being ready in just a day, while others require the full seven days. If you choose to quickly complete the prep portion, please read *all* Paleo-Wise sections in Prep A - G. This information supports conscious, educated dietary choices rather than reverting to old habits.

The Paleovation Workbook is designed to follow a Strict Paleo Protocol which admittedly, can be difficult during holidays or vacations. Therefore, success may improve by delaying your start date until after those obligations are satisfied. In the meantime, consider implementing dietary baby steps described here:

⌐ᵻ Paleovation Baby Steps.

Resource Section

Additional material such as the Group Manual, summary guides, extra copies of charts, key graphics, recipe suggestions, nutritional supplement information and more are located at the back of the book.

The Benefits of Strict Paleo for a Month

A stressed, sick and fatigued body desperately needs a period of rest. This is what a detox/elimination diet is designed to do. Just one month eating a disciplined anti-inflammatory diet jumpstarts your personal health transformation, prompting your body to heal, rebuild and quickly transition from relying on sugar for energy to becoming a fat-burner. Additionally, you will develop lifestyle habits that set the stage for long-term success:

- ➤ Incorporate nutrient-dense foods that minimize hunger and sugar cravings
- ➤ Create new go-to recipes
- ➤ Learn how to identify and shop for anti-inflammatory foods
- ➤ Formulate a plan for restaurants and other social situations
- ➤ Identify personal trigger foods which are not compatible with your digestive system
- ➤ Experiment with and develop long-range strategies for permanent dietary change

> It's beyond amazing how just a few weeks eating the Strict Paleo Protocol reduces *decades of damage* from an unhealthy diet!

Recommended Reading

The world of Paleo is loaded with people who were dissatisfied with their health and had difficulty finding appropriate medical treatment; they eventually decided that the Standard American Diet (even a healthy version of it) was to blame, then wrote about their success. Because it takes a leap of faith to give up staples like "healthy" whole grains or to eat more Paleo-friendly fats, it might be helpful and inspirational to peruse similar elimination-style diet books (additional book recommendations available at ⌐ Paleovation).

Suggestion: Library systems have many Paleo Diet and Lifestyle books available. Contact your library to have a cookbook on hand throughout our program.

Again, there is no shortage of Paleo information. This small sample of popular books offers some direction, but is certainly not exclusive. Feel free to use your preferred Paleo resources. Direct links to all recommendations at ⌐ Paleovation.

Elimination-Diet Books:
- 📖 *It Starts with Food,* by Melissa Hartwig and Dallas Hartwig
- 📖 *21-Day Sugar Detox,* by Dianne Sanfilippo, BS, NC
- 📖 *The Wahls Protocol,* by Terry Wahls, MD
- 📖 *The Paleo Cure* or *Your Personal Paleo Code,* by Chris Kresser
- 📖 *The Autoimmune Solution,* by Amy Myers, MD
- 📖 *The Hormone Reset Diet,* by Sarah Gottfried, MD
- 📖 *The Bulletproof Diet,* by Dave Asprey
- 📖 *Wired to Eat,* by Robb Wolf

Cookbooks (you still need to watch for added sugars):
- 📖 *Practical Paleo,* by Dianne Sanfilippo, BS, NC, and Robb Wolf
- 📖 *Well Fed,* and *Well Fed 2,* by Melissa Joulwan
- 📖 *21-Day Sugar Detox Cookbook,* by Dianne Sanfilippo, BS, NC
- 📖 *The Whole30,* by Melissa Hartwig and Dallas Hartwig
- 📖 *Against All Grain,* by Danielle Walker
- 📖 *Paleo Perfected: A Revolution in Eating Well,* by America's Test Kitchen
- 📖 *Everyday Paleo,* by Sarah Fragoso

Specialty Topic Cookbooks (you still need to watch for added sugars):
- 📖 *Make Ahead Paleo,* by Tammy Credicott
- 📖 *Frugal Paleo,* by Ciarra Hannah
- 📖 *Paleo Comfort Foods,* by Julie and Charles Mayfield
- 📖 *Paleo Meal Planning on a Budget,* by Elizabeth McGaw
- 📖 *Ready or Not: 150 Make-Ahead, Make-Over and Make-Now Recipes,* by Michelle Tam and Henry Fong

---

✦ Master Preparation Checklist (use with Prep A-G)

Flag /dog-ear this page. Return often to check off completed tasks and monitor preparation progress:

- ☐ Located copies of Paleo cookbooks or placed library requests (optional)
- ☐ Kitchen emptied of non-Paleo foods
- ☐ Kitchen stocked with Paleo-friendly foods
- ☐ Found 5 Foundation Recipes and stocked ingredients
- ☐ Invited a friend to join you (Group Manual in the Resource Section)
- ☐ Pre-Paleo Check-in Form completed and scored
- ☐ Body Metrics Form completed
- ☐ Preliminary lab work completed (optional)
- ☐ Fresh cut veggies are stocked in the fridge
- ☐ Freezer or fridge have prepared meals
- ☐ Craving and withdrawal strategies are handy
- ☐ Prepared strategies for a grouchy day
- ☐ Bones purchased for Bone Broth Cooking Assignment
- ☐ Discussed anti-inflammatory eating with healthcare professional (optional)
- ☐ Discussed current medical treatment plans with healthcare provider (required)
- ☐ Eating Plan for Outside-of-the-Home completed (travel, social situations, etc)

Building Your Paleo Foundation

Track Your Paleo Protocol Progress

Use the calendar on the next page to X off your Paleo progress through the program. Fill in the boxes as follows:

1. In the small boxes, write the calendar dates.
2. In the larger area, record numbers 1-28 to identify the 28 days of the Strict Paleo Protocol.
3. Deadlines for Cooking Assignments may be marked on the following days:
   - ➢ Before you begin – Batch cook at least one recipe
   - ➢ Day 3 – Bone Broth
   - ➢ Day 7 – Paleo Mayo
   - ➢ Day 10 – Paleo Comfort Food (optional)
   - ➢ Day 12 – Veggie as a Grain Substitute
   - ➢ Day 19 – Paleo Jerky *or* Paleo Granola
   - ➢ Day 23 – Roast a Whole Chicken

EXAMPLE - PALEO PROGRESS

Sunday	Monday	Tuesday	Wednesday	Thursday	Friday	Saturday
20	21	22 Batch cook a recipe or two	23 ⊠1	24 ⊠2	25 ~~Bone broth~~ ⊠3	26 ⊠4
27 ⊠5	28 6	29 Mayo 7	30 8	31 9	1 Optional 10	2 11
3	4	5	6	7	8	9

Tear out / copy the following calendar. Place inside the front or back cover or magnet to your fridge.

⚡ *The Paleovation Workbook*

Success is no accident. It is hard work, perseverance, learning, studying, sacrifice and most of all, love of what you are doing or learning to do. ~Pelé

PALEO PROGRESS

Sunday	Monday	Tuesday	Wednesday	Thursday	Friday	Saturday

Cooking Assignment deadlines may be marked on the following days:

☐ Before you begin – Batch cook at least one recipe
☐ Day 3 – Bone Broth
☐ Day 7 – Paleo Mayo
☐ Day 10 – Paleo Comfort Food (optional)

☐ Day 12 –Veggie as a Grain Substitute
☐ Day 19 – Paleo Jerky *or* Paleo Granola
☐ Day 23 – Roast a Whole Chicken

The best preparation for tomorrow is doing your best today. ~H. Jackson Brown, Jr

Additional notes or inspiration:

_____

_____

_____

~ This page intentionally left blank ~

Prep A

Today's Topics:
1. Paleo-Wise: Chronic Inflammation Causes Disease
2. How is Chronic Inflammation Affecting You?
3. Foods that Contribute to Chronic Inflammation
4. Kitchen Cleanout: Remove Inflammatory Foods from Your Kitchen

Section I – Paleo-Wise: **Chronic Inflammation Causes Disease**

When the body becomes stressed from an outside stimulus or foreign invader, our immune system reacts with a series of physical symptoms designed to fight, neutralize, then heal any damage incurred in the process. These reactions evolved as a natural defense mechanism for bodily protection and preservation.

Acute Inflammation – Ouch!
Acute inflammation is the initial response to a harmful stimulus like a cut, burn, sprain or insect bite. The body wisely responds with bruising, pain, itching, heat, swelling and loss of function.
- ➤ *Swelling* **Creates Quarantine:** a thick barricade of inflammatory tissue prevents exposure to infection, the spreading of an invading substance, and/or blood loss
- ➤ *Inflammation* **Triggers Pain:** a protective mechanism to reduce use of the injured area while the body actively repairs the damage

Acute inflammation is a short-term process, usually appearing within a few minutes or hours of exposure and dissipating as the body gradually eliminates the source of harm.

Chronic Inflammation = Gradual Deterioration
It's easy to explain *acute inflammation* because we visually and physically observe its symptoms. On the contrary, *chronic inflammation* happens deep inside the body, invisible to external senses – and because we don't see it occur, we rarely connect the dots between its symptoms and the original triggers.

Any irritant we consume or absorb can elicit a subtle, minor immune response. However, regular exposures to irritants gradually inundate the body's healing capacity. These minor inflammatory responses accumulate and fester like hundreds of smoldering embers. Our bodies harbor decades of these exposures, one on top of the next, that slowly deteriorate bodily structures and disrupt major functions. Without a proper chance to heal, the damage intensifies, inflammation creeps through the system and the continual assault eventually produces symptoms of chronic disease.

New Variety of Invaders
Historically, foreign stimuli included items such as splinters, bacteria, viruses, plant toxins or venom. However, in our modern world, the range of what the body perceives as 'foreign invaders' has exponentially exploded:
- ➤ Foods high in sugar, starches and processed fats
- ➤ Manufactured/processed chemicals in foods and personal care or household products
- ➤ Prescription and over-the-counter medications
- ➤ Air pollutants, heavy metals, PCBs, plastics

These modern contaminants repeatedly stress the immune system and trigger inflammatory responses. Not only do these exposures contribute to cumulative damage from inflammation, they can accelerate the process!

You're Not Just Getting Old!
The warning signs of chronic inflammation have manifested insidiously and are so widespread that they have been *accepted as normal aging!* Common indicators of chronic inflammation include aches, pains, weight gain, low energy levels, insomnia, arthritis, brain fog and other characteristics that surface in aging populations.

> **Key Point:** Just because symptoms are common does *not* mean they are normal!

Chronic inflammation is the beginning of a downward spiral that can lead to serious metabolic breakdown and is *a proven risk factor* for a host of chronic diseases. Mark an "x" on those that apply to you:

- ☐ Diabetes
- ☐ Metabolic Syndrome X
- ☐ GERD / Heartburn
- ☐ Diverticulitis
- ☐ Gastritis
- ☐ Gall Stones
- ☐ Colitis
- ☐ Irritable Bowel Syndrome
- ☐ Crohn's Disease
- ☐ Arthritis
- ☐ Osteoarthritis
- ☐ PMS
- ☐ Menopause Symptoms

- ☐ Osteoporosis
- ☐ Cancer
- ☐ Asthma
- ☐ Allergies
- ☐ Bronchitis
- ☐ Acne
- ☐ Eczema / Psoriasis / Dermatitis
- ☐ Depression
- ☐ Anxiety
- ☐ Alzheimer's / Dementia
- ☐ Parkinson's Disease
- ☐ Multiple Sclerosis
- ☐ Infertility

- ☐ Rheumatoid Arthritis
- ☐ Gout
- ☐ Obesity
- ☐ Low Testosterone
- ☐ Hypothyroid
- ☐ High Blood Pressure
- ☐ Heart Disease
- ☐ Peripheral Vascular Disease
- ☐ Stroke
- ☐ Kidney Stones
- ☐ Macular Degeneration
- ☐ Gingivitis / Tooth Decay
- ☐ Stomach Ulcers

> **Key Point:** Chronic inflammation is an *underlying cause of chronic disease*!

Section II: How is Chronic Inflammation Affecting You?

What is your body currently telling you about your overall health? Analyze this list of symptoms linked to chronic inflammation and mark an "x" on all that apply to you.

X	Symptoms of Chronic Inflammation
	Chronic aches and pains – sore muscles, achy joints, back or neck pain, headaches
	Mood swings, irritability, anxiety/depression
	Difficulty losing weight
	Low or erratic energy levels, such as a usual afternoon slump
	Difficulty recovering from physical activity
	Seasonal allergies, phlegm build up, itchy/waxy ears
	Bloating, diarrhea, constipation, irritable bowel syndrome
	Aged appearance
	Diminished range of motion
	Brittle nails or cracking skin
	Regular need for anti-inflammatory medications such as ibuprofen, acetaminophen or other over-the-counter drugs; or prescriptions anti-inflammatory steroid medications
	Difficulty remembering or concentrating
	Cravings for sweet foods or grain-based foods
	Difficulty healing from injury or overuse
	Insomnia
	Weight-gain around the waist
	Low immune system often fighting a cold
	Suffering from one or more of the '-itis' conditions: Arthritis, bursitis, tendonitis, gingivitis, ulcerative colitis sinusitis, plantar fasciitis, etc
	Suffering from one or more of the following conditions: Asthma, acne, chronic fatigue syndrome, fibromyalgia, digestive disorders, hypertension, osteoporosis, heart disease, cancer, pre-diabetes/diabetes, Parkinson's, MS, Hashimoto's Thyroiditis, rheumatoid arthritis, lupus, psoriasis, scleroderma or other autoimmune disorders

Are you surprised with your list? Had you considered that these symptoms are your body's way of *sending a message related to your diet?* Specify two ways your quality of life would benefit if your current symptoms of chronic inflammation were reduced or eliminated:

1. _____

2. _____

The habits below fuel chronic inflammation and general dis-ease. Check-off those in your current lifestyle:

X	Habits/Behaviors that Provoke Inflammation
	I consume grain products (even whole-grain) bread, pasta, cereal, tortillas, crackers, chips
	I regularly eat sugary items like desserts, sweetened yogurt, jam, dried fruit
	I drink sweetened beverages such as juice, soda, diet soda, sports drinks, sweet tea, blended coffee drinks, hot chocolate, protein shakes, sweetened coffee creamers, flavored water
	I rely on convenience foods such as fast food, frozen dinners or pre-packaged items
	I consume processed gluten-free products such as GF pasta, bread, cookies, crackers, chips
	Agave nectar is my sweetener of choice
	I eat or use highly processed oils (vegetable, canola, sunflower, safflower, soybean, corn)
	I eat hydrogenated oil products such as margarine, Cool Whip™, Crisco™ or deep-fried foods
	I follow a low-fat or low-cholesterol diet
	I regularly consume dairy products including milk (even low-fat), yogurt, cheese, whey protein
	I consume products made with soy or its derivatives (tofu, soy burgers, soy protein, soy sauce)
	I consume products made from corn or its derivatives (corn chips, cornstarch or corn syrup)
	I eat less than six vegetable servings per day
	My animal proteins come from factory-farmed animals (eggs, meats, dairy, seafood, bouillon)
	I consistently sleep *less than 8* full hours per night
	I regularly take over-the-counter or prescription medications
	I have elevated stress levels
	I do not read labels
	I do not concern myself with food additives such as MSG, food colorings, preservatives, etc
	I do not exercise regularly
	I am a smoker
	I don't know about anti-inflammatory supplements like omega-3 oils, vitamin D or turmeric

Unfortunately, modern dietary advice often promotes inflammatory choices! The information within this book offers solutions. Was there anything surprising about this list? Notes and other observations:

_____

_____

_____

_____

How to Heal Chronic Inflammation

Since chronic inflammation is an underlying source of chronic disease, reducing overall inflammation levels is essential for healing. The best opportunity for the body to begin the healing process is when all inflammatory foods are removed simultaneously. Without the perpetual assault, damage repair will be initiated by the natural healing mechanisms of the body – there is no magic pill.

*The best six doctors anywhere
And no one can deny it
Are sunshine, water, rest, and air
Exercise and diet.
These six will gladly you attend
If only you are willing
Your mind they'll ease
Your will they'll mend
And charge you not a shilling.*

*~Wayne Fields,
What the River Knows*

9

Section III: Foods that Contribute to Chronic Inflammation

We know it's hard to give up 'comfort foods' that make up the bulk of the typical western diet, but these foods are responsible for the majority of chronic inflammation and ill health. The best approach is to use a positive mindset:

1. These foods are not banned forever, they're just not for now.
2. For one dedicated month, you make the choice to *not* consume these foods. That's all. One month.

When told that we "can't have this" or "don't eat that," our subconscious naturally rebels...no one likes being told what to do. That's the essence of the pink elephant analogy – when told not to think about pink elephants, suddenly that's all you can think about. To use this natural tendency to your advantage, choose to focus on a vibrant body and good health. Consciously think about your food choices with a positive spin:

> ☺ Every time you eat or drink, you are either feeding disease or fighting it. ~Heather Morgan
> ☺ Nothing tastes as good as being healthy feels. ~Author unknown
> ☺ Don't dig your grave with your own knife and fork. ~English proverb
> ☺ Eating crappy food isn't a reward, it's a punishment. ~Drew Carey
> ☺ Eat less sugar. You're sweet enough already. ~Author unknown
> ☺ You can't expect to look like a million bucks if you eat from the dollar menu. ~Author unknown
> ☺ Food can be the greatest form of medicine, or the slowest form of poison. ~Ann Wigmore

Not-For-Now Foods

- **Grains** – wheat, rice, corn, millet, oats, bulgur, rye, barley and pseudo-grains such as amaranth, chia, buckwheat and quinoa (to clarify: if it acts like a grain, remove it for the month)
- **Dairy*** – milk, cheese, butter, yogurt, sour cream, kefir, ice cream, casein, lactose, whey
  - *Exception: *Grass-fed* sources of butter, clarified butter and ghee are allowed during the program
- **Legumes*** – any bean or pea such as soybeans, green peas, garbanzo/chickpeas, pinto beans, lentils, black beans, kidney beans, mung beans, peanuts
  - *Exception: Beans consumed *in the pod* are allowed (snow peas, green beans and sugar snap peas)

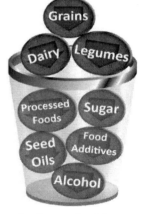

- **Sweeteners*** – all forms of natural or artificial sweeteners: cane sugar, corn syrup, agave nectar, honey, maple syrup, molasses, sucralose, Splenda®, NutraSweet®, Equal®, aspartame, or any sneaky names used in labeling such as fructose, dextrose, maltose, maltodextrin, malitol
  - *If a sweetener is absolutely unavoidable, pure stevia is acceptable
- **High-Sugar Fruits*** – Most fresh/canned fruits, all dried fruit and all fruit juices
  - *Acceptable low-sugar fruits are identified in Prep B
- **Industrialized Oils (seed oils, crop oils and hydrogenated oils)** - canola, soybean, cottonseed, corn, safflower, sunflower, grapeseed, peanut, vegetable oils, shortening, margarine or spreads
- **Chemicals and Preservatives** – In general, if *you* don't recognize an ingredient, your body won't either. These chemicals include FD&C food colorings, MSG, carrageenan, sodium benzoate, sulfites, etc, etc, etc. Also avoid all soy-derived and corn-derived products.
- **Alcohol** – wine, beer, malt beverages, distilled liquor, mixers

What Foods Are Left?!?

At first glance it may be quite depressing to discover that so many foods are pro-inflammatory. "Don't these foods comprise the vast majority of the modern western diet?" Yes! That's precisely why there's an epidemic of poor health today. "But, what's left to eat?" LOTS! But it's probably different than you're accustomed to. Don't despair – we'll guide you to healthier *and tasty* anti-inflammatory food choices. The Prep Section exercises will help you replace Not-for-Now Foods with easily-digestible, nutrient-dense and delicious Paleo options.

[👆] PilatesNutritionist Top 10 Elimination Diet Mistakes

Practice Removing Not-for-Now Foods

Consider a hypothetical day of typical western diet meals. Use the Not-for-Now Food list to determine the items to remove during the program. The foods remaining will be Paleo-friendly (don't worry, a thorough description of Paleo foods is coming up in Prep B):

1. Cover the *Keep*, *Ditch* and *Substitute* columns
2. Read through the example meals
3. Decide which foods to *keep* and which to *ditch*
4. Check your answers and browse our suggestions in the *substitute* column (Day 6 contains a thorough list of Paleo substitutions)

	Example Meal	Keep	Ditch	Substitute
Breakfast	Coffee w/cream & sugar Cereal with milk Toast w/butter and jam Orange juice	Coffee Butter if grass-fed	Cream (dairy) Sugar Cereal (grain) Milk (dairy) Toast (grain) Butter (dairy) Jam (sugar) OJ (sugar)	Coconut milk in coffee Veggie and ham omelet, cooked in grass fed butter
Snack	Apple w/peanut butter	Apple if it's a green one (they're lower in sugars)	Peanut butter (legume)	Use a true nut butter: almond, hazelnut, macadamia, etc
Lunch	Cheeseburger w/the works French fries Diet soda	Burger Bacon Lettuce Tomato Onion Pickles Mustard	Bun (grains) Cheese (dairy) Ketchup (sugar) Mayo (oils) Fries (oils) Soda (sugar)	Use a lettuce wrap, red pepper half or portabella mushroom as the bun Top with guacamole or salsa or grilled veggies Unsweetened tea
Snack	Crackers with cheese and lunch meat	Lunchmeat* *check for sugar or additives	Crackers (grain) Cheese (dairy)	Roll lunchmeat around a pickle
Dinner	Rotisserie chicken Green beans Rice Milk	Chicken* Green beans *Note: most rotisserie chicken contains chemicals in the seasoning mix as well as industrial oils	Rice (grain) Milk (dairy)	*Request a "naked" chicken from your grocer; bonus if you can get free-range or antibiotic-free; or roast one at home Cauliflower rice Unsweetened almond milk

How did you do? Did you correctly identify which foods to keep and which to ditch?

☐ Got them all   ☐ Missed a few   ☐ Need to reread the Not-for-Now Foods and try again

If you stumbled on this exercise, can you pinpoint your slip-ups?

_____

Are the suggested substitutions appealing to you?   Yes   No   Sometimes

Why or why not? _____

Now try this exercise with *your* typical day's meals - include beverages. Learning what foods to ditch is the goal for now; in Prep B you will learn appropriate Paleo substitutions.

	Typical Meal	Keep	Ditch
Breakfast			
Snack			
Lunch			
Snack			
Dinner			

This exercise is repeated several times for practice during Paleo Prep. If you feel frustrated, remember you do not have to reinvent the wheel. Many have already succeeded in the transition to Paleo and their tips and suggestions are logged online. ✋ Search "Paleo substitution for [*insert food*]" for inspiration or fresh ideas.

The food you eat today is walking and talking tomorrow. ~Jack Lalanne

Section IV: Kitchen Clean-Out

It is time to tackle the kitchen. A simple and effective way to eliminate some inflammatory habits is to remove those foods from the equation. The items in the following guide need to be removed from your main cooking and prep areas: quickly use them up, donate them, set aside for the next month or toss. An additional copy of the following clean-out pages is in the Resource Section – tear it out for easy reference.

To-Do List:
- ☐ When you've completed the Kitchen Clean-Out, check it off in your Master Plan.

Coming Up in Prep B:
- Stock the kitchen with foods that nourish and heal (they are also delicious)!

FOODS TO ELIMINATE – from pantry, refrigerator, freezer and spice cupboard

These foods must be avoided during your first Paleo month: No *Exceptions!*

Refined Grains

- ☐ Bread
- ☐ Cereal
- ☐ Tortillas
- ☐ Granola
- ☐ Protein bars

- ☐ Popcorn
- ☐ Crackers
- ☐ Pretzels
- ☐ Cookies
- ☐ Granola bars

- ☐ Pita bread
- ☐ Oatmeal
- ☐ Croissants
- ☐ Muffins
- ☐ Pancake mix

- ☐ Bagels
- ☐ Grits
- ☐ Pasta
- ☐ Rice
- ☐ Starch/Flour

- ☐ Corn chips
- ☐ Tortilla chips
- ☐ Muffin mix
- ☐ Couscous

Whole Grains and Pseudo-Grains

- ☐ Wheat
- ☐ Quinoa
- ☐ Bran
- ☐ Rye

- ☐ Corn
- ☐ Spelt
- ☐ Germ
- ☐ Rice

- ☐ Amaranth
- ☐ Wheat berries
- ☐ Buckwheat
- ☐ Chia

- ☐ Barley
- ☐ Bulgur
- ☐ Groats

- ☐ Oats
- ☐ Millet
- ☐ Teff

Potatoes - Everyone should eliminate processed versions of potatoes for the program. If interested in losing weight, we recommend eliminating *all* potatoes until you have reached your goal weight.

- ☐ White
- ☐ Red
- ☐ Gold
- ☐ Fingerling
- ☐ Chips/Fries
- ☐ Other Processed

Legumes

- ☐ Black beans
- ☐ Refried beans
- ☐ Peanut butter
- ☐ Lima beans
- ☐ Edamame

- ☐ Soybeans
- ☐ Mung beans
- ☐ Kidney beans
- ☐ Soy lecithin
- ☐ Chickpeas

- ☐ Navy beans
- ☐ Pinto beans
- ☐ Tofu
- ☐ Soy sauce

- ☐ Peanuts
- ☐ Lentils
- ☐ Peas
- ☐ Tamari

- ☐ White beans
- ☐ Miso
- ☐ Tempeh
- ☐ Hummus

High-Sugar Fruits (all fruit except those labeled in the low-sugar fruits section in Prep B)

- ☐ Fresh
- ☐ Canned
- ☐ Frozen
- ☐ Dried
- ☐ Juice
- ☐ Jam/Jelly

Dairy Products

- ☐ Cow milk
- ☐ Goat milk
- ☐ Sheep milk
- ☐ Cottage cheese

- ☐ Yogurt
- ☐ Whey Protein
- ☐ Coffee creamer
- ☐ Whipped cream

- ☐ Cream
- ☐ Sour cream
- ☐ Powdered milk
- ☐ Conventional butter (grass-fed is okay)

- ☐ Half & half
- ☐ Ice cream

- ☐ Cheeses
- ☐ Kefir

Beverages

- ☐ Alcohol
- ☐ Sweet teas

- ☐ Soda
- ☐ Diet soda

- ☐ Juice
- ☐ Presweetened coffee drinks

- ☐ Soft drinks

- ☐ Energy/sports drinks
- ☐ Shake or smoothie mixes

Sweeteners

- ☐ Sugar
- ☐ Corn syrup
- ☐ Sweet'N Low®

- ☐ Brown sugar
- ☐ Honey
- ☐ Agave nectar

- ☐ Maple syrup
- ☐ Coconut sugar
- ☐ Nutrasweet®

- ☐ Molasses
- ☐ Sugar alcohols
- ☐ Splenda®

- ☐ Dates
- ☐ Equal®

Fats and Oils

- ☐ Canola oil
- ☐ Soybean oil
- ☐ Coffee creamer

- ☐ Safflower oil
- ☐ Margarine
- ☐ Whipped topping

- ☐ Grapeseed oil
- ☐ Vegetable oil
- ☐ Shortening

- ☐ Sunflower oil
- ☐ Butter spreads

- ☐ Corn oil
- ☐ Crisco

Questionable Foods – Examine Ingredients

READ LABELS! The following items may be perfectly acceptable *if they have clean ingredients*. However, these products typically contain non-Paleo additives, so you must read EVERY LABEL. If the following ingredients are present, remove the item from your kitchen.

Chemicals and Additives to Avoid:

MSG, carrageenan, food colorings, sodium benzoate, soy ingredients, casein/whey, corn-derived additives, wheat-derived ingredients, grains, dairy, sweeteners, industrialized oils, sulfites and anything you can't pronounce or don't recognize. Check Pinterest.com/Paleovation Sneaky Food Additives

---

Reading the Ingredients Label: Just because a product is organic or gluten-free does not mean it is anti-inflammatory. In this example Sauce #2 is the clear winner.

Marinara Sauce 1: Organic Tomato Puree (Water, Tomato Paste), Organic Diced Tomatoes in Juice, Organic **Soybean** Oil, Organic **Sugar**, Organic Extra Virgin Olive Oil, Organic Onions, Sea Salt, Organic Garlic, Organic **Romano Cheese** (Organic Cultured Part Skim **Milk**, Salt, Enzymes), Organic Basil, Organic Black Pepper

Marinara Sauce 2: Imported Italian Plum Tomatoes, Extra Virgin Olive Oil, Onions, Garlic, Basil, Salt

---

PANTRY

- ☐ Gluten-free goods (often contain other grains)
- ☐ Canned goods like fish, sauce and vegetables
- ☐ Boxed/canned broth or stock
- ☐ Bottled items such as marinara sauce
- ☐ Premade or boxed meals/mixes
- ☐

- ☐ Nut butters (legumes, sugar, veg oil)
- ☐ Nuts roasted in seed oils
- ☐ Soups / soup mix
- ☐ Boxed drinks and drink mixes
- ☐ Sauce mixes
- ☐

FRIDGE/FREEZER

- ☐ Salad dressing
- ☐ Ketchup
- ☐ Mustard
- ☐ Teriyaki sauce
- ☐ Hot sauce
- ☐ Olives
- ☐ Other condiments
- ☐

- ☐ Marinades
- ☐ Nut milks
- ☐ Barbecue sauce
- ☐ Salsa
- ☐ Mayonnaise
- ☐ Pickles
- ☐ Pre-made meals
- ☐

SPICE CUPBOARD

- ☐ Table salt (dextrose and anti-caking ingredients)
- ☐ Bouillon cubes
- ☐ Soft drink mixes
- ☐ Vanilla extract (contains alcohol)

- ☐ Seasoning mix packs (taco, onion soup mix)
- ☐ Baking powder (contains corn starch)
- ☐ Purchased seasoning salts
- ☐

OTHER

- ☐ Prepared tea and coffee drink mixes (watch for sugars)
- ☐ Kombucha (no added sugar)
- ☐ Dried tea (some have soy or wheat)
- ☐

Prep B

Once you replace negative thoughts with positive ones, you'll start having positive results.
~Willy Nelson

Today's Topics:
1. Identifying Paleo Foods
2. Special Dietary Considerations
3. Paleo-Friendly Foods and Recipes
4. Finding Appropriate Recipes
5. Stocking a Paleo Kitchen

Section I: Identifying Paleo Foods

Paleo-Approved Foods

Introducing...the foods you can eat in abundance! Paleo is not about counting calories or carbs, it's about providing nutritional building blocks for the body's total health. These foods are the base of the Paleo Pyramid. Eat them in any quantity to satisfy your needs.

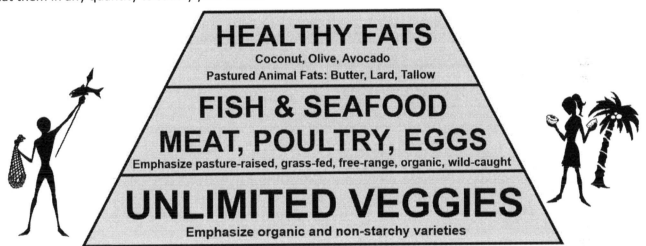

✓ **Unlimited Veggies** – Every day. Every meal. Every color. Your mother would be proud. Fresh, frozen and pesticide-free are best; dehydrated and canned are okay. Consume all vegetables except corn (it's a grain) and legumes (okay to eat snow peas, sugar snap peas and green beans – the ones in the pod).

  Note: Limit white potatoes and select more colorful veggies whenever possible, especially for weight loss.

  Someone has to stand up and say the answer isn't another pill. The answer is spinach. ~Bill Maher

✓ **Safe Protein Sources** – Grass-fed and pasture-raised (or 'pastured' *not* 'pasteurized') animal products and eggs, wild-caught fish, wild game, organ meats or shellfish. If these are out of your budget, then consume the leanest factory-farmed animal products and drain all fat. Fresh, frozen, canned or dried are acceptable.

✓ **Healthy Fats** – Select fats that nature provided long before industrialization: extra virgin olive oil, olives, coconut oil, coconut products, avocados, avocado oil, pastured/grass-fed animal fats (lard, tallow, duck fat, bacon drippings) and grass-fed butter products (including clarified grass-fed butter or ghee).

> **Butter Clarification:** Grass-fed butter is generally well-tolerated by most individuals. However, some Paleo reset programs require clarified butter or ghee. These butter products specifically remove the milk solids to preserve the pure dairy fat. You may select ghee and/or clarify your own butter during the program, especially if you have an autoimmune condition or suspect dairy sensitivities. If you choose to include butter, clarified butter or ghee, make sure it's from a grass-fed source. Kerrygold is a popular choice.

Paleo-Cautionary Foods

These are limited in daily servings because they either contain sugars which spike insulin and feed bad gut flora or contain compounds which make large quantities difficult to digest.

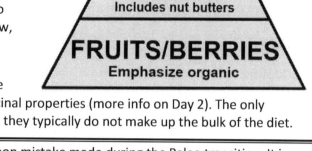

✓ **Low-Sugar Fruits** – For the first 3 weeks, limit fruit to one daily serving of low-sugar fruits. Select berries, grapefruit, Granny Smith apple or a not-quite-ripe banana.

✓ **Nuts and Seeds** – Limit these to one serving daily – a handful is reasonable. Nuts and seeds are calorie-dense, plus large quantities are difficult to digest. Expand your Paleo horizons with other snacks such as vegetables. Select raw, in-the-shell or dry roasted nuts.

   <u>Tip</u>: Soak and dehydrate nuts to boost digestibility.

✓ **Herbs and Spices** – Eat as much as you want. Many are anti-inflammatory, contain antioxidants and offer medicinal properties (more info on Day 2). The only reason they appear at the top of the pyramid is because they typically do not make up the bulk of the diet.

Going Nuts over Nuts: Over-consumption of nuts is a common mistake made during the Paleo transition. It is so easy to let one handful turn into three or five. Furthermore, Paleo baked goods often use nut flours, so almond meal pancakes or muffins count toward a daily nut/seed serving.

Section II: Special Dietary Considerations

Autoimmune Disorders

If you have an autoimmune condition, there are further dietary restrictions which facilitate faster healing. This is known collectively as the Auto-Immune Protocol (AIP).

The AIP takes Paleo-eating one step further, eliminating common triggers such as eggs, nuts/seeds, nut- and seed-based spices, nightshade vegetables (tomato, eggplant, peppers, potatoes), nightshade seasonings (chili, paprika), coffee and chocolate. This strict therapeutic protocol is temporary until the gut heals.

It is not necessary to immediately adopt the AIP – transitioning to Paleo is often enough of a challenge. Many find that eating 'straight-up' Paleo initiates the healing process, so start here using this guide. The next step we recommend is an egg-free Paleo Protocol. Eventually you may experiment with the full AIP elimination, but it is completely your choice if or when you commit.

The full AIP Guidelines are in the Resource Section. The Veggie and Spice Guides also identify AIP omissions.

Vegetarian/Vegan

If you are leery about incorporating animal proteins and fats, know that you are in good company. Many big names in the grain-free world are former vegetarian/vegans who eventually came face-to-face with the fact that their bodies function better with some animal products: Robb Wolf, Michelle Tam, Dr. Terry Wahls, Liz Wolfe, Dave Asprey, Dr. Amy Myers, Mickey Trescott, Dr. William Davis and many more.

Even the Dalai Lama eats some meat because the principle of *ahimsa*, to do no harm, also applies to our bodies. Sacrificing our own health by avoiding animal products does not make the world a better place.

   📖 *The Vegetarian Myth,* by Lierre Keith (also a former vegetarian) is an excellent book to review

➢ **Soy**

   If you prefer to use plant-based protein, proceed with caution using organic, non-GMO soybeans. Soy must be properly prepared by soaking, sprouting, boiling or fermenting. Use non-GMO miso, natto, tempeh and edamame. Additionally, please realize that soy contains phytoestrogens and can interfere with proper hormonal signaling...it is not an ideal protein.

> ➢ **Gentle Introduction of Animal-Based Products**
> Technically the body can put together amino acid sequences from plant protein sources, however the process demands a lot of energy. It's much more efficient to assimilate amino acids from animal sources. If you are feeling sluggish, please consider consuming some animal protein. If you are willing to gently introduce some animal products, start with bone broth, eggs, fish, ground meats or thinly-sliced deli meats (these softer textures may be better tolerated than chewier meats).

It still took me a couple of weeks to actually work up the courage to do it. I began by putting meat into soup, in small amounts and in tiny pieces. Gradually, as I got used to the taste, it began to taste better to me and I began to feel stronger. Eventually, I transitioned to a Paleolithic-style diet. ~Terry Wahls, MD

Pregnant/Lactating

This program is designed to feed your body all the essential building blocks necessary for health – that also includes the health of your baby. However, pregnancy is a unique situation and, depending on the health status of the individual, may not be the best time for a complete dietary overhaul. If this is your situation, consider a less-stressful 'baby steps' approach found at ⌐⊕ Paleovation Baby Steps.

A Paleo template can be followed by pregnant and lactating mothers, but understand you may need more calories and/or more carbohydrates. Unlimited starchy vegetables like sweet potato, carrot, beet, winter squash, sweet peppers or root vegetables and deeply-colored, low-sugar fruits like berries or fresh figs are Paleo-friendly carbohydrate sources.
> 📖 *The Perfect Health Diet,* by Paul and Shou-Ching Shih Jaminet is a good reference for those desiring to increase "safe starches"

Children

The Paleo Diet is a healthful regimen for children. However, children are active and growing with higher energy demands. Do not limit carbohydrate consumption to single-source foods such as vegetables or fruits. Yet, it is completely acceptable to make a rule that children need to eat another vegetable before they get a 2nd or 3rd fruit serving.
> 📖 *Eat like a Dinosaur,* by the Paleo Parents is a kid-friendly cookbook
> 📖 *Paleo Pals,* by Sarah Fragoso is a storybook

Elite Athletes

This program is effective for high-intensity athletes with a few modifications. If you currently use a whey protein supplement*, replace it preferably with whole food proteins (such as a piece of chicken or steak) or as a second choice, protein powders from egg, hemp, collagen or gelatin. To refuel muscles with glycogen, select carbs from starchy vegetable sources such as sweet potato, potato, other root vegetables and winter squashes.
> 📖 *The Paleo Diet for Athletes,* by Loren Cordain and Joel Friel
> 📖 *The Art and Science of Low Carb Performance,* by Jeff Volek and Steve Phinney
> 📖 *The Performance Paleo Cookbook,* by Stephanie Gaudreau includes both pre- and post-workout recipes
> 📖 *Primal Endurance,* by Mark Sisson
> *⌐⊕ RobbWolf Wheying In Are Protein Powders Paleo discusses the necessity of whey supplements. After completing this program, whey can be reintroduced to test your tolerance.

These elite endurance athletes have pushed away the time-honored plate of pasta in favor of a "paleo" approach to nutrition. They've dialed down the carbohydrates and replaced them with copious amounts of healthy fat... (and anecdotal evidence suggests) this may be the key to optimizing performance. ~Dorsey Kindler in Men's Journal

Section III: Paleo-Friendly Foods and Recipes

To start stimulating diverse Paleo culinary ideas, the following table lists a few delicious Paleo YES foods you can enjoy this month. Remember though, there are some rules about ingredients and sourcing (no grains, meats should be sugar-free, fatty cuts from pastured animals, no soybean oil). Circle or highlight a few favorites.

Paleo YES Foods				
Jerky	Grilled salmon	Guacamole	Sweet potato purée	Salmon cake, no grain
Olives	Deviled eggs	Chicken curry	Coconut butter	85%+ dark chocolate
Lobster	Steak kebabs	Tuna salad	Roasted broccoli	Peel-and-eat shrimp
Bacon	Lamb chops	Almond butter	Paleo mayonnaise	Butternut squash soup
Sashimi	Blackberries	Macadamia nuts	Crust-less quiche	Sauteed mushrooms
Kombucha	Coffee/tea	Burgers, no bun	Caramelized onions	Roasted pumpkin seeds
Cocoa nibs	Fresh herbs	Hot sauce and salsa	Approved lunchmeat	Roasted Red Peppers

Paleo Meal Practice

The Keep-Ditch-Substitute exercises show how to identify non-Paleo foods and conscientiously modify or replace them with anti-inflammatory Paleo foods. If you need a reminder of the foods to remove, review the Not-for-Now foods in Prep A: grains, dairy, legumes, industrial oils, sweeteners, high-sugar fruit, alcohol.

1. Cover the *Keep, Ditch* and *Substitute* columns
2. Decide which meal items to keep and which to ditch
3. Choose appropriate Paleo substitutes – <u>hint</u>: use the Paleo YES Foods from the above chart

	Meal	Keep	Ditch	Substitute
Breakfast	Tea w/cream and honey Breakfast sandwich with English muffin, bacon, cheese and egg	Tea Bacon and egg	Honey (sugar) Muffin (grain) Cheese (dairy)	Use coconut milk in the tea, maybe a little stevia Double the portions of bacon and eggs, add some roasted peppers and caramelized onion
Snack	Pita chips and hummus	Nothing! ☹	Pita (grains) Hummus (legume)	Deviled eggs Fresh cut veggies and cashew hummus or olive tapenade
Lunch	Salad topped with grilled salmon Iced tea	Salmon Greens Veggies Tea (unsweetened is perfect)	Salad dressing (oils and sugars) Sugar in tea	Dressing of lemon juice, salsa, guacamole or olive oil and vinegar
Snack	Banana	Banana – only if it's still a bit green	Yellow, ripe banana (sugar)	Make it fun and dip in almond butter
Dinner	Steak Potatoes Dinner roll Glass of wine	Steak Potato* *White potatoes are only for occasional use	Bread (grain) Wine (alcohol)	Alternative veggie side – Select a color you have not eaten today. Broccoli? Radishes? Butternut squash soup? Beets? Mushrooms? Glass of kombucha

Was this exercise any easier than the example from Prep A?   Yes   No

Which non-Paleo foods are easy for you to spot? _____

Are there any non-Paleo foods that are tricky for you to remember? _____

Continue to practice Paleo-tizing your typical meals (if you are short on time, you can use the info you provided in Prep A's example meals and just fill in the substitution column).

	Typical Meal	Keep	Ditch	Substitute
Breakfast				
Snack				
Lunch				
Snack				
Dinner				

Delicious Paleo Foods

The number one way to stay on track for the next month is to populate your kitchen with Paleo foods that you love. Paleo meals are more nourishing and just as delicious, if not more so, than typical western foods. When a recipe includes quality ingredients (especially fats), the results are robust, full-flavored, satisfying meals.

Batch-Cooking Ideas (also known as Cooking in Bulk or Planned-Overs):

The following recipes either freeze well or last a few days in the fridge. Select a few 'batch-able' items that sound good to you. Expect to make a double or triple batch of one of them later this week.

- ☐ Meatballs
- ☐ Roasted veggies
- ☐ Bacon
- ☐ Salmon or tuna cakes
- ☐ Fajita steak/chicken & veggies
- ☐ Mason® jar salads
- ☐ Roast beef, pot roast
- ☐ Stew, soup, chowder

- ☐ Meatza (Paleo pizza)
- ☐ Paleo pumpkin pancakes
- ☐ Egg salad
- ☐ Paleo muffins, unsweetened
- ☐ Pulled pork
- ☐ Taco meat
- ☐ Burgers
- ☐ Whole roasted chicken

- ☐ Shredded beef
- ☐ Tuna salad
- ☐ Cauliflower rice
- ☐ Chili
- ☐ Stir fry
- ☐ Nut/seed granola
- ☐ Sausage patties
- ☐ Baked salmon

Recipe Ideas (Random collection to stimulate ideas and to plan leftovers)

This smattering of ideas proves Paleo can be delicious *and* satisfying. All recipes can be found online; be sure to specify 'paleo' in the search bar. We don't expect your first month to have this much variety; it's just to show plentiful ideas exist. Circle or highlight 5-10 meals that interest you most (and dog-ear this page for the future):

		28 Days of Paleo Meals		
	Breakfast	**Lunch**	**Dinner**	**Snack**
1	Homemade nut and seed granola with coconut milk	Grass-fed sausage and sauerkraut	Baked salmon w/ roasted broccoli	Roasted pumpkin seeds
2	Veggie omelet	Salmon cakes	Cilantro lime chicken	Deviled eggs
3	Pumpkin pancakes w/ crushed berry topping	Sautéed cabbage w/ ground beef	Grilled chicken and veggie kabobs	Cashew hummus and veggies
4	Sausage patties w/ sautéed greens	Chicken and sweet potato hash	Steak with roasted veggies	Grass-fed beef jerky
5	Quiche cups (make in a muffin tin lined w/ bacon)	Tuna salad in cucumber boat	Stir fry w/ cauliflower rice	Dill pickles wrapped in lunch meat
6	Muffin in a mug	Paleo French onion soup	Meatballs in marinara	Olives
7	Steak and eggs	Taco salad	Paleo turkey chili	Deli meat
8	Bacon wrapped green beans	Bunless burger w/ sweet potato chips	Pork chops w/ baked apples and onions	Fresh or dried coconut
9	Almond meal porridge	Egg salad in red pepper	Paleo Irish beef stew	Fresh fruit/berries
10	Frittata w/ veggies and bacon	Frozen turkey burger w/ guacamole	Meatloaf w/ mashed cauliflower	Marinated mushrooms
11	Paleo breakfast pizza	Crab cakes on greens	Grain-free jambalaya	Handful of nuts
12	Poached eggs & asparagus	Fish & coconut milk soup	Crockpot pulled pork chili	Sweet potato fries
13	Crust-less quiche w/ sausage and mushroom	Spinach salad w/ grilled chicken breast	Beef tenderloin w/ braised Brussels sprouts	Celery sticks w/ almond butter
14	Omelet with sautéed spinach and onion	Lunch meats wrapped in romaine leaves	Almond-crusted fish and sautéed greens	Hard boiled eggs w/ guacamole
15	Cucumber boat w/ lox and almond milk 'cheese'	Veggies and sausage baked in acorn squash half	Sweet potato smashed and topped like pizza	Olive tapenade w/ veggies
16	Pumpkin porridge	Oysters on the half shell	Curried coconut shrimp	Paleo granola
17	Turkey and kale breakfast hash	Cobb salad (minus cheese)	Crock pot chicken with sweet potato mash	Tin of baby shrimp w/ salsa
18	Paleo zucchini fritters	Chicken apple stir fry	Caribbean seafood stew	Bone broth in a mug
19	Butternut squash soup w/ bacon bits	Cabbage slaw w/ grilled shrimp	Dry rubbed ribs with mashed cauliflower	Chicken fingers in almond flour
20	Eggs and bacon	Pizza spaghetti squash pie	Lamb and vegetable curry	Freeze dried berries
21	Zucchini pancakes/latkes	Crockpot chicken fajita	Paleo shepherd's pie	Paleo trail mix
22	Paleo veggie Benedict	Coconut lime shrimp	Bacon wrapped chicken	Kale chips
23	Bowl of berries w/ coconut milk and nuts	Taco meat w/ guacamole rolled in cabbage leaves	Macadamia crusted halibut w/ asparagus	Smoked salmon on cucumber slices
24	Easy paleo crockpot breakfast pie	Salmon, tomato and cucumber salad	Beef, bacon and plantain casserole	Guacamole on bacon "crackers"
25	Egg scramble w/ smoked salmon and red pepper	Creamy cauliflower soup with bacon bits	Roasted whole chicken and wilted cabbage	Grass-fed hot dog
26	Sweet potato hash w/ ground chicken	Sausage, bacon and Brussels sprout stir fry	Balsamic roast beef and braised snow peas	Nuts w/ berries
27	Sausage stuffed apples	Marinara chicken thighs	Curry turkey meatballs	Bacon
28	Spaghetti squash crusted quiche	Pork, shrimp and chicken gumbo	Bacon and spinach stuffed chicken	Apple slices with nut butter

Foundation Meals

It's critical to have appropriate food on hand *all the time* for a successful transition: at home, in the freezer, in your bag, at the office, in your locker, in the glove box, in the desk drawer, in your pocket and on the nightstand.

Review all the above meal suggestions and select 5 recipes to rotate for your initial Paleo introduction (including at least one batch-able recipe). These will be your go-to meals for the first couple weeks. As you become more familiar with Paleo cuisine, your repertoire will naturally expand.

A. Foundation Meal Selections:

1. _____

2. _____

3. _____

4. _____

5. _____

B. Locate Recipes for These Five Meals:

Carefully select Paleo recipes from cookbooks, websites and apps* (a few recommendations are listed below). Paleo recipes occasionally include not-for-now foods such as high-sugar fruits, dried fruits, applesauce, honey, maple syrup, coconut sugar, etc – either omit them from the recipe or find another version. Paleo "treats" are high in sugar and are not allowed until after the program.

*Helpful Tip: Establish a time limit per recipe to avoid spending hours browsing online

C. Suggested Foundation Recipes

If you are strapped for time, the Resource Section contains the following foundation recipes to get you started:

Paleo Foundation Recipes	
1. Paleo Turkey Chili	6. Roasted Chicken
2. Fish Cakes/Casserole	7. Roasted Veggies
3. Paleo Burgers	8. Cauliflower Rice
4. Tuna Lettuce Wraps	9. Guacamole
5. Coconut Curry	10. Paleo Seasoning Salt

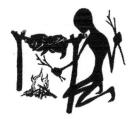

Section IV: Finding Appropriate Recipes (Direct links to all recommendations at ⌐ Paleovation)

Books – Low-sugar Paleo cookbooks with their (⌐ corresponding website recipe archive):
- 📖 *The 21-Day Sugar Detox Cookbook,* (also called 21DSD), by Dianne Sanfilippo (⌐ BalancedBites Recipes)
- 📖 *Whole30,* and *Whole30 Cookbook,* by Melissa and Dallas Hartwig (⌐ Whole30 Category: Recipes)
- 📖 *Well Fed,* and *Well Fed 2,* by Melissa Joulwan (⌐ MelJoulwan Recipe Index)

Online – Paleo blogs, recipe banks, meal planners, grocery list generators and apps; the options are plentiful. Here are a few popular websites to get you started, continue to watch for sugars:

⌐ StupidEasyPaleo   ⌐ ThePaleoMom   ⌐ PaleOMG   ⌐ CulinaryNutrition Top 50 Paleo Blogs

⌐ NomNomPaleo – the app contains pictures, especially helpful if you are not 'handy' in the kitchen

⌐ PrimalPalate myKitchen free menu planner allows recipe filtering like sugar-free, egg-free, etc

Meals for Purchase (optional): Purchase pre-made Paleo meals – search online to find a delivery service near you. These are handy in a pinch, but not all companies are created equal. Notable businesses:

⌐ PreMadePaleo has both Whole30® and autoimmune-friendly (AIP) options

⌐ PetesPaleo has seasonal menus and options for 21DSD or Wahls Protocol® (which is AIP friendly)

⌐ PaleoOnTheGo has seasonal menus and options for sugar-free Strict 30 and AIP

Tip: Paleo Blogs often rate pre-made meals. Example: ⌐ PaleoHacks Paleo Meal Delivery

Section V: Stocking the Paleo Kitchen

Start assembling your Paleo kitchen. Use the following guide to purchase items you want, need and *will actually use* in the next month. Just because they're on the list doesn't mean you have to buy them. An extra tear-out copy is located in the Resource Section. Read labels carefully – common non-Paleo additives are noted.

VEGETABLES

Fresh, frozen, dehydrated and organic are preferred. Nearly all veggies are a thumbs up! Remember, no corn (it's a grain) or legumes (except snow peas, sugar snap peas and green beans – the ones you eat raw in the pod). If weight-loss is a goal, no white, yellow, or red potatoes. Veggie Guide is located on Day 1.

PROTEINS

Emphasize quality sourcing when possible: grass-fed, pastured / pasture-raised, free-range and wild-caught.

➢ **Meats** – (Careful! Processed meats often contain sugar and preservatives – select products with less than 1g of carbohydrate per serving, 0g is best) Beef, pork, veal, buffalo, lamb, venison, goat, wild game, bacon, jerky, ground sausage, soup bones, grass-fed (pastured) hot dogs, organ meats

➢ **Poultry / Eggs** – (Read labels, poultry lunch meats often contain carrageenan) Chicken, turkey, duck, goose, Cornish hens, game birds, eggs from well-raised birds (pasture-raised)

➢ **Seafood** – Salmon (sockeye red salmon is always wild-caught), cod, perch, whitefish, snapper, halibut, tilapia, herring, grouper, trout, catfish, tuna, lobster, shrimp, mussels, clams, scallops, oysters, calamari, sardines, anchovies, caviar, other shellfish/seafood

NUTS and SEEDS

Dry roasted, in the shell or raw. Macadamias, cashews, hazelnuts, almonds, pecans, pistachios, pumpkin seeds, walnuts, pine nuts, sunflower seeds, sesame seeds, nut butters (no peanut products – legume).

PANTRY

☐ Canned fish in 100% olive oil or water (watch for soy, even if packed "in water")
☐ Canned vegetables like pumpkin, tomatoes
☐ Tomato paste
☐ Canned coconut milk
☐ Dried seaweed
☐ Vinegars (avoid malt, sulfites and sweetened)
☐ Coconut butter

☐ Broth or Stock (Most have sugar; Imagine® or Costco® organic is okay)
☐ Raw or dry roasted nuts and seeds
☐ Nut/seed butter (not peanut)
☐ Nut flours/meal
☐ Arrowroot or tapioca starch/flour (occasional use)
☐ Unsweetened applesauce (occasional use in cooking, not as a low-sugar fruit serving)

OILS/FATS

☐ Extra virgin coconut oil
☐ Extra virgin olive oil (dark bottle and bold taste)
☐ Pastured animal fats – lard, duck fat, tallow
☐ Drippings from pastured bacon or meats
☐ Avocados and avocado oil

☐ Olives
☐ Grass-fed butter or ghee
☐ Unsweetened coconut flakes
☐ Walnut, macadamia nut or toasted sesame oils (small amounts occasionally, keep refrigerated)

LOW SUGAR FRUITS

☐ Strawberries
☐ Raspberries
☐ Blackberries
☐ Blueberries

☐ Lemon
☐ Lime
☐ Grapefruit
☐ Green apples

☐ Unripe banana
☐ Fresh figs
☐ Unsweetened applesauce (occasional use)

SPICE CUPBOARD

☐ Salt – Himalayan, Celtic, Real Salt® or sea salt
☐ Pepper
☐ Sugar-free and additive-free spice mixes
☐ Dried herbs
☐ Cinnamon

☐ Bouillon – Rapunzel® is okay (low-sugar)
☐ Onion powder
☐ Garlic powder
☐ Seaweed flakes
☐ Dried mushrooms

FRIDGE

- ☐ Fresh cut veggies, ready to eat
- ☐ Eggs - preferably raised on a pasture
- ☐ Sugar-free mayo like Primal Kitchen® Mayo or Chosen Foods® Avocado Mayo (minimal sugar)
- ☐ 100% olive oil dressings – Tessamae's®, Whole Foods 365® Herbes de Provence, Bolthouse® has one
- ☐ Guacamole – most prepackaged are fine
- ☐ Nut milk, unsweetened (avoid carrageenan, soy lecithin) Silk® or Whole Foods 365® organic are okay
- ☐ Dill pickles (often contain coloring), Vlassic Market® pickles, Bubbies® are okay
- ☐ Fresh herbs (dill, parsley, rosemary, thyme, basil, oregano, chive, etc)
- ☐ Garlic, horseradish or ginger root
- ☐ Sauerkraut (buy refrigerated to preserve healthy bacteria, read label carefully for active, live cultures)
- ☐ Kimchee (watch out for MSG)
- ☐ Fish Sauce like Red Boat® brand
- ☐ Hot sauce (watch for colorings), Cholula® is okay
- ☐ Coconut aminos to replace soy sauce
- ☐ Ketchup by Tessamae's® has a little bit of dates for sweetener (use sparingly)
- ☐ Mustard (most are okay)

FREEZER

- ☐ Frozen burgers (chicken, grass-fed beef, turkey, bison, salmon) for quick protein
- ☐ Other frozen meats (whole chicken, ground beef)
- ☐ Veggies w/no additives
- ☐ Cauliflower rice
- ☐ Puréed veggies to add to soups and sauces
- ☐ Frozen berries
- ☐ Guacamole – purchased guacamole servings can be frozen to put in lunch bags
- ☐ Sausage, easy to make your own and freeze (raw or pre-cooked)
- ☐ Homemade freezer meal
- ☐ Herb purées or minced herbs
- ☐ Soup bones

OTHER

- ☐ Herbal tea
- ☐ Root teas (ginger, turmeric)
- ☐ Other teas
- ☐ Coffee, preferably organic
- ☐ Coconut water (occasional)
- ☐ Kombucha, no sugar added to final product
- ☐ Sparkling water
- ☐ Dark chocolate, soy-free 85%+, (occasional treat)

To-Do List:

- ☐ Locate recipes for your 5 foundation meals
- ☐ Stock up your kitchen with Paleo-friendly foods (it's helpful to know what ingredients will be needed for those recipes first)
- ☐ Sometime before Day 1, prepare a large batch of a foundation recipe so you have easy-to-grab leftovers
- ☐ **Check off your completed tasks on the Master Plan**

Coming Up Soon:

- • You'll document your current level of health in the next Prep section
- • Prep C and D contain tips for creating new healthy habits and getting mentally prepared

Prep C

Today's Topics:
1. Paleo-Wise: All About Sugar
2. Check-in: Markers of Current Health
3. Creating New Healthy Habits
4. Set Appropriate Goals
5. Success Strategies for a Non-Compliant Household
6. Contemplate Excuses that Inhibit Success

Section I – Paleo-Wise: All About Sugar

Food is medicine. We can actually change our gene expressions with the foods we eat.
~David Perlmutter, MD, author of <u>Grain Brain</u>

It shouldn't be surprising that our first discussion is about sugar. There's a remarkable amount to learn about this seemingly simple topic. Despite the universal understanding that "excess sugar is not healthy," discrepancy exists in the definition of 'excess' and what genuinely qualifies as sugary food.

Blatantly sweet foods like candies or desserts are easy to identify, but sugar also abounds in palatable, savory items like bread, pasta, oatmeal, sauces, processed meats, peanut butter, soups and beverages. The sheer volume of sugar and starches in the modern diet has displaced nutritious, wholesome food and has contributed to nutritional deficiencies. Compound this malnutrition by the fact that sweet and starchy foods are easy to overeat...and the chronic disease and obesity epidemics are not surprising.

> **Bottom Line:** Sugar and starch cannot replace real food without creating health consequences.

Glucose – Fast Facts

Technically, glucose is a single molecule and is the primary sugar in blood. The generic term 'sugar' is often used to reference glucose but it's also used interchangeably to identify white table sugar which is actually a 50/50 combination of glucose plus fructose. Glucose is essential for life – it is the universal energy source of every living cell on the planet. It is so easily assimilated that digestion starts in mouth!

> **Food for Thought:** Starchy foods are equivalent to sugar – *starch is simply a string of glucose molecules connected together*. Bread, french fries, pasta, rice, chips and other starchy, processed or refined carbohydrates have nearly identical effects on blood sugar as pure glucose.

Humans are Engineered for a Low Sugar Diet

High concentrations of glucose rarely occur in nature so historically, sugar was impossible to over-consume. To satisfy glucose needs, most mammals (including humans) evolved the ability to manufacture glucose in their own liver, not *by eating it*! Modern humans, however, have deviated significantly from that genetic design. Our industrialized food supply is so brimming with sugar that our metabolism is simply not prepared for the 150 pounds of sugar an average American consumes annually!

Sugar is sneaky, seductive, sentimental, and passionate. And sugar is everywhere.
~Kristina Turner, author of <u>The Self-Healing Cookbook</u>

Every culture, upon adopting the western diet, records increased rates of obesity and disease. This fact alone demonstrates how devastating excessive sugar and starch consumption is to the human body.

> **Key Point:** The number one enemy of vitality, health and longevity is not saturated fat – it's sugar! Sugar's effect on hormones, moods, immunity and weight is enormous...and it's all negative. Of course there are many other destructive components to the modern diet and lifestyle, but sugar and starch are major contributors.

Excess Sugar = Body Fat

Glucose has *no nutritional value* – it simply serves as an immediate energy source and is quickly absorbed into the blood. "Immediate energy" generally means dietary glucose rushes into the bloodstream and is depleted within a few hours. Unfortunately in this case, what goes up quickly comes down quickly – when available glucose is exhausted, a rebound energy crash occurs and sparks the need for a snack, coffee or nap. These energy crashes initiate a cycle of sugar cravings as the body desperately attempts to maintain energy levels.

> *Sugar is a type of bodily fuel, yes, but your body runs about as well on it as a car would.* ~Terri Guillemets

Glucose consumed at one sitting is not evenly distributed for energy throughout the day. Once eaten, part of the glucose supplies energy needs for the next few hours, but any extra glucose is *immediately packaged into fat* for future energy needs (the amount of extra varies between individuals and activity levels). Modern diets promote regular sugar/starch consumption at levels typically exceeding needs. This perpetual overabundance of glucose shifts metabolism toward ongoing fat production and storage – easily contributing to weight gain and obesity.

> **Bottom Line:** No matter how much glucose is consumed at one meal, when the body has sufficient dietary sugar to satisfy *short-term* energy needs, excess sugar is converted into fat.

How Much is Too Much?

The term *excess* is an over-used quantitative phrase that's never defined, not unlike *in moderation*. The truth is that *excess* is conditional and not an exact amount. Some individuals can tolerate more sugar with no obvious adverse health consequences while others are extremely sensitive and develop consequential symptoms like headaches, hyperactivity, acne, stomach aches or insomnia. These tolerance levels can change over time.

> **Eye Opener:** A healthy individual's body needs a little less than one teaspoon of glucose dissolved in the entire blood pool (~5 quarts)! Maintaining this level does not require much sugar in the diet.

Generally, the tipping point between consuming sugar in *moderation* versus *excess* depends on the sugar source, individual health, lifestyle factors and, of course, the quantity eaten:

1. **Source of the Sugar**
   a. **Refined/Processed** – Has no vitamins or minerals and is often accompanied by unpronounceable chemicals and additives. *Any amount of refined sugar is excessive!*

   > *If it came from a plant, eat it. If it was made in a plant, don't.* ~Michael Pollan

   b. **Naturally-Occurring** – Accompanied by valuable vitamins, minerals and fiber: for example, one orange contains 12 grams of sugar (that's 3 teaspoons) but also boasts significant amounts of vitamin C, folate, calcium, potassium and fiber.

> **Beware of "Natural" Sugars on Labels:** The FDA definition of "natural" only requires that the end product does not contain man-made chemical *additives* (such as food coloring). Therefore, high fructose corn syrup is considered a natural sugar even though it is impossible to find it in nature.

2. **State of Health**
   a. **Healthy** – People with an active, unimpaired metabolism may not experience any overt problems digesting moderate amounts of naturally-occurring sugar
   b. **Health-Compromised** – The upper boundary of sugar tolerance is much lower for those with *any kind of metabolic problems*, especially those who are diabetic or obese
3. **Activity Level**
   a. **Sedentary** – Over-consumption of sugar is easy due to low metabolic demands
   b. **Vigorous** – Highly active individuals tend to have higher sugar tolerance
4. **Genetic Predisposition** – Some people naturally have a 'higher metabolism' than others, allowing a higher intake before glucose is metabolized into fat for storage

Sugar Addiction

Sweet tastes are strongly tied to the brain's reward centers and have been shown to relieve pain and reduce symptoms of depression and stress.

Sweetness, however, is not simply an innocent source of pleasure – our brains are hard-wired to purposely hunt for sweet foods. Historically, the sweet taste was one way our ancestors could identify safe, non-poisonous foods with a high energy storage value (a desirable combination, perfect to pack on a few pounds before winter arrived). Natural sweetness generally signifies a safe fuel and a *lack* of toxins.

> **Sweet Vice:** Sugar literally stimulates opioid receptors, just like heroin or cocaine! The reward center of the brain releases dopamine, whose powerful, pleasurable effects can lead to symptoms of addiction.

Unfortunately, exposure to sweet sources in contemporary cultures is unnaturally extreme – exponentially higher than amounts found in any wholesome, real food. Over time, the brain becomes desensitized to high sweetness levels and requires increasingly more sugar to stimulate the same sense of reward.

> **Endless Cycle:** The more sugar we eat, the less we taste it – the less we taste it, the more sugar we eat!

Find the Sugar, Sherlock

Sugar is ubiquitous in our culture – it's commonly used as a stealth flavor enhancer. We expect sugar in desserts, but few realize how much sugar is contained in yogurt, ketchup, salad dressings, pasta sauces, protein bars, juices or sports drinks. This is called *added sugar*. Most people have no clue as to just how much sugar they are actually eating.

It is important to distinguish *added sugars* from sugars that occur naturally in foods. When sugar is added to a food over-and-above the natural carbohydrate content, it provides *nothing* nutritionally and displaces more nourishing foods in the diet, such as vegetables.

Our bodies were never designed to have access to this much quick and easy sugar. ~Ellen Vora, MD

Problems with Added Sugar:
- No physiological need for this extra calorie load
- Contributes to disruption of insulin metabolism and chronic inflammation
- Leads to nutritional deficiencies
- Leads to unnecessary weight gain

> **Fat Fact:** On average, Americans get *350 calories per day* from hidden, <u>added</u> sugar in the diet (not even including glucose consumed in the form of starches and grains). This is equivalent to a daily covert sugar consumption of 22 teaspoons, totaling up to 35 pounds of *unintentional* sugar eaten every year!

Label Deception

Food and beverage manufacturers currently utilize over 60 names for sugar on food labels and they're in search of more. In general, if an ingredient ends in a *-ose* it's a sugar. Yet there are many other names for sugar including syrups, fruit juices, malt or even names denoting the sugar's geographical source like Panocha (Philippines), Demerara (South America) or Muscovado (Barbados).

Why So Much Added Sugar?
1. **Camouflage** – Cover up the taste of chemical additives, preservatives, colorings or poor-quality food.
2. **Profit** – People crave sugar, plain and simple – if we eat more, they sell more!

> **Marketing Magic:** Manufacturers deceptively use several types of sugar in the same product to augment the health appeal. Nutritional labels list ingredients by quantity, from highest to lowest. By utilizing multiple types of sugar in a product, the total sugar load can be spread across several ingredients so that each of those names appears much further down the list.

Complex versus Simple Carbohydrates

In biological terms, sugars are the building blocks of carbohydrates. The following table provides a quick lesson on the breakdown of sugar. Although this may appear technical, it's helpful to recognize these terms because they're commonly used on product labels to camouflage sugar content.

Chemistry Corner: Carbohydrate = Sugar			
Simple Carbohydrates Easy to digest, the body can use these immediately for energy (like a "sugar rush" after eating too much candy).		**Complex Carbohydrates** Strings of three or more sugars; the body must first break them down into their simple sugar components before utilizing them.	
<u>**Single Sugars**</u>	<u>**Double Sugars**</u>	<u>**Digestible**</u>	<u>**Non-Digestible**</u> <u>**Fiber**</u>

• **Glucose:**
  o Occurs naturally in plants; byproduct of photosynthesis
• **Fructose:**
  o Found only in fruit
  o Sweetest natural sugar
• **Galactose:**
  o Found in dairy
  o Less sweet than glucose
	• **Sucrose:**
	  o White table sugar
	• **Maltose:**
	  o Formed when certain grains germinate (like barley 'malt' in beer)
	• **Lactose:**
	  o Found in milk
	  o Those who cannot digest it are *lactose intolerant*
		• **Starch:**
		  o Strings of glucose found in grains and root vegetables
		  o Enzymes break these into simple sugars
		• **Glycogen:**
		  o Strings of glucose found in some organ meats and shellfish
		  o The body's storage form of glucose
			• Not broken down with digestion
			• The body lacks the enzymes to digest
			• Examples include:
			  o **Cellulose**
			  o **Pectin**
			  o **Inulin**

Bittersweet Truth: Most people assume that sugar must taste sweet. Unfortunately, *sugar doesn't always taste like sugar.* Complex carbohydrates such as breads or rice or corn flakes rarely taste as sweet as their simple sugar cousins – but they're still digested into glucose. As far as the body is concerned: sugar on your cereal is the same as cereal on your sugar!

Ill Effects of Sugar

Numerous studies show that excess sugar (and starch) compromise health more than any other dietary component. Modern quantities of concentrated sweeteners have eroded our bodies, altered our eating patterns, produced excess fat baggage and left us nutritionally-deficient. Other consequences include:

- **Appetite Disruption** - Excess sugar confuses our natural appetite regulation systems
- **Chronic Inflammation** - Metabolic processing of excess sugar drives systemic inflammation
- **Digestion Difficulties** - Excess sugar disrupts the balance of friendly and not-so-friendly gut flora resulting in digestive complications and *more* inflammation
- **Immune Compromise**
  - o Reduces production of antibodies
  - o Interferes with vitamin C transport, an important nutrient for immune function
  - o Contributes to mineral imbalances and allergic reactions; both weaken the immune system
  - o Neutralizes action of essential fatty acids, making cells more permeable to invasion by allergens and micro-organisms
- **Chronic Conditions Exacerbated** with sugar intake:

o Obesity	o Cancer	o Cardiovascular disease	o Macular degeneration
o Diabetes	o Dementia	o Immune dysfunction	o Chronic kidney disease
o Elevated triglycerides		o High blood pressure	

Though it is not our fault we gravitate toward sweet and starchy foods, we can no longer blindly consume excess sugar and starch while blaming ill health on bad luck. It's time to take responsibility for dietary sugar overload.

Artificial Sweeteners

'No calorie' sugar creations have only existed about 100 years. However, 'no calories' doesn't mean 'no problems.' Many types of zero-calorie sugar substitutes contribute to metabolic problems, even weight gain, despite touting no direct caloric value. Essentially, when a sweet taste is sensed, the pancreas expects to digest sugar and releases some insulin. Even if the sweet taste is not followed with any calories, this sudden and repeated insulin stimulation contributes to hormonal signaling confusion which can prompt overeating later.

If you must, *pure stevia* powder or drops is an acceptable sugar substitute to be used as a crutch until complete sweet withdrawal can be achieved (avoid brands laced with dextrose, common in individual packets).

Artificial Sweeteners	
NutraSweet® **(aspartame)**	Contains aspartate, a neurotoxin similar to MSG; produces formaldehyde when metabolized which may not be effectively detoxed; phenylalanine breaks down to a known carcinogen when heated
Splenda® (sucralose)	Chlorinated sugar; toxicity concerns; not safe for cooking because heating it releases dioxin (yet it's marketed to be heat safe); destroys gut bacteria; modifies glucose and insulin levels
Sugar alcohols	These do not elicit an insulin response; includes xylitol, sorbitol, maltitol and erythritol; can cause gas and bloating; erythritol is the sugar alcohol least likely to cause gastrointestinal problems
Stevia	Herbal extract; available in liquid or powder (sold under several brand names, including Truvia®); the jury is still out on whether it interferes with insulin response
Sweet 'n Low® **(Saccharine)**	A coal tar product; cross-sensitivity with sulfonamides has been demonstrated so people with "sulfa" allergy should avoid
High fructose corn syrup (HFCS)	Industrial sweetener comprised of fructose and glucose; it comes with its own unique problems (more on HFCS on Day 22)

> **Paleo Advantage:** Metabolism *can* be changed! Paleo-eating limits regular glucose consumption from sugar and grains, encouraging our bodies to become increasingly more efficient at burning fat for fuel rather than sugar.

Section II: <u>Check-in</u>, Markers of Current Health

This will give you an overview of your current health status. None of these measurements deem that you are healthy or unhealthy but just provide a benchmark to record progress over time.

👆 <u>MayoClinic</u> Tests and Procedures for standard blood work ranges

Blood Work Options:

🔸 **Lipid Panel:** Cholesterol is a necessary component in a healthy body and brain. High *total cholesterol* does not necessarily indicate poor health (just as *too low* total cholesterol does not indicate good health; levels below 150 or 160 are problematic for brain health). General recommendations for a healthy cholesterol panel:
  - **HDL:** >50 but in general, more is better
  - **Triglycerides:** <150, but the lower the better; high levels indicate other problems such as insulin resistance (with risk of diabetes) or inflammation (and risk of heart disease); Ideally <100
  - **Useful Lipid Ratios:** The ratios below indicate a healthy lipid profile and lack of inflammation:
    - ✓ **Total cholesterol ÷ HDL** Ideally <3.5
    - ✓ **Triglyceride ÷ HDL** Some sources say <3, but ideally <2
  - **LDL-P (particle count):** LDL comes in different sizes so particle size matters: large, fluffy LDL particles are healthy and desirable, but the small dense ones are not. The LDL-P test measures the total number of LDL particles and a high count suggests excessive, unhealthy, small LDL particles and is ideally <1000.
    Note: The LDL-C number on a typical cholesterol test is an estimate of how much LDL is present, it does not correlate with the particle size.
    👆 <u>DocsOpinion</u> The Difference between LDL-C and LDL-P

📖 *Grain Brain*, by David Perlmutter, MD

📖 *Cholesterol Clarity*, by Jimmy Moore and Eric C. Westman, MD

📖 *The Wahls Protocol,* by Terry Wahls, MD

⚡ Cholesterol and Heart Disease are covered in detail on Days 17 and 18 including other testing and resources to understand and predict heart disease risk.

♦ **Fasting Blood Glucose Level**: Best to keep this less than 100; over 100 indicates pre-diabetes and over 120 indicates diabetes. <90 is desirable.

♦ **A1C**: This measures blood sugar level over time and is a more accurate picture than the Fasting Blood Glucose which is just a one-moment snapshot. The A1C measurement averages ~3 months of blood sugar levels, so do not retest this until after you have been eating Paleo-style for at least three months. A 'normal' score is between 4.5 and 5.6 percent; 5.7 - 6.4 percent indicates pre-diabetes and two separate test results of 6.5 or higher indicates diabetes. Optimal levels are 5.0 and below.

♦ **CRP**: C-Reactive Protein measures the amount of inflammation currently in the body. Some drugs can affect levels (birth control pills, NSAIDS like ibuprofen, Tylenol, etc) so advise your healthcare provider accordingly. The higher the score, the more systemic inflammation present. Ideal results are < 0.8 mg/L.

♦ **Vitamin D Levels**: Ideal scores for the 25-OHD test range from 40-60mg/mL. Vitamin D fluctuates with sunshine exposure. It's common to take a supplement in the winter.

Medical Caution: If you follow a medical regimen (any doctor-monitored medications or treatments), please tell your healthcare provider(s) that you intend to eat an anti-inflammatory, nutrient-dense diet for 4 weeks to observe how your body responds. Also address concerns about prescriptions that may need adjustment during the next month. Fantastic information here: ⚡ Whole30 Talk to your Doc: Prescription Medications

---

Body Metrics Chart

Record any current test scores or measurements in the following table (we'll revisit these on Day 28).

Body Metric Benchmarks				
Suggested Blood Work			**Physical Measurements** (Measure at the fullest point)	
Test	**Ideal**	**Test Result**		
HDL	> 50		Chest	
Triglycerides	< 100		Waist	
Total ÷ HDL	< 3.5		Hips	
Triglycerides ÷ HDL	< 2		Arm	
LDL-P	< 1000		Thigh	
Fasting glucose	< 90		Neck	
A1C	< 5.0		Weight	
CRP	< 0.8		Blood	_____
25-OHD (vit D)	40-60		Pressure	

Picture Time (front and side views)

Take a "before" picture in revealing clothing, like swim wear or workout attire, so you can see the not-quite-firm sections of your body (a bare midriff). This photo is only for you – but it's a marker for your accomplishment. It's quite amazing to see the difference one month can make! You do not need to share it with anyone...until you're ready to show them who you used to be!

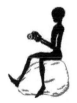

Check-in Questionnaire: How Vibrant is Your Current Health?

The following questionnaire is an opportunity to establish general health parameters and will provide a snapshot of your overall health prior to starting the Strict Paleo Protocol. Questionnaire scores are explained on the subsequent page. You'll retake this quiz at the end of 28 days to compare results.

ꙮ Pre-Paleo Check-in

Date: _____

*Please record any specific observations or clarifications in the notes below.	Strongly Disagree -2	Disagree -1	Neutral 0	Agree +1	Strongly Agree +2
I have even energy levels throughout the day.	☐	☐	☐	☐	☐
I fall asleep easily and sleep soundly.	☐	☐	☐	☐	☐
I rarely have food cravings.	☐	☐	☐	☐	☐
I'm satisfied with both my hunger levels and my response to hunger.	☐	☐	☐	☐	☐
My joints and tendons are comfortable and work smoothly.	☐	☐	☐	☐	☐
I am satisfied with my range of motion (flexibility) throughout my body.	☐	☐	☐	☐	☐
I have relatively few aches or pains (including neck, back, headache, joint, muscle, etc).	☐	☐	☐	☐	☐
I am satisfied with my athletic performance and body's response to physical activity.	☐	☐	☐	☐	☐
My body heals quickly from overuse or injury.	☐	☐	☐	☐	☐
My immune system functions properly (rarely catch a cold, recover from illness well, etc).	☐	☐	☐	☐	☐
My skin, complexion, hair, nails, teeth and gums are all healthy and strong.	☐	☐	☐	☐	☐
My moods are stable and easy to control.	☐	☐	☐	☐	☐
I am satisfied with my mental clarity and ability to focus.	☐	☐	☐	☐	☐
In general, I am able to calmly respond to stressful situations.	☐	☐	☐	☐	☐
My digestion functions properly (no stomach cramps, heartburn, bloating, painful gas, etc).	☐	☐	☐	☐	☐
My elimination function is normal and comfortable (no diarrhea, constipation, etc).	☐	☐	☐	☐	☐

Additional Notes:

Score Your Check-in:

All statements on the *Pre-Paleo Check-In* are made in the positive form so a "strongly agree" response scores +2 points, a "strongly disagree" is -2 and neutral is zero. This is not a perfect science (there really is no way to compare the value of sleeping well to having a full range of motion) but this gives a general idea of your current health status and some parameters to monitor for changes.

Pre-Paleo Check-In Score: _____ (The best possible score is +32)

Don't despair if your number is negative (typically it is at the start of the Paleo Protocol) – this gives you more room to improve! How would it feel if one or two of those items moved from the negative side to the neutral or positive side? Our clients average an improvement of +17 points!

Section III: Creating New Healthy Habits

Much of this transition to the Paleo Lifestyle is about creating new eating patterns and healthier habits. Take a moment to record some healthy habits you already possess:

☐ Non-smoker   ☐ Take time to de-stress   ☐ Maintain a healthy weight
☐ Avoid fast food   ☐ Eat home-cooked meals   ☐ Have a solid social support network
☐ Read labels   ☐ Practice gratitude   ☐ Practice good posture and breathing techniques
☐ Eat lots of veggies   ☐ Spend time in nature   ☐ Avoid high fructose corn syrup
☐ Limit sweets   ☐ Sleep a solid 8 hours   ☐ Committed to improving health
☐ Exercise daily   ☐ Avoid trans fats   ☐ Limit alcohol over-consumption

What else do you do to stay healthy?

_____

How quickly were these healthy habits created? By a slow transition? By starting up cold turkey?

_____

What influenced you to start or maintain your current healthy habits:

☐ Understanding the danger of poor habits   ☐ Feel healthier when I follow these habits
☐ Health scare, illness or life-changing event   ☐ Motivational material (book, testimonial, video)
☐ Other: _____   ☐ Other: _____

Will these factors also help you commit to this program?   Yes   No

What else will help you complete this program?

☐ Creating a strong support network   ☐ Committing to one day at a time
☐ Having a buddy join me   ☐ Creating strategies for restaurants
☐ Completing thorough prep-work   ☐ Addressing my concerns ahead of time
☐ Understanding the science behind Paleo   ☐ Adding new Paleo habits before Day 1

Five New Habits

Here are five habits that will be encouraged during the program. Consider beginning some now!

1. **Keep fresh cut veggies in the fridge**, replenish frequently – to save prep time visit the salad bar for chopped veggies or purchase pre-made party platters and remove the dip
2. **Replace sweetened beverages** with sparkling water, spa water, herbal tea or occasional kombucha
3. **Replace bread** with a vegetable: red pepper halves, lettuce/cabbage leaves, cucumber boat, jicama slices
4. **Avoid industrial crop and seed oils** and use coconut oil, extra virgin olive oil or grass-fed butter instead
5. **Take a walk** every day, perhaps after dinner or before lunch to set a habit

Check the healthy habits you are already utilizing 5-7 days per week:

☐ Fresh-cut veggies   ☐ Unsweetened beverages   ☐ Bread replacement   ☐ Better fats/oils   ☐ Daily walk

Which of the 5 healthy habits are you able to include in your daily routine starting today:

☐ Fresh-cut veggies   ☐ Unsweetened beverages   ☐ Bread replacement   ☐ Better fats/oils   ☐ Daily walk

Speaking of healthy habits, continue to practice converting typical western meals into Paleo-friendly ones. Cover the three right-hand columns while you think it through in your head:

	Example Meal	Keep	Ditch	Substitute
Breakfast	Ham and cheese omelet Toast with butter Café mocha	Ham Eggs Grass-fed butter Espresso	Cheese (dairy) Toast (grain) Factory farmed butter (dairy) Chocolate sauce (sugar) Milk (dairy)	Ham and veggie omelet cooked in grass-fed butter Sweet potato hash Mix coconut milk and cinnamon into espresso
Snack	Trail mix	Nuts Seeds *check added oils	Dried fruit (sugar) Chocolate chips (sugar, dairy)	Add some coconut flakes
Lunch	Fajitas with all the toppings Lemonade Fried ice cream	Meat Veggies Olives Salsa Guacamole	Tortillas (grain) Cheese and sour cream (dairy) Refried beans (legume) Rice (grain) Lemonade (sugar) Fried ice cream (sugar, fat)	Make a taco salad or fill lettuce wraps Sparkling water with lemon Apple slices dipped in coconut butter
Snack	Granola bar	Nothing!	Granola bar (grains, sugar, oils)	Cocktail shrimp or fresh cut veggies dipped in guacamole, jerky
Dinner	Meatloaf Mashed potatoes Sparkling water	Meatloaf (omit flour) Mashed potatoes (grass-fed butter) Sparkling water		Add a salad If potatoes are your go-to veggie, replace with more colorful vegetables

If these were your meals for today, what seems to be an easy swap for you?

_____

What would the typical *western diet eater* find most challenging to change?

_____

What two thoughts could you share with this western dieter to help them swap out those items?

1. _____

2. _____

Section IV: Set Appropriate Goals

Attaining the Perfect Weight is NOT the Goal

Nearly everyone is dissatisfied with their weight. Most want to shed pounds; a few want to pack on more muscle. Will that happen throughout this program? Perhaps. However, total health encompasses more than merely gaining or losing weight.

Re-focus the goal toward supporting better overall health. Reflect on how a healthier body would feel. What aspects of your health would define a healthier you? Do your desires include having abundant energy, reduced brain fog or enjoy a good night's sleep *every single night*?

What 'Good Health Results' Do You Desire Most?

☐ Sound sleep ☐ Fluid joints ☐ Fewer headaches ☐ Not hunger-driven ☐ No energy crashes
☐ Clear skin ☐ Less aches ☐ Thinking clearer ☐ Healthy libido ☐ Lower blood pressure
☐ Soft stools ☐ Less snacking ☐ Range of motion ☐ Body composition ☐ Quick recovery times
☐ No reflux ☐ Easy digestion ☐ More active ☐ Better lipid panel ☐ Better performance

All these results are possible with Paleo, but to get there, the number one goal must be to take care of yourself, every day, for a month, with no cheating! Check this box if you are ready.

☐ **Take care of yourself for 28 days in a row** – you have waited a long time [you must check this one!]

> **Wake-up call:** This sounds divine, but there is a long road ahead!
> *Good news* – the physical preparation is quite easy
> *Not-so-good news* – the mind is stubborn and tends to need some serious convincing
> *Best news* – the transition progressively gets easier as your body begins to feel healthy again!

Section V: Strategies for Success in a Non-Compliant Household

It happens…resistant spouses, roommates or children. If you have politely discussed your plans for anti-inflammatory eating, your job is done, although they may or may not act on that request. Regarding children, as the adult, you get to help them make healthy choices at a pace you deem necessary. Not everybody is ready for this transition at the same time and that's okay. *You* are ready – *you don't need to wait.* In fact, please don't!

Here are some strategies to be successful on your first month:

1. **Prime Kitchen Real Estate:** Because you are taking the step toward better health, you earn all the prime food spots: eye-level shelves in the cupboards, open counter space, a favorite shelf in the fridge, etc. Your food gets to live where you see it first and foremost. All junk foods or non-Paleo foods are hidden in a separate area.
2. **Toaster-Free Counter:** Some appliances may trigger a craving for you: a toaster, smoothie blender, juicer, pizza oven, ice cream maker, popcorn popper, etc. Out of sight means out of mind. Kindly ask housemates to hide these appliances for a while – make it easy for them by creating accessible space elsewhere (in the pantry or cupboard).
3. **Agree on a Joint "Baby Step":** Maybe not everyone is ready to jump into full-blown Paleo, but perhaps they will try snacking on veggies instead of chips, going gluten-free or eliminating dairy for a month. Discern how household eating plans can overlap. Each negotiation improves the likelihood of success.
4. **Remove Yourself from Temptation:** Not everyone is willing to compromise and that's okay. You are still in charge of you. When you are done eating dinner, leave before dessert is served. If popcorn comes out during a movie, skip the movie and read a book, take a walk or call a friend or family member. When temptation is around, then you don't have to be.
5. **Find Some Paleo Support:** Having a friend along on the Paleo journey is always a good idea – use the Group Manual in the Resource Section to guide your experience together. If none of your friends are interested, consider a Paleo meet-up group in your area (🖱 MeetUp), join Paleo groups on Facebook, look for Paleo events on 🖱 EventBrite or sign up for newsletters at a Paleo blog. You are not alone – it's a big world out there and the Paleo Diet and Lifestyle are here to stay.

Jot down more ideas to transform your household into a Paleo-friendly zone:

1. _____

2. _____

3. _____

> **Bottom line:** You are responsible for your decisions. No one will make you eat the pasta, snack on candy or drink the wine…that is your choice: a choice that's already been decided for the next month.

Section VI: Contemplate Excuses Inhibiting Success

Other Obstacles to a Successful Paleo Implementation

The mind will find many excuses justifying why you should not start this program. This is a distraction from your goal of renewed health. Mull over the list below to consider what you personally may need to address before beginning. Each individual *is* individual...focus on your personal issues and brainstorm a solution.

We are going to do our best to assist you in your physical and mental commitments. *In Prep D we will give you our suggestions for creating specific strategies to neutralize these concerns.*

Where do you think you could stumble? Mark any that apply:

Common Concerns During a Paleo Transition	
☐ Missing a favorite non-Paleo food	☐ Feeling comfortable with Paleo logic
☐ Getting a doctor on board	☐ Locating quick recipes
☐ Stocking a kitchen	☐ Having support of a friend
☐ Working within a budget	☐ Abstaining from alcohol
☐ Making a travel plan	☐ Making a restaurant plan
☐ Coping through withdrawal or cravings	☐ Having snacks on hand

What else may be problematic at a personal level?

1. _____

2. _____

3. _____

Can you think of specific strategies to address any of the above concerns?

_____

_____

_____

To-Do List:

☐ Find your 5 foundation recipes if you haven't already
☐ Make a double batch of something yummy before Day 1
☐ **Check off the completed tasks in the Master Plan**

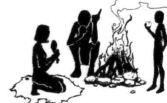

Coming Up Soon:

- In Prep D we'll discuss how to keep you on track when you eat outside of the home

Prep D

Today's Topics:
1. Paleo-Wise: Grains Part I, Why Giving Up Grains is Hard
2. Remove the Excuses, Prepare for Opportunity
3. Planning Social Situations: Traveling, Eating Out, Visiting Friends and Attending Celebrations

Section I – Paleo-Wise: Grains Part I – Why Giving Up Grains is Hard

Whether you eat sugar or starch, in the end, your body absorbs sugar.

Common Grains
🌾 Wheat
🌾 Corn
🌾 Rice
🌾 Oats
🌾 Barley
🌾 Rye
🌾 Millet
🌾 Buckwheat
🌾 Sorghum

Many people don't understand why grains, a food that they've eaten their entire lives, suddenly became *bad*. Although the *awareness* that grains are a problem is relatively recent, the truth is the *compatibility* of grains in human digestion has never existed.

To put the history of grain consumption in perspective, humans evolved eating a hunter-gatherer type diet (Paleo) for greater than one million years. Grains did not become a highly-available food source until agriculture was introduced only six to ten thousand years ago – which is less than 1% of our time on earth!

There simply has not been enough time for human digestive systems to genetically adapt to this food group. This doesn't even account for the modern manipulation of grain during the last hundred years which has also magnified digestive incompatibility.

> **Point to Ponder:** In the spectrum of human existence, grains didn't suddenly become bad; they've never been good in the first place. Recent history is the first time, ever, that grains have been labeled *heart-healthy*.

Grain Changers in Modern Society
Modern grains have been hybridized and manipulated for mass production to the point that today's grains are only distant cousins to the historical grains available to our ancestors. Unfortunately, eating grains is culturally "ingrained." As a food group, they comprise the largest percentage of the western diet and they are marketed as a key to heart health. However, modern grains present major concerns:
1. **Hybridized and Genetically-Manipulated** – Modern grains of the past 50 years are especially controversial since they're bred and manipulated for commercial gain, including faster growth and higher yield. This inadvertently increased starch and gluten content while decreasing the protein and fiber content, all of which amplify digestive distress.
2. **Compatibility with Agricultural Chemicals** – Some of the genetic modifications involve splicing in genes from unrelated species to create herbicide resistance or "built-in" insecticides. This means fields can be doused with weed-killing chemicals without destroying the plant. These crop-preserving practices are intended to kill weeds and insects; however, when eaten, the grain's "built-in" insecticides *plus* chemical residues from excessive herbicide use can damage human digestive bacteria.
3. **Increased Availability** – The portion of our diet consisting of grain products has steadily increased – currently over 50% of the typical western diet is composed of starchy grains. In fact, many people have never gone a *single day* without some grain-derived foodstuff as part of meals or snacks.

Eliminating Grains is like Moving a Mountain
Many people break into a sweat with the mere thought of giving up grains! Why the attraction?
➢ **Habit** – Grains are a staple. They infiltrate our diets in the form of cereals, breads, pasta, rice, tortillas and snack items. We consume these foods by default, so *eliminating grains requires a conscious choice*.
➢ **Price** – Grains are relatively cheap, especially when compared to quality proteins and fats. It is human nature to be frugal and 'get a deal' but that means grains are often substituted for healthier, more expensive food options by both consumers and food manufacturers.

> ➤ **Convenience** – Grains are easily accessible and have a long shelf-life (especially with added preservatives). This handiness often places grain foods as a first choice for modern grab-&-go lifestyles.
> ➤ **Addiction** – Despite their destructive nature, we crave grains. The glucose content of starchy grains is certainly a factor, but that's not all. ⏻ WheatBellyBlog Bread is My Crack
> > • **Physical Addiction** – On top of the addictive glucose load, the protein structures in some grains create morphine-like compounds which stimulate the same brain centers as cocaine or heroin. In fact, many people exhibit classic addiction-denial behavior at the thought of eliminating grains from their diets. Rationalizing the need for grains is common strategy to justify an addictive dependence!
> > • **Emotional Addiction / Habit** – The sad reality is that most emotional 'comfort foods' are grain-based, and habits are difficult to break. Unfortunately, we are accustomed to the convenient, mass-produced, chemically-laden and nutritionally-deficient breads and baked goods prevalent today.

Grain's Anatomy

To better grasp the issues with grains, a basic understanding of the components is helpful. Grains are the seeds of grasses with a protective layer of bran surrounding the endosperm (starch) and the germ (the part that sprouts). Two types of grains are typically incorporated in foods:

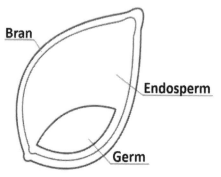

Whole Grain Seed

Bran

Endosperm

Germ

> ➤ **Whole Grains**
> > • Contain all three parts, *whether intact or processed*
> > • Commonly referred to as 'complex carbs'
> > • Legally defined as "any mixture of bran, endosperm and germ *in the proportions one would expect to see in an intact grain*" (the parts are often processed separately, then reassembled as "whole grain flour" – more on the next page)
> ➤ **Refined Grains**
> > • Made of the starchy endosperm only – stripped of bran and germ
> > • Few nutrients remain after processing – classic "empty calories"

> *Swapping refined grains for whole grains has no significant reductions in body fat or other risk factors for metabolic syndrome.* ~Mike Sheridan, Eat Meat and Stop Jogging

Starch – A House of Carbs

Grains are composed predominantly of starchy carbohydrates with some meager amounts of protein and fat, all protected by an outer shell of fiber. Starches are technically called 'polysaccharides' which literally translates to 'many sugars' – and that's exactly what grains are: numerous glucose molecules weakly bound together and easily broken apart. *Sugar by another name is still sugar.*

> **Reality Check:** There are 8-9 teaspoons of sugar in two slices of allegedly healthy whole grain bread! Some people don't dare put a teaspoon of sugar in their coffee, yet proceed to eat bread thinking it's a healthy option.

| **Paleo Isn't Necessarily Low Carb, It's Low Crap!** | Just because the body can endure high percentages of carbohydrates doesn't mean it *should* – there will be health consequences. It's not that all carbs are bad, but they're certainly not necessary to the degree currently in the western diet. The Paleo Diet includes carbs but prioritizes *nutrient-dense* sources like vegetables. |

Carbohydrate Source Matters

Processed carbohydrates made from grains lack nutrients and satiety (the feeling of being full); this makes them incredibly easy to overindulge. Refined and processed grains are far more palatable than fruits and vegetables ever could be. For example, it's not uncommon to consume enormous amounts of pasta in one sitting – but in contrast, a person seldom overeats nutrient-dense carbohydrate sources such as vegetables or fruit (exorbitant pile of broccoli, anyone?).

> **1200 Calories** = 10 ½ cups of sweet potato = 12 ½ medium apples = *just 1 box of macaroni & cheese*

Processing Increases Starch Availability

When ground into flour, the surface area of a grain's contents is exponentially increased up to 10,000 times! This means the starch is completely exposed for rapid digestion. Though cloaked under a deceptive "whole-grain" label, flour-based foods such as bread, pasta or cereal are truly no different than consuming pure glucose.

Point to Ponder: Starch = glucose. Starchy flour is often mixed with sugar to create baked goods (then called "breakfast!"). In reality, a 'healthy' bran muffin is just starch + sweetener…a double-dose of sugar in disguise.

Fortified is Glorified

Processed grain products are often 'fortified' or 'enriched' with select artificial nutrients to replace those that were stripped out during processing. Although that sounds thoughtful from a marketing standpoint, this is a case of "what you *don't* see is what you *don't* get." Here are problems with fortification:

1. **Cherry-Picked Vitamins and Minerals** – Only a few select nutrients are chosen to be replaced, neglecting many other micronutrients.
2. **Poor Bioavailability** – Replaced nutrients are often artificially-manufactured in chemistry labs and the body doesn't always absorb them well.
3. **Poor Functionality** – Of those nutrients that do get absorbed, the function of many is suboptimal when compared to their naturally-occurring counterparts, especially in the absence of other coexisting nutrients that were discarded.

Show me a serving of "healthy whole grains" that can compete nutrient-, vitamin- and mineral-wise with a big-ass salad. What's that? Can't do it? Thought so. ~Mark Sisson, author of Primal Blueprint

Food for Thought: Just because you can eat it doesn't mean it will nourish you. There is a big difference between swallowing nutrients and actually absorbing and utilizing them.

Whole Grain-Wreck

The definition of "whole grains" has been watered down to a point where it is virtually meaningless and purposely confusing. To be labeled *whole*, grains do not actually have to be *intact,* but just need to reflect the three anatomical components in the same proportions naturally found in the seed.

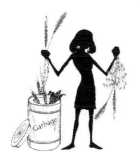

To grasp the difference between intact and whole grains, examine the whole grain milling process:

1. Grain seeds are separated into their three individual parts (bran, germ and endosperm)
2. Each part is independently ground then pulverized into fine flour, destroying fiber and nutrients
3. The naturally-occurring oil is removed to extend the product's shelf life
4. The ground components are then reassembled into foods and called "whole"

Normally, when eating unadulterated *intact* grains, digestive enzymes are required to break down the outer bran layer before accessing the starch. However, in milled whole grains, the bran is pulverized and can't provide that metabolic damper, so the starch in whole grain flour is as *directly accessible as it is in refined flour.*

There is simply no such thing as 'whole' grain bread, pasta or breakfast cereal. These foods are all processed in some way. Don't kid yourself and say, 'it's healthy because it's brown bread.' It's still just flour! I dare you to go to a paddock of wheat and eat the 'whole grain.' I think you would chip a tooth! ~Stephen Eddy, PhD

What about Fiber? Whole Grain Fiber Fail

Fiber plays a very important role in proper digestion and admittedly, whole grains do contain fiber. Advertisers are quick to point out that whole grains have more fiber than refined grains – but *more* doesn't mean *most.* The flaw in that description is the insinuation that whole grains are the best source of fiber, but they're not. What foods have the *most* fiber? Vegetables!

When compared to vegetables, grains fail miserably. Vegetables have 8 times more fiber than intact whole grains and up to 30 times more than refined grains! Even fruits have up to 7 times more fiber than refined grains. If the goal is to increase fiber, simply eat more vegetables. Without the fiber argument, there is no nutritional justification for whole grains, even if intact.

> *Eating whole grains to get more fiber is like eating carrot cake to get more vegetables!* ~Unknown

High Calorie-Load for Minimal Fiber

It's tempting to use a grain's fiber content to justify eating absurd amounts of grain. Ironically, the extra starches and calorie load undermine the benefits of fiber and undeniably lead to weight gain.

> **Eat Paleo for Weight Loss – it's a 'No-Grainer':** Eat lots of vegetables and get butt-loads more fiber (literally) while acquiring far more nutrients with way fewer calories!

> *No one dies of a bread deficiency. We do not need flour in our diets. They are dead foods that contribute nothing more than empty calories and soaring obesity.* ~Neander-Steve.blogspot.com

Tip of the Iceberg

If it weren't bad enough that grains are heavy in starches, nutrient-poor, low in fiber, addictive, highly-processed and much too convenient…grains also directly damage the intestine, disrupt proper digestion and prevent nutrient absorption. More details coming in Prep E's Paleo-Wise section: Grains Part II.

Further Reading:

- WellnessMama The Real Problem with Grains
- WheatBellyBlog Wheat is an Opiate

Section II: Remove the Excuses, Prepare for Opportunity

The person who says it cannot be done should not interrupt the person doing it. The sentiment from the first quote today fully applies to that doubting, criticizing voice in your head…self-doubts need to be addressed.

We understand that extinguishing the inflammatory and addictive western diet is a giant undertaking. Rather than addressing this as an uphill battle, *embrace it as an opportunity.*

> *Healing is a matter of time, but it is sometimes also a matter of opportunity.* ~Hippocrates

Before you embark on your journey to break dietary habits, heal your body and realize optimal health, thorough preparation is necessary. This includes overcoming mindsets that interfere with taking the first step. What's holding you back? Dig deep…what excuses need to be quashed to put forward your best effort?

1. _____
2. _____
3. _____
4. _____
5. _____

> *If you don't want to do something, one excuse is as good as another.* ~Yiddish Proverb

Some common concerns for planning a Paleo Transition were highlighted in Prep C. Do not allow excuses like these to delay implementation. Keep reading to learn how to address those concerns, dispel common anxieties and solidify mental commitment (it's okay to skip any of the following suggestions that don't apply to you).

> **Rachel's Journey:** I researched Paleo eating for over 9 months before I was ready to shed 10+ years of vegetarianism. There's no reason it needed to take that long – I was stalling with multiple excuses.

I Don't Want to Give Up [...fill in the blank...]

- **Specific Favorite Food** – Sometimes the foods we resist giving up are the ones hurting us the most. The good news is you only avoid them for a month; the bad news is you may discover those favorite foods trigger a negative response when you add them back in. Stick with us here...no one wants to lose their favorite foods, but entertain the possibility that by the end of the program, you may not even miss them. Until you know how good your body feels without your trigger foods, you will never understand their true impact on your health and happiness. Prepare to be amazed!
  P.S. Fortunately, not every single favorite food turns out to be a trigger food!

> **Kelly's Experience:** I love popcorn! Still do. When I felt ill constantly, I didn't realize popcorn was a contributor. However, even after years of eating Paleo, popcorn still causes digestive upset, despite being organic, popped in healthy coconut oil and topped with pastured butter and Celtic sea salt. No, I didn't *want* to give it up, but now I know when I indulge, I will feel ill for a few days.

- **Low-Fat Diet** – If low-fat diets worked, then we would already be our perfect, energetic, lean, muscular selves. But look around – recommendations based on the 'grain pyramid' have been followed for decades, yet obesity and diabetes continue to escalate. Even though avoiding fat is not the solution, many are afraid to add fat back into the diet. Disregard that *big fat fear* for just one month to discover how good you feel and how delicious food tastes when it includes healthy, traditional Paleo fats. Don't worry, future Paleo-Wise sections elaborate on multiple fat topics, plus explain why *essential fats* are...um, essential.
- **Convenience** – Admittedly, many commercial foods are cheap, convenient and tasty – designed to capture our bliss point. Giving up convenience is difficult BUT there is nothing convenient about feeling bloated, lethargic, achy, depressed or forgetful. For one month, with just a little forward planning, you can create Paleo convenience by batch-cooking and freezing meals, having veggies ready to eat and purchasing some high quality convenient Paleo foods like pre-made guacamole or pasture-raised jerky.
- **Alcohol** – Our society and culture uphold alcohol as a key component of celebrations and relaxation. The downfall of alcohol consumption is well known – loads of calories, burdensome on the liver, highly addictive. Ask yourself this question: Have you ever gone a full month without drinking alcohol? If yes, then you know you can. If not, then maybe it's time.

> *How strange to use "You only live once" as an excuse to throw it away.* ~Bill Copeland

I Don't Feel Prepared

- **My Kitchen isn't Paleo-Compliant** – Designate a kitchen area and fill it with Paleo foods using the Clean-Out and Stock-Up lists. Explain to your housemates that this is important to you and you'd appreciate their help keeping non-Paleo foods out of eyesight. You could even offer to cook dinner to make the deal more attractive. If your kitchen won't be Paleo-safe, then carve out a place in your closet, buy a dorm fridge or just forge ahead with your plans in a non-Paleo kitchen (it can be done).
- **I Don't Know Where to Buy Paleo Foods** – Local grocery stores, health food stores, farmer's markets and online grocers carry many Paleo foods. Check items for added sugars even at these online Paleo markets:

  ⬧ ThriveMarket*   ⬧ BarefootProvisions   ⬧ OneStopPaleoShop   ⬧ PaleoFoodMall

  * Visit ⬧ Paleovation for direct links to ThriveMarket and all other recommended sites and reading

- **I Need Some Go-To Meals** – We supply easy starter meals (Prep E), offer a few foundation meal recipes (Resource Section), breakfast ideas (Prep F) and snack recommendations (Day 2). More to come.
- **I Need a Stocked Freezer** – Leftovers frozen in single serving sizes make a quick meal. Here are other tips:
  - ➤ The Kitchen Stock-Up form (Prep B) has some Paleo-friendly freezer-filling suggestions.
  - ➤ Many 'tedious' Paleo foods are increasingly available in grocer freezer sections including squash purees, chopped spinach, cauliflower rice or pre-measured herb packets.
  - ➤ Search ⬧ "OAMC Paleo" (meaning Once-A-Month-Cooking) to find some prep-ahead recipes.
  - ➤ Consider purchasing a few pre-made Paleo meals to keep in the freezer (suggestions in Prep B).

I'm Second-Guessing this Paleo Commitment

- **Don't I Need Dairy for Calcium?** Simply stated, no. We specifically address dairy, calcium and bone health in the Paleo-Wise topics on Days 7 and 16.
- **I Feel All Alone in this Decision** – Ask a friend to join you…the more the merrier (also good for inspiration and commiseration). Use the Group Manual in the Resource Section to guide your support for each other. Or find someone at the gym, the library, the health food store, start a meet-up group, ask your social media friends, a colleague, a spouse, a parent, your neighbor's kid. You won't know until you ask. Even if no one joins you, they'll know your intentions and will be watching your transition to Paleo.
- **I Need More "Proof" that Paleo Works** – Get online and search "Paleo + [insert your health problem here]." Read thousands of testimonials: diabetes, ADHD, high cholesterol, high blood pressure, brain fog, tendonitis, ulcerative colitis, MS, eczema…success stories abound. Our bodies *will* heal when we remove destructive foods and consume nourishing foods compatible with human digestion.
- **Will I Be Ready for Withdrawal Symptoms or Cravings?** – Yes, you will. We detail numerous tips, tricks and strategies throughout these Prep segments as well as during the first days of the program.

> *The only limit to our realization of tomorrow will be our doubts of today.* ~Franklin D. Roosevelt

I Don't Think Eating Paleo Fits into My Lifestyle

- **I Travel a Lot** – Travel is no excuse. Bun-less burgers on salad greens are perfectly acceptable. Hard-boiled eggs and berries work in a pinch. Stock your hotel room with Paleo foods – it may be even easier to stay compliant on the road because the typical temptations from home aren't around. Surround yourself with healthy foods and you will eat healthy foods (more travel solutions are detailed next).
- **Can I Eat Paleo in a Restaurant?** – Yes, keep reading. Restaurant strategies are discussed next.
- **Social Obligations** – You have no bigger obligation than to your own health, so plan wisely. Eat healthy before attending gatherings – snack on the fresh veggies or shrimp (cocktail-less). When at a dinner, eat the protein and salad and skip the starch. Everyone drinking? Have sparkling water with a twist of lime. If you must scrape the breading off the chicken, so be it. It's doable and is only for one month.

I'm Concerned About What Other People Will Say

- **People Think It's Crazy to Give Up Grains** – Yep. The three givens in life are death, taxes and cynics. No matter what your decision, someone can claim it's flawed. Yet if you make the opposite choice, someone else will criticize that as well. The truth is, people are afraid of change. Your willingness and resolution to explore dietary choice may be threatening to them (perhaps they don't want to feel pressured to give up grains). Sometimes others just aren't ready to support you. Continue to educate yourself and reassure concerned individuals that this is just for a month (and no one has died from a grain deficiency…or dairy or legume deficiency either). Stay confident and resilient – you'll shine through this!

> *You can make excuses, or you can get the job done, but you can't do both.* ~Hap Holmstead, The Biggest Loser

- **I Feel Like I Should Have my Doctors' Approval** – Great. Tell your doctors you intend to eat nutrient-dense, anti-inflammatory foods for one month to see how you feel, though take any dietary advice with caution. Realize that medical doctors are indispensable for trauma care and surgical intervention. They are well educated about medicines most appropriate for a particular condition or symptom set. However, in general, doctors lack nutritional education. Furthermore, it's highly likely that their dietary knowledge consists of conventional wisdom promoting the low-fat diet (also endorsed by national and state medical associations, organizations, foundations and societies). Return to the doctor after your first month of Paleo to get updates on lab tests, readjust any medications and report your personal experience.
  - ☞ Whole30 Talk to your Doc: What to Do if your Doctor Says "No"
- **I Need a "Cheat Sheet" to Quickly Address Any Questions about Paleo** – We have one! Look for the "Science-Behind-Paleo Cheat Sheet" in the Resource Section.

I Cannot Afford Paleo Food

"My budget doesn't allow me to eat Paleo" – That hits the nail on the head...except it's a nail in a coffin.

Excuses are the nails used to build a house of failure. ~Don Wilder and Bill Rechin

Your hard-earned money can purchase vegetables, quality meats and coconut oil or it can pay for doctors, hospitals and drugs. A healthier you will save medical expenses in the long run. Pay it forward to yourself. Budget quality food for just one month then re-evaluate...these may be small sacrifices for renewed health!

1. If grass-fed or pasture-raised animal products are too expensive, choose lean factory-farmed meats.
2. If organic produce is unaffordable, select conventional vegetables.
3. Purchase meats on the bone. It's less expensive per pound, plus the meat is more nutritious when cooked on the bone...and you can use the bones for making broth.
4. Begin incorporating organ meats, they're inexpensive and extremely nutritious, regardless of sourcing.
5. Squeeze every nutrient out of your purchases:
   - A whole chicken? Roast it, eat the meat and skin, use the bones and giblets for 2-3 batches of broth.
   - Swiss chard? Sauté the greens like spinach, chop the stems to use like celery.
   - Roasting beets? Save the greens for a salad or sauté them into an omelet.
6. Reallocate entertainment and restaurant funds for quality home-cooking and consider inviting friends. Start entertaining yourself with free Paleo podcasts while you chop veggies:
   - 🎧 BalancedBites Podcast
   - 🎧 Bulletproof Radio
   - 🎧 PaleoMagOnline Paleo Radio PMR
   - 🎧 MarksDailyApple 9 Primal/Paleo Podcasts You Should Be Listening To
7. Put the price difference in perspective: grass-fed ground beef will only cost a few extra dollars per week, less than the cost of a fast food value meal (more price comparisons on Day 19).

Don't just bargain for success. Pay the price! ~Israelmore Ayivor, Become a Better You

8. Grow vegetables and herbs or visit a you-pick farm to harvest vegetables in the field at a reduced price.
9. Forage for free! Many public places allow foraging – dandelion greens, berries, garlic mustard, hazelnuts, purslane, morels, truffles, lamb's quarters, etc. Need a guidebook?
   - 📖 TheAtlantic 11 Books for Foragers
10. Do you hunt or fish or know someone who does? Inquire if they have meat to share.
11. Purchase food in bulk via the internet, wholesalers or at local farms (both vegetables and meats).
12. Offset the expense of meat with loads of vegetables. For example, 1 pound of ground beef can be mixed with 2 ½ lbs of minced vegetables to make a giant meatloaf.
13. Find a local farm that will swap vegetables for manual labor. Local CSAs often do this.
14. Quit the $4-per-cup fancy coffee drink and make your own with coconut milk and cinnamon.
15. Remember the alcohol budget will be $0 – this frees up money for extra fresh veggies and quality meats.
    - 📖 *Frugal Paleo,* by Ciarra Hannah, is a great resource for stretching your food dollar.

My Mindset Isn't Ready

- **"I Could Never Do That"** – Yes, you're right. You have already made your decision. Hundreds of thousands of people have revived their health with Paleo, but you've defeated your desires, willpower and resilience before even beginning. You can put this book away right now. Better luck next time.
- **"I Can Probably Do That"** – Yes, you're right! You *probably* can ☺.

Whether you think you can or think you can't, you're right. ~Henry Ford

Understanding Mental Commitment

The bottom line is that thousands of excuses exist whether you make a change or not. It is a conscious choice to release excuses and proceed on the Paleo journey. *Your mind has everything to do with your success.*

In the book, 📖 *Rise of Superman*, author Steven Kotler cites a study in grip strength. Each participant is randomly assigned a group; their grip strength is measured at the beginning and end of the study:

The Random Groups	Increase in Grip Strength
1. Performed grip-strengthening exercises	56% increase
2. Only *visualized* grip-strengthening exercises (did *not* physically practice the exercises)	34% increase
3. Performed *arm*-strengthening exercises	23% increase
4. Did nothing (the control group)	No change

Notice that Group 2 improved without even physically training! Their improvements came by only *visualizing* the grip-strengthening exercises. We've all heard "mind over matter," but it truly makes a huge, tangible difference. Get your mind in the right place, visualize your future health and your commitment will be solid.

Everything you can imagine is real. ~Pablo Piccaso

Please look at the apprehensions you noted in Prep C. Which items still concern you?

1. _____

2. _____

3. _____

If you need further assistance addressing concerns, go online to find a Paleo forum. In these groups, you can search previous entries and/or ask your specific question to receive feedback from others with similar situations.

Section III: Planning Social Situations (An Eating Outside-of-the-Home Master Plan)

How do you remain Paleo-successful outside of your controlled home environment? **Preparation!**

Social Obligations

Expect to stay on track no matter where you roam. Many ideas overlap so we will start with the basics:

Meal Strategies	Celebration Strategies
• Eat ahead of time • Bring your own meal • Bring a Paleo dish to pass • Offer to host the dinner • Suggest a potluck • Suggest grilling-out or a picnic • Follow restaurant strategies (below)	• Come and go as you please (leave before dessert, come after dinner finishes) • Skip dessert • Offer to bring a fruit salad for dessert • Drink sparkling water with lime/lemon • Bring along a jug of kombucha

Packable Foods

Highlight your favorite ideas – you need to plan leftovers for some of these (Day 2 has more snack ideas):

Room Temp		Keep Cool	
• Jerky (beef, turkey, salmon) • Cured meats (whole salami, beef sticks) • Roasted nuts or trail mix • Plantain chips fried in coconut/palm oil • Paleo muffins or crackers (homemade, unsweetened)	• Nut butter (pouch) • Baked veggie chips • Fresh fruit • Baby food pouches/jars • Canned fish, shrimp • Olives (single serve pouch) • Paleo protein bar (Day 2) • Freeze-dried fruit / veggies	• Guacamole (individual serving) • Salmon/fish cakes • Fresh cut veggies • Paleo sushi with cauliflower rice • Grass-fed hot dogs • Hard-boiled eggs	• Deviled eggs • Lunch meats • Paleo waffles • Frittata slices • Leftovers • Liverwurst • Bacon • Pickles

Restaurant Strategies

- Selecting a Restaurant:
    - ✓ Search words that imply quality meat: grass-fed, local, wild-caught, artisan, farm-to-table
    - ✓ Seek styles that easily convert to Paleo by omitting grains and dairy: burgers, fajitas, curries, omelets, salads, steaks and most poached, steamed or grilled entrées
- Choosing Your Meal:
    - ✓ Browse a gluten-free menu to remove items with hidden gluten such as soups, sauces or meatloaf
    - ✓ Omit anything deep-fried – the fryer has rancid oil as well as gluten from other items
    - ✓ If high quality meat is not available, select lean proteins
    - ✓ Salad bar is a good option – dress with straight olive oil and vinegar
- Modifying a Meal:
    - ✓ Let your server know you are "working around food sensitivities"
    - ✓ Request no bread bowl or tortilla chip basket
    - ✓ Request "cracked eggs" in an omelet (versus omelet mix that often contains flour for added fluffiness)
    - ✓ Ask for your food to be cooked in butter instead of industrial oils
    - ✓ Order your entrée without dairy, legumes or grains:
        - ▪ Order a sandwich in a lettuce wrap versus a bun
        - ▪ Order nacho fixings on top of salad greens versus tortilla chips; hold the cheese and sour cream
        - ▪ Request extra steamed veggies to replace entrée sides such as french fries, chips or rice
        - ▪ Request fresh fruit to replace breakfast sides such as toast, pancakes or muffins

    > *When in doubt, add bacon.* ~Unknown

- Other:
    - ✓ Do not agonize if you consume a little canola oil at a restaurant, just continue to avoid it at home
    - ✓ Use caution with Chinese restaurant food (generally contains many additives and soy sauce has wheat)
    - ✓ When your server helps guide you to an appropriate meal decision, tip well
    - ✓ Almost every Paleo blog has a Restaurant Guide for more suggestions

Describe your favorite restaurant meal and how to modify it to be Paleo:

_____

_____

Other restaurant strategies that would work for you:

_____

Travel Strategies

- **In Your Luggage**
    - ✓ Reusable containers to fill along the way (they can hold non-perishable foods like jerky when packed)
    - ✓ Paring knife, can opener, plate for microwave, set of silverware (plastic and paper often work well)
    - ✓ Use a small cooler as carry-on luggage
    - ✓ Individual guacamole servings can be frozen and used as ice packs (but remember to place them in your liquids bag for TSA screening)
    - ✓ Consider taking desiccated liver pills (Day 23) during travel for high quality protein and vitamins
- **At the Hotel**
    - ✓ Use your fridge for leftovers, fresh veggies and coconut milk (for coffee/tea)
    - 📖 *Make Ahead Paleo,* by Tammy Credicott includes recipes to cook in a hotel microwave
    - ✓ Choose a room with a kitchenette when possible – bring seasonings if you'll be cooking
- **On the Road**
    - ✓ Pack a Paleo picnic (use packable foods on previous page)
    - ✓ Utilize restaurant strategies above

- **At the Grocery Store or Farmer's Market**
  - ✓ Purchase veggies, hard-boiled eggs, berries, baby carrots, pickles, canned tuna, lunchmeats, fruits, nuts and olives
  - ✓ Visit the salad/cold bar or deli for prepared veggies and salads
  - ✓ Stock up on sparkling water, kombucha and herbal tea bags to avoid sugary drinks

> *Inaction breeds doubt and fear. Action breeds confidence and courage.*
> *If you want to conquer fear, do not sit home and think about it. Go out and get busy.*
> ~Dale Carnegie, author of <u>How to Stop Worrying and Start Living</u>

Section III: Practice Eating Outside-of-the-Home

The following Quick Paleo Reference Guide can be carried in your wallet, car, briefcase, purse, etc. Another copy is located in the Resource Section to tear out.

Quick Paleo Reference Guide

Foods to Eat

Meats: Beef, poultry, pork, lamb, bison, venison, wild game (grass-fed, pastured, pasture-raised or organic preferred...if factory-farm raised then trim/drain off fat)

Eggs: Chicken, duck, quail – look for antibiotic-free, free range or pasture-raised (be generous with the serving size, 3-5 eggs per serving is perfectly acceptable)

Seafood: Salmon, herring, cod, tilapia, halibut, perch, whitefish, trout, tuna, shrimp, lobster, crawdads, clams, mussels, oysters, scallops, caviar, etc (canned, fresh, or frozen; wild-caught is best...farm-raised are often fed grains, hormones or other chemicals, though some Scandinavian companies are quite strict with sustainably-raised farmed fish and sockeye red salmon is always wild-caught)

Veggies: All vegetables except corn (a grain) and white/yellow/red potatoes (if weight loss is a goal); Fresh, frozen, dehydrated or organic are best, canned is okay

Low-Sugar Fruits: Raspberries, blackberries, cranberries, blueberries, strawberries, green apples, fresh figs, grapefruit, lemons, limes or not-quite-ripe banana - **One serving daily**

Oils: Extra virgin olive oil (for cold or medium heat), coconut oil or avocado oil (for high heat), macadamia oil (cold use only)

Fats: Grass-fed butter (or ghee), avocado, coconut, pasture-raised tallow, lard or duck fat

Nuts/Seeds: Dry-roasted, sprouted, in-the-shell, raw or butter, **one serving daily,** *no peanuts (legume)*

Foods to Avoid - Read labels!

Grains: Wheat, rice, corn, barley, oats, amaranth, millet, buckwheat, sprouted grains, bulgur, etc, plus pseudo-grains such as quinoa (if it acts like a grain, omit for the program)

Dairy: Yogurt, cheese, cream, whey protein powder, sour cream, cottage cheese, kefir, ice cream, casein, lactose, factory-farmed butter (only grass-fed butter or grass-fed ghee is allowed)

Industrialized seed oils: Canola, corn, soybean, sunflower, safflower, vegetable, shortening, grapeseed, cottonseed, margarine, spreads

Legumes/Beans: Soy, pinto, black, garbanzo/chick peas, hummus, refried beans, lentils, peas, peanuts (green beans, sugar snap peas and snow peas are fine to consume because the whole pod is eaten)

High-sugar fruits: Most fresh/canned fruits, all dried fruits, fruit juice

Sweeteners: Honey, maple syrup, corn syrup, sugar, aspartame, Equal®, Splenda®, agave nectar, dates, etc (stevia is acceptable in controlled amounts – avoid brands that mix stevia with dextrose)

Chemical additives: MSG, carrageenan, food colorings, soy products, corn products, sulfites and other preservatives (check 🖑 Pinterest.com/Paleovation Sneaky Food Additives for specifics)

Sweetened Beverages: Soft drinks, juices, drink mixes / shakes

Alcohol: Spirits, wine, beer, alcohol extracts like vanilla

> *The best day of your life is the one on which you decide your life is your own. No apologies or excuses.*
> *No one to lean on, rely on, or blame. The gift is yours — it is an amazing journey — and you alone*
> *are responsible for the quality of it. This is the day your life really begins.* ~Bob Moawad, <u>Whatever it Takes</u>

Paleo Meal Practice

Using the Restaurant Strategies and Quick Paleo Reference Guide for ideas, fill in typical meals you would order in a restaurant and how you can make them appropriate for this program:

	Typical Meal	Keep	Ditch	Substitute
Breakfast				
Snack				
Lunch				
Snack				
Dinner				

Until someone launches a Paleo Pizza Parlor, pizza is the hardest meal to replicate in a restaurant. As a worst-case scenario, you can request to have the veggie and meat toppings baked with marinara sauce (which likely has sugar). It is best to have a back-up plan for other options to order at your favorite pizzeria:

1. _____

2. _____

3. _____

> *A year from now you will wish you had started today.* ~Karen Lamb, <u>I Felt My Wings</u>

Your Last Exercise for Prep D: Write down some Paleo-friendly foods for these situations:

Eating Outside the Home	
Situation	**Paleo-Friendly Option**
Picnic food	
In carry-on luggage through TSA screening	
Something to keep in your gym bag	
Fast food restaurant option	
Family restaurant option	
Quick lunch at a grocery store	
Replacement for sandwich bread	
Beverage	
Snack to bring for game day	

When you are satisfied you have strategies for eating-outside-of-the-home,

    ☐ **Mark it off on the Master Preparation List**

To-Do List:

    ☐ Finish locating 5 foundation recipes.
    ☐ Is that batch cooking job done?
    ☐ Are you including new healthy habits (veggies, unsweetened beverages, no bread, better oils, walk)?

Coming Up Soon:

    • Tweaking meals to make them Paleo and some quickly-prepared meals

Remember: *The person who says it cannot be done should not interrupt the person doing it!*

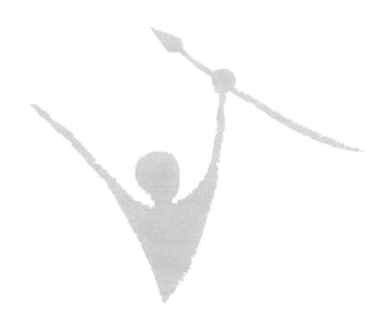

Prep E

Today's Topics:
1. Paleo-Wise: Grains Part II, Gluten, Anti-Nutrients and Obesity
2. Low-Carb Flu and What to Do
3. Meal-Tweaking Strategies
4. Solidify Mental Preparation
5. Quick-Meal Ideas
6. Tips for a Successful Transition

What are some Paleo foods you're already adding to your repertoire?

Breakfast: _____

Lunch: _____

Dinner: _____

Snacks: _____

Beverages: _____

Section I – Paleo-Wise: Grains Part II (Gluten, Anti-Nutrients and Obesity)

The increase in commercially-available gluten-free products creates general awareness that there's something bad about gluten, but many still don't understand exactly what gluten is and why it's unhealthy.

Gluten generically refers to part of the protein that grass plants build into their seeds to support future growth (remember, grass seeds are 'grains'). The most familiar type of gluten is found in **wheat**, **rye** and **barley**, and is responsible for the chewy, doughy, elastic texture in food (*and* wallpaper paste by the way – the word *gluten* is literally Latin for glue!). Over the years, increasingly more gluten invaded the daily diet.

> **Marketing Magic:** Because gluten is a protein, bread marketed as 'high protein' is often higher in gluten.

Gluten – We Can't Stomach it…
Gluten by nature is sticky. So in essence, it sticks to the digestive tract lining, contributing to damage, erosion and potentially significant health problems (explained further in the Lectin section next). Even individuals who thought they tolerated gluten well report relief of multiple ailments after eliminating gluten for a month.

Symptoms of Gluten Intolerance:
➢ Gastrointestinal (GI), stomach and digestive issues including gas, bloating, cramping, constipation, heartburn (GERD or acid reflux), diarrhea or IBS
➢ Headaches or migraines
➢ Fibromyalgia or chronic fatigue
➢ Sudden mood shifts, irritability, anxiety or depression
➢ Dizziness or balance problems
➢ Tingling or numb hands and feet
➢ Hormonal imbalances or unexplained infertility
➢ Inflammation, swelling or joint pain
➢ Autoimmune disease (Celiac Disease, Hashimoto's Thyroiditis, Multiple Sclerosis, Rheumatoid Arthritis, Lupus, Psoriasis, Scleroderma, Ulcerative Colitis, etc)

> **Be Aware:** Gluten intolerance may indicate sensitivities to other similarly-shaped proteins. Those with known gluten sensitivities have a high probability (~50% chance) of cross-reactivity to casein, a protein found in dairy.

Gluten-Free Caution

Although *wheat* contains the most notable aggressive gluten, other "gluten-free" grains have similar glutinous compounds, plus they still carry all the destructive elements of high starch. The gluten-free label deceptively lulls us into a false sense of security, essentially justifying consumption of highly-processed, insulin-stimulating foods. Furthermore, it's difficult to prevent cross-contamination between wheat and non-gluten grains as they commonly are grown in the same fields or processed with the same equipment.

Gluten-Free: "Out of the Frying Pan but Into the Fire"

Gluten-Free is NOT PROBLEM-FREE! For those considering *only* eliminating gluten-containing grains, gluten-free does not translate to healthy. Problems with gluten-free grains include:

- **Starch-Heavy** – Gluten-free grains like rice, corn, oats and pseudo-grain quinoa have the same starchy effect on blood sugar as their wheat-based counterparts.
- **Trigger Insulin Response** – Excess insulin harms blood sugar regulation, promoting obesity and making weight-loss very difficult.
- **Low Nutritional Value** – Many gluten-free products are highly-refined which destroys any potential nutrition. Most flour-based food can be classified as 'empty calories.'
- **Contain Other Harmful Ingredients** – Palatability and shelf-life is often enhanced with sugars, high fructose corn syrup, artificial sweeteners, colorings, preservatives, etc.

Just because gluten-free grains are *less bad*, doesn't mean they're ideal – it's bad if you fracture both ankles; it would be *less bad* if you only fractured one ankle, but that's certainly not ideal!

> **Paleo Version of "Gluten-Free"**: Enjoy foods that never had gluten in the first place! Choose vegetables, animal proteins, fruit and healthy fats (coconut, avocado, olives and nuts).

Anti-Nutrients: Trojan Horses of Grains

As a survival mechanism, plants protect their reproductive seeds via toxic molecules which preserve and safeguard nutrients essential for seed growth. These toxins are designed to resist digestion for two reasons:

1. **Propagation:** Whole undigested seeds will grow when excreted in a pile of manure (fertilizer)
2. **Deterrent:** Toxins upset digestion to protect the seed from predators (including humans)

 Although grains taste delicious, their protective toxins act like Trojan horses. Once these compounds arrive in the digestive tract, they inflame the gut lining, trigger immune reactions (like allergies) and prevent absorption of essential nutrients. Because they contribute to *nutrient* deficiencies, these plant toxins are therefore called *anti-nutrients*.

> **Key Point:** The miniscule amount of nutrients potentially attainable from grains is irrelevant if anti-nutrients encage them and make them inaccessible.

Absorption: It's Not Really in Your Body Until It's in Your Blood

Before delving into anti-nutrient details, a brief explanation of digestive absorption is helpful to grasp how consuming these toxins disrupts health.

The digestive tract is a 30ft-long gut tube extending from the mouth to the anus. Food in the tube is technically not inside the body – yes, it's in your intestines but it hasn't yet left this enclosed tube. Before the gut contents are allowed access to the bloodstream, they must first filter through the intestinal wall. This selective membrane is tightly lined with cells that screen digestive tract contents. Like checkpoint guards, these cells selectively absorb nutrients while simultaneously blocking dangerous particles, like parasites or toxins, from entering the bloodstream.

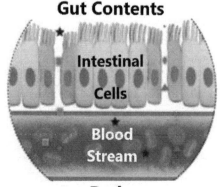

Gut Contents

Intestinal Cells

Blood Stream

Body

Types of Anti-Nutrients

Grains are not the only foods with anti-nutrients, but they are a dense source of these damaging plant toxins. The following types of anti-nutrients have the highest potential for digestive distress.

Lectins

Lectins are toxic compounds found in all plants, but particularly potent varieties abound in grains and legumes. The most familiar aggressive lectin is found in gluten (WGA – Wheat Germ Agglutinin) but known toxic varieties also exist in soy and peanuts. *All grains AND legumes contain lectins.* The major issues with lectins include:

- **Resist Digestion** – Humans do not have the necessary digestive enzymes to break down lectin protein structures. Lectins remain largely intact throughout the digestive tract, causing trouble along the way.
- **Contain Enzyme Inhibitors** – Foods with lectins also contain compounds that prevent digestive enzymes from breaking down other proteins, further disrupting the digestive process.
- **Damage Gut Lining** – Lectins can harm the intestinal lining, especially the 'brush border' (the microvilli are finger-like projections that extend into the gut tube – see image on previous page). Each meal containing grains/legumes repeatedly introduces more destructive lectins which provokes cumulative damage, interrupts proper nutrient absorption and never gives the digestive tract the chance to heal.
- **Generate Immune Response** – When consumed, lectins are rightly identified as foreign invaders – an immune response to create antibodies is activated. Because lectins imbed into the digestive lining, the body's attempt to attack the lectin also destroys adjacent normal cells. Eventually, gaps/holes develop in the digestive lining (Leaky Gut Syndrome) allowing undigested food particles, bacteria, toxins and other invasive substances to pass through the protective barrier directly into the blood.

> **Leaky Gut Carpet Analogy:** The 'brush border' lining of the intestine resembles a shag carpet. Chronic destruction from lectins erodes the yarn-like fibers (microvilli)...so over time, that shag carpet begins to resemble Berber, making nutrient absorption much more difficult. With ongoing onslaught, holes develop in the Berber and foreign particles can no longer be stopped from entering the body.

- **Harm Other Body Systems** – Once in the blood, lectins have the potential to bind to almost any structure in the body, continuing the assault elsewhere: organs (brain, heart, kidneys, eyes, etc), glands (thyroid, adrenals, pituitary, reproductive, etc), nerves, muscles, cartilage or skin. Damage includes inflammation, chronic joint pain, hormonal disruption, mental health conditions and even allergies.
- **Trigger Autoimmune Conditions** – Because lectins often resemble normal body proteins, the same antibodies created to attack a lectin can also attack similar body structures. This is referred to as an autoimmune response – when the body mistakenly attacks its own tissues.

Phytates

Phytates are a storage form of minerals, primarily phosphorus, preserved for seed growth. They're concentrated in the hull (bran) of grains and legumes as part of the protective shell. Problems arise because the phytate form of minerals cannot be digested by humans without help from enzymes produced by good gut bacteria.

Unfortunately, prevalent antibiotic use (both intentionally via prescriptions and inadvertently by eating animal products from farms that medicate confined livestock) has altered digestive bacteria. This diminishes our ability to break down phytates. The encased minerals stay trapped and can potentially result in mineral deficiencies.

- **Enzyme Interference** – Phytates prevent enzymes from breaking down (digesting) the seed. This also makes enzymes less effective for any other foods present, resulting in additional digestive distress.
- **Snare Other Minerals** – Besides phosphorus, phytates engulf other minerals like a cage, preventing their absorption, especially iron and zinc but also magnesium, calcium, chromium and manganese.

Food for Thought: Although marketed as healthy, bran cereal has one of the highest concentrations of phytates, consumption of which leads to mineral deficiencies (including calcium in the accompanying milk).

Proper Preparation is Critical – Phytate levels can be reduced by using a combination of soaking, sprouting, fermenting, pounding and cooking. However, the degree of phytate reduction is highly variable. Legume anti-nutrients tend to respond positively to these preparation methods, but whole grains aren't typically prepared in these manners so high phytate levels remain a concern.

Key point: E*ven when consuming quality vegetables or nutritional supplements, minerals like calcium, zinc, magnesium, phosphorus and iron will be difficult to absorb if phytates are present to trap them.* Grains are a concentrated source of phytates. Bottom line: High-phytate, grain-based diets result in mineral deficiencies.

Grain Gain – Obesity Linked to Grain Consumption

High-grain diets contribute to obesity in many mammals, including both ends of dietary extremes: herbivores and carnivores. As omnivores, humans fall between the two and are likewise vulnerable to the obesity influence of grains.

- **Herbivores** – Beef cattle are purposely *grain-fed* or *grain-finished* to increase fat content, especially desirable for well-marbled, juicy steak. Feeding grains to herbivores like cattle makes them fatter, not dissimilar to their effect on humans.
- **Carnivores** – Dogs and cats are carnivores, yet many commercial pet food formulas use grains as primary ingredients. A simple observation of the obesity epidemic among domestic dogs and cats demonstrates the fact that grains, as a dietary staple, are incompatible in carnivores.

Grains are "For the Birds": Many birds, including chickens, are *granivores* (grain-eaters). Their anatomy includes a *crop* to store and moisturize grains prior to digestion, a *gizzard* to grind the outer seed shell, and pouches called *ceca* to ferment any course material remaining at the end of the small intestine. Until we evolve these extra organs, humans are not designed to digest grains!

No Grain = No Pain

We've established that human physiology suffers when grains are consumed, resulting in digestive and nutritional consequences. We can survive but *will never thrive* on grain-based diets. Grains provide no unique nutritional value that cannot be attained from non-destructive sources: quality produce and animal products.

Paleo Advantage: When grains and legumes are removed from the diet, nutrient absorption increases! That's because these problematic, anti-nutrient foods are replaced with anti-inflammatory vegetables, animal proteins and healthy fats with increased nutritional density and bioavailability.
The Paleo Diet Supplies Increased Nutrient Content with Less Digestive Interference.

Are Paleo Foods Free from Anti-Nutrients?

Many foods contain lectin or phytate anti-nutrients, including Paleo foods such as nuts, eggs and nightshade vegetables (tomato, eggplant, potato, peppers). For folks with leaky gut syndrome, offenders in these foods can sneak into the bloodstream and cause damage. This explains why some individuals have additional sensitivities to these food groups (read more about Autoimmune Protocol recommendations in the Resource Section).

The main distinction between the anti-nutrients of grains/legumes and those in Paleo-approved foods is that grains and legumes tend to have high concentrations of types that are more resistant and damaging. Specifically eliminating grain and legume sources of anti-nutrients for a month gives the body an opportunity to heal digestive damage, restore gut barrier integrity and encourage healthier habits by swapping nutritionally-dense foods for nutritionally-poor grains.

- ThePaleoMom Are All Lectins Bad?
- *Grain Brain,* by David Perlmutter, MD

Section II: Low-Carb Flu and What to Do

Eating Strict Paleo for an entire month is a big undertaking. Though it's tempting to stray off the program or cut it short, stay vigilant! In order to reap the full health benefits of Paleo-eating, committing for only a week or two is not nearly long enough – the body truly needs a full month for amazing things to happen internally:
- ✓ Reset the hormonal signaling network
- ✓ Clear out built-up toxins in the system
- ✓ Adjust metabolism to use fat as a fuel (rather than sugars and starches)
- ✓ Rebuild the cells in the digestive tract
- ✓ Heal damage and inflammation throughout the system

The good news is that once these tasks are underway, your body *will* start burning your stored fat for energy! However, because burning sugars is easier than burning fats and starchy carbs have been generously available (until now), your body *will resist* this change.

> *The culprit is sugar and the refined carbohydrates that break down into sugar once inside your body.*
> *If we were addicted to real food...we wouldn't be talking about addiction.*
> ~Daniel Amen, MD, author of <u>Change Your Brain, Change Your Life</u>

Sugar Withdrawal – The Low-Carb Flu

The high amounts of glucose (from starches and sugars) in the typical western diet stimulate opioid receptors in the brain. That's right...opioid. Those same receptors are triggered by morphine, heroin, opium, codeine and other narcotics. Sugar is addictive. That means when sugar is removed, the Paleo transition may generate withdrawal symptoms similar to those from opiates. A cascade of effects ensues:
- Yeast organisms in the body will starve without sugar...flooding the body with die-off toxins
- The body starts burning fat stores...toxins stored in the fat will be released into the system
- Opiate receptors are left empty...causing cravings, headaches, irritability, etc

> *Sugar lights up the addiction center in the brain like the sky on the Fourth of July.*
> *Think cocaine cookies, morphine muffins or smack sodas!* ~Mark Hyman, MD, <u>Eat Fat, Get Thin</u>

There will be a natural influx of toxins into the blood and lymph as your body starts to heal...and potentially, you may not feel very good. This experience is known as the "low-carb flu."
- ➤ **The Good News:** It's temporary!
- ➤ **The Bad News:** The intensity and duration in your situation is unknown – it's highly individual and depends on current health status, degree of toxin accumulation, metabolic sensitivity, prior carbohydrate consumption and other factors.
- ➤ **The Remedy:** The best approach is to anticipate a slump and have good food ready to eat, just in case.

Common Symptoms of the Low-Carb Flu and Detoxification Period:

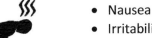

- Nausea
- Irritability
- Increased allergy sensitivity
- Low energy
- Stool fluctuations
- Disrupted sleep

- Headaches
- Acne, zits and pimples
- Low immune system
- Loss of hunger
- Ravaging hunger
- Intense cravings

> *Here's another shocking fact: Sugar is eight times as addictive as cocaine.* ~Mark Hyman, MD

How to Physically Deal with the Low-Carb Flu

Toxins are flushed into the body's lymph system...which has no pump! If you are sedentary, the lymph remains stagnant – the toxins accumulate and will prolong uncomfortable detox symptoms, making you feel lousy longer. The body can be encouraged to rid these toxins more efficiently by sweating or moving lymph through the body (strategies to do so are listed in the following table). Highlight or circle those that appeal to you:

> [On the low-carb flu]: *It is a withdrawal syndrome, a good thing, a transitional phase as your body tries to return to its normal state.* ~William Davis, MD, author of <u>Wheat Belly</u>, <u>Undoctored</u>

Low-Carb Flu Relief Strategies	
Deep tissue massage	Gentle exercise like walking
Sauna	Deep breathing exercises
Steam room	Hot bath with Epsom Salts (helps remove toxins)
Supplement with liver support nutrients*	Gentle movement like Tai Chi
Hot, steamy showers	Stretching exercises
Dry brushing	Drinking fluids especially tea, aloe and bone broth
Activated charcoal supplements	Liberally consume salt or coconut aminos
Mud or clay baths and masks	Use herbs like ginger, turmeric, peppermint, rosemary, saffron, parsley and horseradish
Consume ketone-generating fats like coconut oil and grass-fed butter/ghee (ketone info in Prep G)	Consume algae, kelp and seaweed or apply to skin (may be contraindicated if on thyroid meds)

*N-Acetyl L-Cystine (NAC), milk thistle (silymarin), broccoli sprouts (sulphoraphane), turmeric (curcuminoids), selenium, dandelion

Can I Expedite the Low-Carb Flu?

This is a common question...the low-carb flu is not comfortable. In addition to the strategies above, it's possible to take a detox support supplement. Our favorite is made by Pure Encapsulations, a pharmaceutical-grade supplement company. Their comprehensive detox supplement contains hard-to-obtain vitamins, trace minerals, liver support and other detoxification nutrients; it's sold in a one-month supply. Though it's not required to take a supplement to complete the program, it may help relieve symptoms faster.

* Visit ⌐ PureRXO.com/Paleovation to research/purchase these detox support options:
  ➢ **"Detox Pure Pack"** by Pure Encapsulations – 8 capsule packets, 1 per day (30 packets)
    Tip: If desired, the Detox Pure Pack may be taken as a long-term daily nutritional supplement
  ➢ **"Detoxification Support Packets"** by Designs for Health – 5 capsule packets, 1 per day (60 packets)
  ➢ **"Detoxification Factors"** by Integrative Therapeutics – 1-2 individual capsules, 3x/day (60 capsules)

> **BEWARE:** You cannot supplement your way out of a poor diet!

Advocate for a Potential Low-Carb Flu Episode

Because there is no way to predict your individual manifestation of the low-carb flu, it is best to set up precautionary strategies prior to starting the program. Circle or highlight any that appeal to you.

- Inform your colleagues you may be grouchy
- Take a 2-week break from high-intensity workouts
- Limit social engagements to avoid temptation
- Schedule time for a hot bath or two (try Epsom salts)
- Continue eating three daily meals, even if small
- Consider a reduced work schedule or vacation day(s)
- Arrange some daily nap time
- Have food prepared ahead of time
- Stock up on Paleo convenience foods
- Ask for childcare help
- Make some bone broth
- Plan a spa treatment, like a massage

Thoughts on the low-carb flu? Do you anticipate this will be an issue for you? Other strategies appealing to you?

Section III: Meal-Tweaking Strategies

Going Paleo doesn't always mean giving up favorite foods – sometimes it's just finding suitable substitutions for the dishes you love. Fortunately, there are workarounds for many Not-For-Now foods. So...what if you wanted to eat pasta alfredo? Clearly the noodles and cream sauce are out, but what's in? How can it be transformed into an anti-inflammatory Paleo-compatible meal? There are two options:
1. Make a homemade Paleo version of the Not-For-Now items
2. Omit those ingredients completely and substitute a Paleo-friendly food instead (see example next)

Example: Tweaking Pasta Alfredo	
Pasta Tweak ✓ *Homemade* ___zucchini noodles (zoodles)___ ✓ *Substitute* ___chicken strips___	**Alfredo Tweak** ✓ *Homemade* ___Paleo coconut milk alfredo___ ✓ *Substitute* ___marinara sauce___

Ingredient Subtitution Practice

Using this *Homemade-or-Substitute* system, revamp the following western diet meals. Hints are offered below each category. Learning these strategies will also help with menu planning for future get-togethers and entertaining. Practice makes perfect!

Tweaking Breakfast: Pancakes with Blueberries and Whipped Cream	
Pancake Tweak ✓ *Homemade* _____ ✓ *Substitute** _____	**Whipped Cream Tweak** ✓ *Homemade* _____ ✓ *Substitute** _____
*What can be fried instead of a pancake?	*What other toppings are good on pancakes?

Tweaking Lunch: BLT Sandwiches	
Bread Tweak ✓ *Homemade* _____ ✓ *Substitute** _____	**Mayonnaise Tweak (industrial oils)** ✓ *Homemade* _____ ✓ *Substitute** _____
*What else can hold this filling?	*What other food gives a creamy texture?

Tweaking Dinner: Chicken Enchiladas	
Tortilla Tweak ✓ *Homemade* _____ ✓ *Substitute** _____	**Cheese Topping Tweak** ✓ *Homemade* _____ ✓ *Substitute** _____
*What can be used to wrap the enchilada filling?	*What other garnishes are tasty with Mexican food?

Tweaking Dessert: (Green) Apple Pie	
Crust Tweak ✓ *Homemade* _____ ✓ *Substitute** _____	**Added Sugar Tweak** ✓ *Homemade* _____ ✓ *Substitute** _____
*What can the pan be lined with instead of crust?	*What other flavors go well with green apples?

Suggested Answers (only because you asked, not because you needed them...of course):

➢ **Breakfast:**
  ✓ Homemade Paleo pumpkin pancakes, substitute fried sweet potato or plantain slices
  ✓ Homemade whipped coconut cream, substitute whipped grass-fed butter or unsweetened applesauce

➢ **Lunch:**
  ✓ Homemade Paleo almond meal bread, substitute a coconut wrap or make BLT salad
  ✓ Homemade Paleo mayo from avocado oil, substitute guacamole

➢ **Dinner:**
  ✓ Homemade Paleo cassava or cauliflower tortillas, substitute thinly-sliced veggies (eggplant, zucchini)
  ✓ Homemade cashew cheese, substitute pico de gallo, chopped olives or guacamole

➢ **Dessert (reminder, no added sugar until after the program):**
  ✓ Homemade Paleo almond meal crust, substitute crushed pecans
  ✓ Homemade sweet potato caramel, substitute cinnamon for natural sweetness

Section IV: Solidify Mental Preparation

Prep D covered some heavy thought-provoking, excuse-breaking strategies to challenge the stubbornness of the mind. Please take a moment now to re-read those suggestions and solidify your mental commitment.

> *Restoration of your body's healing power is generated by altering what you eat and do each day.*
> ~Terry Wahls, MD, The Wahls Protocol

Why are you beginning this program?

_____

What do you hope to achieve?

_____

How do you expect this program will be different from any other program you have tried?

_____

Do you think your commitment will waiver during the next month? Explain what would trigger changes.

_____

What can you personally do to keep your motivation and commitment levels strong?

_____

Anything else you need to do to be mentally prepared for the next month?

_____

Section V: Quick Meal Ideas

All the following ideas are easy to make, consist of common ingredients, are appropriate for big batches, and leftovers will either stay fresh in the fridge for a few days or will freeze well. Keep necessary ingredients handy and restock the fridge accordingly.

Stir-Fry
Fry sliced meats in coconut oil, avocado oil or grass-fed butter/ghee. Add cut veggies and spices.
* Substitute cauliflower rice for rice (recipe in the Resource Section for Foundation Meals)
* Skip the soy sauce, use coconut aminos, sesame oil, powdered mushroom or bone broth for flavor

Roasted or Sautéed Veggies (directions on next page)
Roast with olive oil + spices; sauté in coconut oil or grass-fed butter/ghee + spices
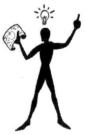
* Make ahead to use as a side or on a salad
* Add to scrambled eggs or cooked meat
* Add to broth for a quick soup
* Chop/purée and mix into meatloaf

Mixed Vegetable Salad
* Top with a protein (tuna/salmon, hard boiled eggs, lox, chicken, pasture-raised bacon pieces)
* Include some fats like olives, avocado, nuts or seeds
* Dress with olive oil and vinegar, salsa, lemon or pureed berries; season with herbs, salt and pepper
* Can prepare in large amounts – for ideas, 🖰 search "Mason® jar salad"

Omelet/Scramble
Sauté cut veggies in coconut oil, avocado oil or grass-fed butter; set aside. Add beaten eggs to skillet and let set for omelet (or scramble). Return sautéed vegetables. Frittatas and quiche are similar, just baked to finish.
* Top with marinara sauce, salsa, guacamole or fresh herbs

Seasoned Ground Meat (example: taco, sausage, or Italian-seasoned – homemade or carefully read labels)
Season and fry up to 4lbs ground meat/turkey (pastured or leanest available). Use extra as planned-overs.
* Eat in a lettuce leaf shell, sandwich between red pepper halves, wrap in coconut wrapper, top a salad, bake in roasted squash or stuff roasted peppers

Restaurant or Eating Out Ideas
* Grilled entrees (steak, chicken, fish) are okay – you can request "naked" cuts to avoid MSG
* Steamed and poached entrees or veggies are typically safe
* Cracked eggs and omelets (avoid omelet mix) can often be ordered any time of day
* Salad bars (dress with vinegar and olive oil or salsa)
* Some grocers now provide grain-free hot bar options

> *It's bizarre that the produce manager is more important to my children's health than the pediatrician.* ~Meryl Streep

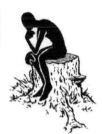

Section VI: Tips for a Successful Transition

The easiest way to stay on track is to **always have proper food options available**.
Here are some ideas to fill your kitchen with healthful ready-to-eat foods.

Tips for Kitchen Stocking

The Paleo transition often means you'll be eating new foods in abundance. In the beginning it's hard to gauge which items will appeal to you the most or how often you'll need to replenish. Here are some popular choices for your kitchen:

Useful Foods to Stock		
In the Fridge	**In the Freezer**	**In the Pantry**
Cut up fresh veggies	Burgers ready to fry	Sugar- and soy- free jerky
Hard boiled eggs	Leftover entrees	Raw nuts and seeds
Salad greens	Cooked taco meat	Freeze-dried berries
Olives	Premade guacamole (freeze ~3mos)	Canned tuna, sardines, salmon
Approved* lunchmeat	Homemade soup/stew	Ripening avocados
Approved* sausage	Berries	Dried seaweed flakes/sheets
Pasture-raised bacon	Veggie Blends or cauliflower rice	Coconut flakes/butter

*Approved meats would be 0-1 g carbohydrates per serving and no additives like MSG, carrageenan, etc.

> *Real food is the stuff that fuels real life!* ~Kristina Turner, Self-Healing Cookbook

Tips for Batch Cooking

Roasting – Consider a Double-Duty Oven: Anytime the oven is on, fill up the extra space with veggies for roasting. Even consider roasting bacon – directions next...

Vegetables for Roasting				Oils
• Sweet potatoes	• Peppers	• Broccoli	• Cabbage	• Coconut
• Onion	• Winter squash	• Cauliflower	• Beets	• Avocado
• Whole carrots	• Okra	• Parsnips	• Turnips	• Olive
• Asparagus	• Garlic Bulbs	• Kohlrabi	• Zucchini	
• Eggplant	• Radishes	• Green beans	• Mushrooms	

* Toss veggies with oil and seasonings; roast between 300°- 375°F until desired tenderness
* Cook-time depends on vegetable size: whole sweet potato = 1-1½ hrs, sliced zucchini = 15-20 min
* To roast garlic: Take a whole bulb, cut off the top half inch, drizzle oil over the cut clove tops, roast ~50min – when cool enough to handle, squeeze out as a paste

- Save prep time…skip the peeling and chopping
  - ✓ Root vegetables can be scrubbed, pricked with a fork and roasted in the skin
  - ✓ Cauliflower and cabbage can be cut in large ¾" slices and roasted flat
  - ✓ Some winter squash (like butternut) has edible peels: scrub, remove seeds, slice/halve and roast
  - ✓ Eat peels when you can – this saves prep time *and* adds fiber and nutrients
  - ✓ Large squashes can be halved and seeded, rubbed with oil, then roasted cut side up or down
  - ✓ Eggplants can be pricked, roasted whole, then scooped out when cool enough to handle

Use extra roasted veggies – on a salad, mixed with ground meat, scrambled into eggs, ground up in meat loaf, covered with marinara, pureed with coconut milk, topped with stir fry, chopped into quiche, etc.

You don't have to cook fancy or complicated masterpieces — just good food from fresh ingredients. ~Julia Child

Roasting Bacon…Who Would've Thought?

Using a baking sheet <u>with a rim</u>, place bacon directly on the sheet or on top of parchment paper. Roast at 300°-350°F until desired crispness. Thin slices take 8-12 minutes, thick slices 20-25 minutes.

Roasting Bacon	
Pros	**Cons**
<ul><li>No slaving over the stove</li><li>All bacon finishes simultaneously</li><li>It's bacon…lots of bacon</li></ul>	<ul><li>You must have a rimmed baking sheet</li><li>DO NOT spill the hot grease when removing the tray from oven, move very mindfully</li><li>Bacon with maple syrup cure tends to burn</li></ul>

Uses for leftover bacon (assuming there are leftovers): crumble on salads, chop into roasted veggies, cut into chip-sized pieces to dip in guacamole, scramble into eggs, eat straight out of the fridge, blend into a sauce, etc. If the bacon is a quality pasture-raised variety, reserve the drippings for a future cooking project.

Bacon is the answer. I don't remember the question. ~Unknown

Double Meats

Assume all your lunches will be leftovers. Prepare double portions of all proteins to keep some planned-overs in the fridge/freezer for a quick meal. Though most meals withstand freezing please note that beef roasts and shredded beef tend to dry out in the freezer. Here are some better freezer options:

Meat Entrees that Freeze Well	
Fish cakes	Seasoned ground meats (taco, sausage)
Meatloaf and meatballs	Pulled pork
Soups and stews	Burgers – can freeze raw, separated by parchment paper
Shredded or roasted chicken	Ham slices

It's better to look ahead and prepare than look back and regret.
~Jackie Joyner-Kersee

A Tale of Two Chickens*: Roasting a chicken? May as well roast two at the same time!
1. Eat a chicken dinner
2. Carve the rest of the birds for leftovers, chicken salad or frozen entrees
3. Make broth with the bones, onions, celery, bay leaves and seasonings, simmer for 4-24 hours
4. Strain the stock and adjust the seasoning (option to start a 2nd batch of broth using the same bones)
5. Save some plain broth to freeze in an ice cube tray for a future dish
6. Return remaining broth to a simmer, add nicely chopped veggies and meat picked off the bones
7. Store a few servings of soup in the fridge
8. Freeze remaining soup in individual bowls, once frozen remove from bowl and place in a freezer bag
   *Cooking Assignment #5 on Day 15 details roasting a whole chicken

Tips for Utilizing Appliances

Slow Cooker: Use this appliance to cook a meal overnight or while you're at work. Meats are tender and juicy when simmered 4-10 hours. It also comes in handy for bone broth or for when it's too hot to turn on the stove.

Pressure Cooker: High-pressure cooking reduces time: 16 hours to slow cook pulled pork translates to 1 ½ hours in the pressure cooker. Large vegetables like whole sweet potato or squash also cook quickly.

Food Processor Efficiency: Process systematically so the flavors do not interfere with the next item to chop, grind or slice. This way you will not have to wash the container between recipes.

Example of Food Processing for the Paleo Overachiever:
1. First use the chopping blade to make nut or coconut butter
2. Next process pre-soaked nuts with water to make nut milk
3. Strain the milk, reserve pulp for baking (almond milk pulp is almond meal)
4. Insert the grating disc and grate a cauliflower for 'rice'
5. Grate some carrots for slaw
6. Insert the slicing disc to slice a cabbage for slaw
7. Slice sweet potatoes and onions to roast – if oven is on for the 'rice,' you'll need more veggies anyway
8. Slice some carrots and celery for a soup, stir-fry or salad (where the onion flavor is fine)
9. Re-insert the chopping blade and chop onions to use or store

---

Overwhelmed? We are just providing ideas to keep you organized and prepared; you get to pick and choose which strategies to use. The more effort you put into the initial preparation, the easier the program is to follow.
Having appropriate food on hand all the time is your best strategy for success!

Instead of counting calories and perfectly partitioned portions (say THAT three times fast), you'll be focusing on eating the right foods instead. ~NerdFitness.com

Which Strategies Will Help You Stay Organized with Food Preparation?
- ☐ Trying Paleo OAMC (Once A Month Cooking) freezer meals
- ☐ Stocking non-perishable Paleo foods
- ☐ Double- or triple-batching a few recipes
- ☐ Ordering pre-made Paleo meals online
- ☐ Visiting the grocery store's salad bar for pre-cut vegetables
- ☐ Always roast veggies whenever the oven is on
- ☐ Locating Paleo recipes for the slow cooker or pressure cooker
- ☐ Using a shopping list app to easily check off items to replenish
- ☐ Ordering a large restaurant meal, saving half of the entrée for lunch or dinner tomorrow
- ☐ Purchasing some Paleo convenience foods to leave in the car, at work, etc
- ☐ Planning a meal-share program with friends, neighbors, roommates, colleagues

What else will work for you specifically?

1. _____

2. _____

Is It Possible to Wing It? Of course – but you may feel discombobulated. A piece-mealed lunch of canned tuna, almonds and broccoli florets is nutritious but not as psychologically satisfying as leftover grilled salmon with roasted vegetables. Much of this transition is about embracing nutrient-dense foods and feeling completely nurtured by them. Plan your meals well during the transition but know you can grab-n-go as necessary.

To-Do List:

- ☐ Prep for Cooking Assignment #1: Bone Broth – find some bones (directions in Prep F)
    - ➢ Just about any bone will work for bone broth, it only needs to fit into your pot. You can freeze bones until you are ready to start creating your broth.
        - • Save bones from ham, T-bone steak, bone-in roasts, wings, chops, ribs or a roasted chicken.
        - • Purchase soup bones, marrow bones, knuckle bones or even chicken feet from a local butcher.
    - ➢ Though pastured and grass-fed sources are emphasized, bone broth made with conventional bones is still packed with hard-to-attain nutrients for healing and overall health.
- ☐ Keep working on the Master Preparation List, get some meals into your fridge / freezer for easy access.
- ☐ Are you sticking with a new healthy habit (from Prep C)? Which one(s)? _____
- ☐ Anything else or any other thoughts? _____
- ☐ **Check off completed tasks on your Master Plan**

Coming Up Soon:

- • Prep F introduces the Paleo Staple recipes– these recipes provide the backbone of the Paleo Diet and are either hard to find or expensive to purchase if you do not make your own.

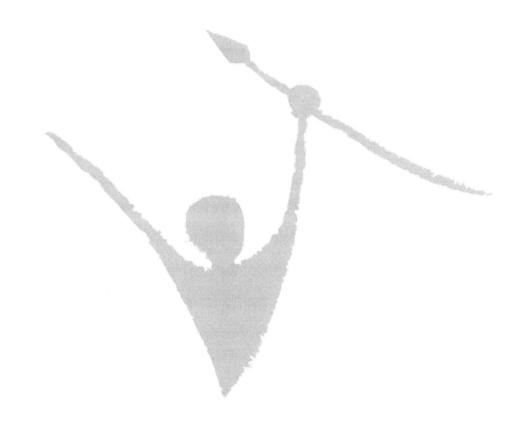

Prep F

> *We may find, in the long run, that tinned food is a deadlier weapon than the machine-gun.*
> ~George Orwell, author of <u>Nineteen Eighty Four</u>

Today's Topics:
1. Paleo-Eating Check-In
2. Paleo-Wise: Insulin and Leptin
3. Explore Breakfast Ideas
4. Quick Quiz: Test Your Knowledge of Paleo Foods
5. Cooking Assignment #1: Bone Broth

Section I: Paleo-Eating Check In

Review your eating habits, especially those that will change for the next month.

Have you modified any eating patterns since you began reading *The Paleovation Workbook*?   Yes   No

In what ways do you already eat in the Paleo-style?

☐ Consume lots of veggies
☐ Use olive, coconut and avocado oils
☐ Use high quality fats like pastured lard
☐ Eat meals at home
☐ Pack a lunch

☐ Limit sweet foods/beverages
☐ Avoid gluten
☐ Avoid dairy
☐ Avoid seed oils
☐ Avoid alcohol

Name two feasible strategies that will help you commit to the rest of the changes:

1. _____

2. _____

Identify a full day of Paleo meals that sound good to you:

✓ Breakfast: _____

✓ Lunch: _____

✓ Dinner: _____

✓ Snacks: _____

✓ Beverages: _____

Section II – Paleo-Wise: Insulin and Leptin (A Metabolic Balancing Act)

Although most people understand that insulin lowers dangerously high blood sugar in diabetics, many imagine that insulin magically 'dissolves' glucose. It's not quite that simple – excess blood glucose doesn't disappear. It must go somewhere, and generally speaking, insulin sends excess into storage (we know it as body fat). The complex hormonal processes that manage glucose and energy reserves are primarily driven by two hormones: insulin and leptin.

> *Insulin shunts sugar to fat. Insulin makes fat. More insulin, more fat. Period.*
> ~Robert Lustig, MD, author of <u>Fat Chance</u>

Part 1: Insulin

The hormone insulin is produced and secreted by the pancreas in response to rising blood glucose levels (this occurs after eating sugar or starch). Glucose is energy – so insulin directs it from the bloodstream into cells to be metabolized either for immediate use or to store for future energy needs.

Insulin: Growth and Storage

Insulin is one of the *key hormones* that regulates human metabolism and energy use. Insulin's major message in the body is growth and storage. Although insulin is *triggered* by blood glucose, its storage effect does not discriminate – when insulin is active, *all* nutrients present in the blood will get the same storage/growth message. This includes amino acids for muscle growth and fats for fat growth (larger graphic in Resources).

Insulin's Effect on Nutrients:

Amino Acids (protein):
1. Immediate bodily needs – in organs, tissues, muscles or enzymes
2. *Excess* protein can be converted to glucose. 'Excess' depends on multiple factors (more about Protein on Day 6)

Glucose (sugar or starch):
1. Immediate energy needs – every cell can burn it
2. Short-term energy storage – a limited amount is stored as glycogen in the muscles and liver
3. Long-term storage – any remaining or excess glucose is converted to fat

Fat (triglycerides, fatty acids):
1. Immediate structural needs – cell walls, nerves, brain
2. Storage – mobilized into fat cells

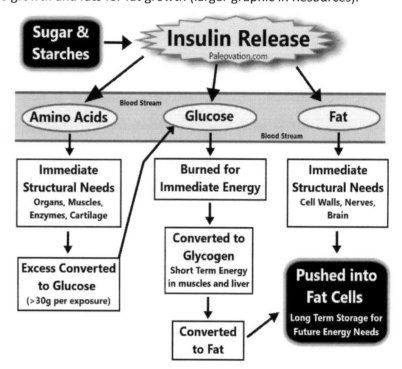

NOTE THAT EXCESS ANYTHING IS EVENTUALLY STORED AS FAT!

Faster Fat: Foods high in glucose AND fat (mac & cheese, potato chips, cheesecake, frosting) create a fat double whammy: insulin, triggered by glucose, sends both excess glucose *and* accompanying excess fat to storage.

Fat Storage – a Survival Strategy

From an evolutionary perspective, fat is precious. Our ancestors' survival relied on fat-preservation to endure periods of famine. On a primitive level, elevated blood glucose indicates an abundance of sugar and starch in the environment – an ideal situation for the body to increase energy reserves for "a rainy day." Insulin's message is:

➤ Convert excess glucose into fat for energy storage
➤ Prevent the body from burning fat; it locks down fat stores for two main reasons:
  • There's no need to burn fat since plenty of glucose is present
  • It is pointless to create a rainy-day energy supply if it's immediately reconverted back into energy

Triglyceride Trigger: Fat compounds called triglycerides are derived from glucose. High blood triglyceride levels indicate chronic inflammation and can be reduced by lowering dietary sugar/starch (not fat).

Snack Attack

Insulin levels normally stabilize a few hours after blood glucose is cleared. The typical western diet, consisting of multiple starchy meals, creates problems. Insulin surges repeatedly though the day, dipping after glucose energy is exhausted. Our natural instinct to replenish energy triggers glucose cravings for high-carb snacks (granola bars, chips, yogurt, pretzels, cookies, candy) – creating a blood sugar roller coaster. Sugar- and starch-based foods guarantee hunger between meals; frequent snacking perpetuates the dilemma. Insulin is always active!

> **Weight-Loss Lesson:** As long as a high-starch grain-based diet is consumed, insulin never rests! Not only does insulin push excess glucose into fat storage, it also protects those stores from being burned. Therefore, when blood sugar drops, fat is not utilized for energy – glucose cravings arise and weight-loss struggles are born.

Insulin Resistance: Crave Sugar ↔ Store Fat

Though insulin is absolutely essential for survival (ask any diabetic), our bodies are not designed to indefinitely sustain insulin in constant action. Eventually cells become numb or 'resistant' to insulin's storage message – forcing the pancreas to produce increasingly more insulin to get the same job done. This results in higher blood concentrations of both insulin and glucose <u>all</u> <u>the</u> <u>time</u>.

The Making of a Couch Potato

The irony with insulin resistance is, although blood glucose is plentiful, cells are not receiving enough because insulin's storage message is being ignored. The brain thinks it's starving because cells are being deprived of glucose! For energy preservation and survival, the brain sends us into sloth mode:

1. Conserve energy by moving less
2. Crave sugar and starches to replenish energy reserves

As insulin resistance progresses, the demand to produce increasingly more insulin just to maintain normal blood glucose levels overwhelms the pancreas. Ultimately, type II diabetes develops.

> **Chronic Insulin Message:** "Eat *more* sugar. *Preserve* fat. *Slow* down."
> Insulin resistance causes obesity.

This process is a leading driver of many diseases including metabolic syndrome, obesity and cardiovascular disease. Ironically, modern 'healthy' diet recommendations to lose weight promote *increasing* whole grains which triggers *more* insulin. That's like using a blow torch to fight a fire!

> **Point to Ponder:** Most westerners *start their day eating sugar* on an empty stomach: cereal, toast, croissants, oatmeal, pancakes, granola, waffles, donuts, fruit juices and even smoothies. This sets the stage for insulin disaster! The mid-morning result: headache, indigestion, energy crash and craving more.

Part 2: Leptin

Leptin is the counter-balance hormone to insulin, secreted by fat cells as they fill so the brain can monitor when enough energy is stored. Put bluntly – leptin gauges when fat cells are fat enough and signals it's time to stop eating. The bigger the fat cells, the more leptin they secrete and the quicker we put down the fork. Since the effects of leptin can be recognized when we feel full (satiated), leptin is called the 'satiety hormone.'

Leptin Prevents Obesity

Leptin is a built-in appetite suppressant but also has other associated messages to prevent over-accumulation of fat:

1. Stimulates burning some of the fat reserves for energy
2. Raises metabolic rate, burning more calories even at rest
3. Promotes movement

> **Leptin Message:** "Eat *less*. *Burn* fat. Move *more*." Leptin promotes a lean, energetic physique!

➤ **The Bad News:** Elevated insulin levels override the leptin signal. In the presence of chronically high insulin (as with the western diet), leptin is suppressed so the constant message is, "Eat more, burn less."

➤ **The Good News:** In a lower sugar/starch diet like Paleo (lower insulin, functional leptin), the balance of insulin and leptin is preserved, naturally preventing obesity!

> **Paleo Advantage:** Want to lose weight? Stop consuming foods that trigger insulin. That's Paleo.

Leptin Resistance

High insulin levels block the signal from leptin so we never feel full despite leptin abundance. At this point, the body becomes both insulin *and* leptin resistant. Obesity and diabetes are inevitable and the nightmare begins...this is what we call the **Sugar UNmerry-Go-Round***.

Key Points:

- Sugar/starch starts the cyclical disaster.
- Diabetes and obesity are perpetually encouraged.
- The foods that cause the problem are craved.
- The "key" to ending the cycle is to remove sugar and starch from the diet.

  * A larger copy is available in the Resource Section

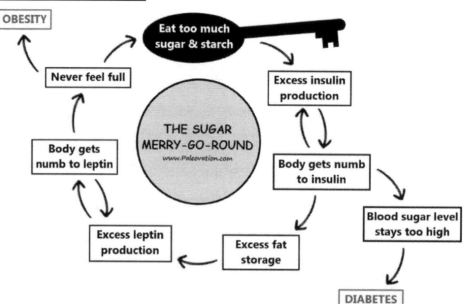

Trying to exert willpower over this powerful insulin-leptin cycle is next to impossible. Even moderate levels of dietary starches/sugars create constant hunger because the body perceives starvation. Simply eating less of them and exercising more is not sustainable long-term – glucose cravings lurk and willpower is constantly tested. Paleo teaches what to eat in order to step off the merry-go-round and finally correct the cycle.

The only way to stop riding the Sugar UNmerry-Go-Round is to address the 'key' – avoiding sugars and starches. When excess insulin production declines, the body resets proper hormonal signaling of both insulin and leptin.

> *Grains are actually nutrient defunct compared to meat, nuts and seeds, and vegetables.*
> ~Mike Sheridan, author of Eat Meat and Stop Jogging

Paleo Advantage: The Paleo Diet minimizes the body's use of insulin. Starchy carbohydrates of grains are replaced with healthy fats, proteins and anti-inflammatory carbohydrates from vegetables and whole fruits. Paleo foods generate slow and limited increases in blood sugar as well as a healthy insulin response. This is the first step in normalizing the interaction between insulin and leptin.

Section III: Explore Breakfast Ideas

Perhaps the biggest change in eating habits is starting the day with veggies, protein and fat for breakfast. Many people love cereal and milk...either because they're addicted to cereal or are just accustomed to eating something mindless early in the morning. If either of those descriptions apply to you, you'll need a new plan.

The Easiest and Fastest Breakfast: *Yesterday's leftovers, of course!*

Egg-Based:

- Mini quiches baked in a muffin pan (line with bacon or sausage) or use a cake pan and cut slices
- Frittatas (lots of Paleo-friendly recipes online)
- Scrambled / fried / hard-boiled / soft-boiled / poached / deviled eggs with guacamole
- Omelets
- Egg baked in a half avocado, half a pepper, half a pre-roasted squash/sweet potato, etc
- Soufflé – Browse ☝ PrimallyInspired for recipes, some are sweetened only with banana
- Flan or custard, omitting sugar from the recipe for a savory and creamy treat (stevia is okay)

Veggie-Based:

- Salad/slaw
- Pumpkin Pancake (✍ BalancedBites *Easy Recipe Pumpkin Pancakes*)
- Veggie latkes – eat plain or as a sandwich, fill w/olives, avocado, lettuce, tomato, pepper, etc
- Fresh cut veggies with guacamole
- 'Cream' of veggie soup or purée
- Mason® jar salad with a protein
- Veggie hash made from grated sweet potato, squash or roots like beets, turnips, parsnips, etc
- Fried rice – use cauliflower rice as the base and sauté with chopped veggies and add an egg

Nut-Based:

- Savory Paleo muffin made with almond meal
- Almond meal or coconut porridge
- Nut and seed Paleo granola
- Nut butter on green apple slices

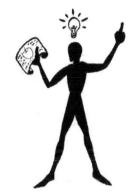

Meat-Based:

- Salmon cakes
- Fried ham
- Sausage cups with egg cooked inside
- Squash halved, stuffed with sausage and baked
- Tuna salad, smoked salmon or lox on greens
- Cold cut plate
- Soup or stew
- Stir fry with cauliflower rice

Fruit-Based (we recommend consuming alongside fat and protein):

- Fresh berry parfait with coconut crème and sliced almonds
- Fresh berries and green apple with prosciutto or bacon

Restaurant- or Store-Based:

- Any of the above options work or opt for the salad bar or hot bar.

"Fun" Breakfast after Strict Paleo Protocol:

- Breakfast ice cream (frozen bananas and berries, almond butter and coconut milk blended in a food processor - freeze remainder in molds for smoothie-cicles)
- Frozen banana bites (thinly sliced banana spread w/almond butter, top w/banana and freeze)
- Paleo breakfast cookie – check recipes online
- Paleo baked good like plantain-based banana bread or almond meal pumpkin muffins

Finding More Breakfast Recipes:

- ✍ Search online "Paleo + [*breakfast idea*]" (example: "Paleo granola")
- ✍ WellnessMama Breakfast – a blog that has a whole collection of breakfast ideas

What breakfast meals will work for you? Anything you need to purchase or prep before Day 1?

_____

_____

> *I went to a restaurant that serves 'breakfast at any time'. So I ordered French toast during the Renaissance.*
> ~Steven Wright

Section IV: Test your Knowledge of Paleo Foods

Quick Quiz – Just for fun, time yourself when answering these questions. Ready, set...go:

1. Name an appropriate Paleo-friendly meal you could order in a restaurant:

_____

2. What is a quick Paleo meal you can make with ingredients currently in your fridge (note: you need to use a veggie, a protein and a healthy fat)?

_____

3. Your favorite Paleo snack is: _____

4. How can you flavor your coffee/tea instead of using cream and sugar?

_____

5. Name a frozen Paleo item that you could prepare and eat in a pinch:

_____

How did you do?

>5 minutes	Time to reread the workbook up to this point
2-5 minutes	Slow and steady wins the race
1-2 minutes	You have the hang of this
<1 minute	Hey, why aren't you writing this book?!

Section V: Cooking Assignment #1 - Bone Broth

What's All the Buzz About Bone Broth?

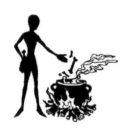

Bone broth is the extremely nutritious, traditional, gelled soup base made by gently simmering bones for many hours. The nutrients extracted from bones and connective tissues are easy-to-absorb and healing for the gut. Cartilage breakdown causes the broth to gel. Compared to other protein sources, cartilage provides a higher percentage of unique amino acids (like proline and glycine). These protein building blocks are assimilated into the musculoskeletal, nervous, digestive and immune systems.

⟨ ThePaleoMom Health Benefits of Bone Broth
⟨ NourishedKitchen Bone Broth: How to Make it and Why it's Good

The collagen in bone broth will help heal the lining of the gut to relieve heartburn, GERD, and other types of intestinal inflammation. On top of that, collagen will support healthy skin to make it supple and strong to reduce the appearance of cellulite. Cellulite comes from a lack of connective tissue. ~Donna Gates, Body Ecology Diet

There is really no right or wrong way to make bone broth, except not making it at all ☺. Fortunately for those with a busy lifestyle, genuine bone broth is now available to purchase. Check local health food grocers (try the freezer section), butcher shops, delis, farmer's markets or online.

Online Broth Sourcing Examples*		
Fresh, frozen and shelf-stable versions available		
Direct Order	**Paleo Markets**	**Meal-Delivery Services**
⟨ KettleAndFire	⟨ ThriveMarket†	⟨ PaleoOnTheGo
⟨ GrasslandBeef	⟨ OneStopPaleoShop	⟨ PetesPaleo
⟨ EpicBar	⟨ BarefootProvisions	⟨ PreMadePaleo

*Visit ⟨ Paleovation for more recommendations,   †Direct link from ⟨ Paleovation

How to Make Bone Broth:

Don't feel intimidated if you have never made broth before – most of the time involved is waiting for it to finish. Here are basic instructions (recipe variations follow):

1. Attain bones
   - Just about any bone will work for bone broth, it only needs to fit into your pot. You can freeze bones until you are ready to start creating your broth.
     - Save bones from wings, chops, T-bone steak, bone-in roasts, ham, fish or a roasted chicken.
     - Purchase soup bones, marrow bones, knuckle bones or even chicken feet from a local butcher.
   - Though pastured and grass-fed sources are emphasized, bone broth made with conventional bones is still packed with hard-to-attain nutrients for healing and overall health.
2. Use a stock pot, a slow cooker or a pressure cooker. As a rule of thumb, the thicker the bone, the longer it simmers. Approximate cooking times for a stock pot or slow cooker: 2-4 hrs for fish, 16-24 hrs for chicken and 24-72 hrs for beef. Cooking times are much faster with a pressure cooker.
3. Slowly simmer the bones in water with a touch of vinegar or lemon juice. Season as you wish: plain, salt, pepper, herbs, spices and/or vegetables (tip: just scrub them, you don't need to peel).
4. Skimming the froth on the surface is optional (it's protein-rich so it can be eaten).
5. When simmering is complete, cool the broth slightly. Strain it *before completely cooled* (if the broth cools all the way, it congeals onto the bones and vegetables you're trying to remove – total mess!)
6. Once cooled, the fat rises to the top. It's okay to leave the fat in the broth if you used quality bones. If you choose to skim off the fat – it can be reserved for cooking or discarded.
   Note: If you did not use high-quality animal bones, we recommend skimming *and* discarding the fat.

Recommended Reading/Recipes:
- Bone broth questions and answers: Whole30 Bone Broth FAQ
- Slow cooker recipe: NomNomPaleo Slow Cooker Beef Bone Broth
- Pressure cooker: NomNomPaleo Quick Pressure Cooker Bone Broth

Storing Your Broth
There are various storage options, depending on how you plan to use the broth.
- Immediate use within 4-5 days: Canning jars are great for storage because they are upright and take up less shelf space in the fridge/freezer.
- Freeze for future use (best to cool the broth in the fridge first):
  - **Ice cube trays** – Freeze in ice cube trays, then dump into a plastic bag or container once set. Add frozen cubes to stir fry, sautéed vegetables or braising meats (browning meat in a skillet with liquid).
  - **Muffin molds** – Various sized tins or silicone molds available. Note the size of your molds; if you have 1-cup tins and a soup recipe calls for 2 cups, then take 2 blocks out of the freezer.
  - **Canning jars** – Quart-sized or smaller are most durable, larger jars risk breakage in the freezer. Jars with straight sides work best, the frozen brick of broth can't be extracted if the jars have 'shoulders.' Leave at least 1 inch at the top for expansion and freeze uncovered. Do not place the lid until after completely frozen (this helps to prevent the jar from breaking).
- Additional tips: NomNomPaleo How to Store Bone Broth

Bone Broth Variations
Once you get the hang of making bone broth, you can customize to personal preference: ✓ Oven-roast the bones first for extra flavor ✓ Reuse bones for your next batch of broth – they can be reused until they fall apart and crumble; they also can be refrozen until you're ready to make a new batch Note: cook subsequent batches extra time (2-3 times longer) and use fresh veggies/herbs ✓ Season well or omit the seasoning for a bland basic broth to flavor later ✓ Add any veggie combination, or no veggies at all ✓ If you use vegetables, blend them into the final broth for a creamier texture ✓ Add bones from different animals into the same batch Tip: keep a bag of bones in the freezer and add to it each time you eat wings, ribs, etc

Bone Broth Uses:

1. <u>Low-Carb Flu Remedy</u> – Especially soothing and healing…drink up!
2. <u>Veggie Purée</u> – Blend some broth with cooked vegetables to make a purée (sweet potato, canned pumpkin, frozen winter squash, roasted cauliflower, steamed broccoli, etc)
3. <u>Creamy Soup</u> – Add more broth to the veggie purée until you reach the consistency of a creamy soup
4. <u>Reheat Leftovers</u> – Place leftovers and 1-2 cubes of bone broth in a skillet, cover and cook on low/med heat, using the steam to heat the food (enjoy the "sauce" with the reheated meal)
5. <u>Paleo French Onion Soup</u> – Use beef bone broth (choose grass-fed butter to caramelize onions):
    - <u>Meatified</u> Chunky Paleo French Onion Soup
    - <u>PaleoGoneSassy</u> Paleo Crockpot French Onion Soup
6. <u>Easy Egg-Drop Soup</u> – Use chicken broth. Gently boil 1-2 cups of broth on the stovetop, stir to give the liquid a swirl, drizzle in a beaten egg or two. When fully cooked adjust seasoning (salt, pepper, coconut aminos for a soy sauce alternative, ginger, splash of sesame oil) and top with scallions

Frequently Asked Bone Broth Questions

What if My Bone Broth Doesn't Gel?

Even if your broth doesn't gel, it's still exceptionally nutritious. The gelling has to do with how much connective tissue was used. Chicken feet or knuckle bones almost always gel, but long beef leg bones sometimes don't. If using long bones, consider sawing or cracking them open to expose more nutrients: after they're softened from a few hours of cooking, place bones on a cutting board and whack with a heavy chef's knife. Return to the pot for the remainder of the cook time.

Why Doesn't Commercial Broth Gel?

Most commercial facilities make non-gelling stock or broth because the cooking time is insufficient for the genuine gelled result. In addition, flavor enhancers like MSG are often added to create an illusionary taste of meat, allowing the broth to be watered down to a point that little gelatin or nutrients remain. If you purchase a pre-made bone broth, seek a brand that explains their cooking techniques.

Why "Chicken Feet?"

We have mentioned chicken feet more than once…feeling squeamish? That's common the first time! But there's good reason for the feet – they contain many bones connected together. Connective tissues, tendons, joint padding and cartilage contain targeted nutrients necessary for our bodies to build tendons, joint padding, etc. The more connective tissue used in the broth, the more nutrients available for your system.

Still squeamish about the feet? Have you ever thought about what goes into commercial broth or bouillon? All the leftover parts that didn't go into sausage…you have been consuming chicken-feet broth your entire life!

> *The best bones for broth are knuckle bones and feet (thanks to their large quantities of gelatin) as well as marrow bones (for their minerals and other nutrients).* ~Greg Cleland, <u>Bone Broth Power</u>

Bone Broth Bouquet: Sometimes making bone broth smells like Grandma's house; other times it emits a strange odor. Both are perfectly normal and healthy. <u>Hint</u>: A pressure cooker can reduce smell.

To-Do List:

- ☐ Planned-overs: are they made? Get them done before Day 1.
- ☐ Prep for Cooking Assignment #1: If you have your bones, you can get started. If you are not ready yet, then plan to have bone broth made by the end of Day 3.
- ☐ Are you keeping up with your new healthy habits? Time to add another: fresh cut veggies, replace the bread with a veggie, use coconut oil or grass-fed butter, replace sugary drinks or take a daily walk.
- ☐ **+Have you completed anything else from the Master Preparation List? Check it off!**

Coming Up Soon:

- Prep G addresses cravings. Before you begin reading, consider strategies that already work for you.

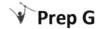 Prep G

Today's Topics:

1. Paleo-Wise: Becoming a Fat-Burner!
2. One Final Temptation?
3. Paleo-Eating Quiz
4. If Cravings Hit…
5. How to Handle a Grouchy Day

Section I – Paleo-Wise: Becoming a Fat-Burner (Fat-Adapted)

> **The Reality:** If you eat abundant sugar or starch, there is no reason to burn fat
> **The Problem:** There is no scarcity of sugar and starch, *and* we crave them!
> **The Goal:** Change metabolism and become a *fat-burner*
> **The Solution:** Stop excessive sugar and starch intake by eating Paleo

Sugar-Burners by Default

Humans have evolved to expect times of food scarcity…such as enduring winter or a season of drought. Self-preservation necessitated that our bodies develop a survival mechanism to accumulate and protect stored energy in the form of fat reserves. These are *only used* when glucose is unavailable in the diet.

The body's preferred fuel hierarchy is clear: Burn glucose first, fat second. When dietary sugar is abundant, the body easily defaults to glucose as its primary energy source *and fat-burning stops!* The form of glucose doesn't matter – whether grain or simple sugar, the message is the same. Even though there's no longer a survival need to accumulate fat, the body hasn't changed its evolved programming. Human metabolism is stuck in *survival auto-pilot*, and the body follows the same basic instructions that have been crucial for the past million years:

> *Preserve stored fat. Crave sugar. Convert excess sugar to fat for survival.* ~Your Brain

Convenience Has Consequence

Modern luxuries guarantee daily food consumption: glucose is readily available in grocers, restaurants, home kitchens, convenience stores, or even home delivery. Civilized cultures rely on an endless grain-based food supply; and because grains are dietary staples and overly-abundant, there's absolutely no reason for our bodies to deplete energy reserves and burn fat. *Every meal, every snack, every day reinforces sugar-burner metabolism.*

Those eating a typical western diet are functioning solely on sugar, not fat. Fast food is indeed fast fat! Whenever glucose is plentiful, the body guards its fat reserves and will not access them until sugars/starches are absent for an extended period of time (minimum 2 weeks).

> **Key Point:** To burn fat, stop eating sugar and starches. Simple concept; not so simple to implement.

Catch-22: Eat Sugar ↔ Crave More Sugar

Sugar consumption generates sugar cravings to sustain the fueling-refueling cycle. Unfortunately, many people are exposed to sugars and starches at a very young age (infants, toddlers) and consumption never stops. Societal norms such as birthday celebrations, pre-packaged snacks, sweet beverages, pizza delivery, holiday festivities, using food as a reward, etc, further encourage regular sugar consumption.

Many have lived their entire lives depending exclusively on sugar for fuel. The longer glucose is relied on for fuel, the stronger the cravings for additional glucose grow. If the body is never given the opportunity to tap into fat reserves, it essentially forgets how to burn fat for fuel!

> **Fat Fact:** Relying on sugar for fuel induces stronger cravings for *more* sugar…to stock pile even *more* fat!

Consequences of Sugar-Burning Metabolism

This is not a carte blanche attack on carbohydrates. In fact, vegetables and whole fruits are *indispensable* carb sources because they provide innumerable nutrients not attained elsewhere. However, 'empty calorie' carbs from sugars, grains and starches are a serious health problem – and they are in virtually every processed food! The low-fat diet is a glucose-based diet. Metabolically speaking, it's highly inefficient and comes with drawbacks:

- Low in satiety and causes persistent hunger
- Provides only short-term energy; glucose is exhausted within 2-3 hours, so the body must frequently refuel to prevent low blood sugar symptoms of irritability, mental fog, fatigue, shakiness, nausea, etc
- Tendency to overeat due to increased craving for more sugar/starch
- Excess fat eaten alongside sugar is *automatically stored* rather than burned due to insulin's influence
- High insulin levels make it impossible to access fat stores for energy

---

Fat-Burner / Sugar-Burner Campfire Analogy

To better grasp the concept of sugar- versus fat-burning, imagine the body's metabolism like a campfire:

Logs: The large foundational logs sustain the fire for extended periods of time. Body fat functions like those big, fat logs – once they are burning, they provide a steady, long-term energy supply.

Kindling: When kindling like sticks or twigs are tossed on the campfire, there's a short-term burst of heat. After it recedes, the underlying logs again provide the primary fuel. Sugar functions like kindling – short-term energy.

Sugar-Burner: Now imagine trying to sustain that fire with no large foundational logs, just twigs. Constantly refueling with kindling is an exhaustive process! Likewise, sustaining metabolism solely on sugar is extremely inefficient – there's constant demand for more fuel to replenish its short-lived energy. This is what happens to our bodies as sugar-burners – *sugar-burners are exhausted, achy and continually craving more sugar.*

Sugar-Burner Weight-Loss ("Skinny Fat")

Simply cutting calories while continuing to consume ample sugar/starch (such as sustaining on rice cakes and air-popped popcorn) *will not allow the body to burn fat*. High insulin levels ensure fat stays stored. If a reduced-calorie diet doesn't provide enough fuel, the body is directed to *break down muscle protein* to convert into glucose. Weight-loss in a sugar-burner happens by sacrificing muscle, not fat – the term 'skinny fat' applies here.

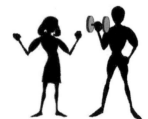

Fat-Burner Weight-Loss

When sugar/starches are removed from the diet, the body *must* fire up its fat-burning mechanism to survive. The longer the duration without glucose, the more dominant fat-burning becomes. *Weight-loss in this case will target fat* while *preserving muscle*!

> *If you are not burning fat, then you have missed the point.*
> ~Mark Sisson, Primal Blueprint, Primal Endurance

The Body Prefers Fat Fuel

Fat for fuel provides some major advantages to the body:

- **Efficiently Stored** – From a survival perspective, fat can supply more than double the calories per gram (9) than protein or carbohydrate (4). More 'emergency energy' is stored in less space.
- **Reliable** – Self-preserving energy is readily available when necessary. Even lean adults easily have 1-2 months of energy stored in their body fat.
- **Steady Fuel** – Body fat burns evenly with none of the highs and lows that occur with sugar rushes
- **Metabolic Flexibility** – A fat-adapted body remembers how to use glucose. It functions mainly on fat but can process a higher carb meal periodically without reverting back to sugar-burning metabolism. This does not work vice versa: when sugar-dependent, the body *never burns fat* due to insulin's storage effect.

Point to Ponder: If the body was designed to run indefinitely on glucose, logic suggests that all energy reserves would be in the form of sugar (glycogen), not fat. The body stores fat because it is well-adapted to utilize it.

Fat-Burning Metabolism	
Facts	**Benefits**
✓ Body fat is simply stored energy ✓ The body burns fat for fuel *only* when glucose is insufficient for sustenance ✓ Fat breaks down to ketones, an alternate energy source the body can use the same as glucose ✓ Burning ketones is the normal, preferred metabolic state of humans ✓ Body fat provides steady long-term fuel, even a lean person has 1-2 months of energy stored	✓ Can easily span several hours between meals without becoming ravenous, nauseas or cranky ✓ Steady, even energy throughout the day, skipping a meal is not a problem ✓ Improved sleep quality and mental alertness ✓ Reduced hunger levels and appetite ✓ Exercise can burn even more fat ✓ No sugar cravings (at least physically – emotional cravings are habits to be modified)

Choosing to Be a Fat-Burner

The primary difficulty in achieving a fat-burning metabolism is that modern diets can be 50-80% carb based. Removing a dietary staple of this magnitude is absolutely a life-changing proposition. Due to inherent cravings, transitioning to fat-burning metabolism must be a conscious choice – you must keep your brain in the game because it won't happen accidentally. Sugar and starches have got to go!

1. You *must* step off the Sugar UN-Merry-go-Round. Once the body stops over-production of insulin, *fat stores will no longer be locked down* and *can finally be accessed for fuel.*
2. Eat healthy fats, especially those that easily produce ketones...like coconut oil, MCT oil and butter.
3. Focus on attaining carbohydrates from vegetables and fruits (low-sugar varieties) that offer fiber and other necessary nutrients.

> **Conscious Commitment:** You *must consciously choose* to remove sugars and starches from your kitchen and diet – it won't happen *accidentally.*

How Long to Become Fat-Adapted?

The fat-adaptation process evolves in a couple of stages but cannot start unless sugars and starches are limited. Glucose consumption must be kept *consistently low* for several weeks to solidify fat-adaptation, otherwise sugar-burning will continue indefinitely.

1. The initial stage of ketone production gradually reaches its maximum in 10-14 days.
2. Long-term efficient ketone usage throughout the body develops over a period of 6 weeks.

> **Key Point:** During the initial phase, eating any more than a small amount of carbs will hinder progression toward fat-adaptation (thus the reason for limiting even fruits during the Strict Paleo Protocol).

Counting Carbs is *Not* Necessary

The Paleo Diet is a naturally fat-adapted diet. By eliminating grains and sugars, carbohydrate content is drastically lower than a typical western diet, prompting the body to burn ketones and whittle away fat stores. Carbohydrates from vegetables and low-sugar fruits are packed with fiber and nutrients. Not only are they difficult to overeat, but their glucose content is slowly released to the bloodstream, averting insulin surges.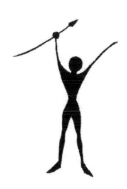

As long as meals are built with vegetables + protein + fat, carbs naturally stay in a manageable range – there's no reason to micromanage every carb morsel. Once fat-adapted metabolism is solidified, the Paleo Diet is a flexible template from which individuals can determine ideal carbohydrate consumption.

> **Note of Caution:** While the body relearns to burn fat and utilize ketones, it's common to temporarily experience flu-like symptoms. Homemade broth is a great supplement (more on Low-Carb Flu Relief in Prep E).

Accelerate the Transition to Fat-Burning (Optional Strategies)

The following options will increase production of ketones and accelerate the fat-adaption process:

1. Utilize coconut oil, MCT oil or grass-fed butter to provide easy-to-burn fats. These short- and medium-chain triglycerides bypass the gallbladder and quickly break down to ketones for immediate energy (the basis of Bulletproof® coffee: ☝ Bulletproof How to Make Bulletproof Coffee). Excess ketones are flushed out in the urine, not stored!
2. Avoid high isolated-protein intake, such as protein shakes. *Excess* protein can be converted to glucose (discussed on Day 6). Opt for a portion of real meat such as fish, poultry, beef, pork, etc, preferably with high-quality fat to slow digestion.
3. Strictly limit carb intake (less than 50g/day), consisting only of non-starchy vegetables and one serving of low sugar fruit; may intensify low-carb flu; diabetics are strongly cautioned to monitor ketone levels.
4. Experiment with intermittent fasting (IF), but *never fast during a time of stress* (this technique is more advanced and may be more appropriate after the Strict Paleo Protocol – read more on Day 27).

Carbohydrate Tolerance Limits

Once fat-adaption metabolism is well established, *some* carbohydrate can be consumed without consequence. The operative question is, "How much?" There's definitely a tipping point for sugar/starch consumption, after which fat-burning stops and the body reverts to sugar-burning, along with increased sugar cravings.

However, there is no one-size-fits-all carb tolerance level because metabolisms vary based on multiple factors, including genetics and activity level. Each individual will need to experiment and determine how much glucose they tolerate without upsetting the fat-burning metabolism (more about Carb Tolerance on Day 24).

> **Carb Benchmark:** According to scientifically-evaluated carb levels, daily carbohydrates should be no more than 1/3rd of daily calories. This translates to a max of 150 g of carbs/day for a 2000-calorie diet.
> 📖 *The Perfect Health Diet*, by Paul and Shou-Ching Jaminet

Ketosis versus Keto*acidosis*

Though these two terms sound similar, they are quite different. Ketosis is the deepest stage of fat-burning – the body is fueled by fat from both diet and body stores. There is nothing dangerous about ketosis in a *healthy* body.

Ketosis† - A normal metabolic state when the body burns ketones for energy

-   Not only is this healthy, but it's *beneficial* to dip into ketosis between meals, overnight or during a fast
-   The trivial glucose needs are maintained via small dietary amounts or by converting protein to glucose
-   Strict ketosis is generally not meant for long-term sustenance, though some individuals use *extended* ketosis for therapeutic purposes

> *The more you use ketones for energy in your lifetime as opposed to glucose, the longer and healthier you will live – BY FAR.* ~Nora Gedgaudas, Primal Body, Primal Mind, Primal Fat Burner

Ketogenic Diet – Designed to keep the body in *sustained ketosis*

-   A very low-carb dietary plan, consisting of less than 20 grams of carbohydrate per day
-   A high-fat diet, not high-protein
-   Ketosis metabolism is most commonly pursued for rapid weight loss, but also has therapeutic value for cancer (most cancer thrives solely on glucose) and brain disorders including epilepsy, traumatic brain injury, bipolar disorder and even Alzheimer's, Parkinson's or autism.
-   Due to rapid loss of water from sustained ketosis, sodium and potassium may be lost as well. Supplemental salts are recommended – another reason to add bone broth!
-   Some individuals respond beautifully to sustained ketosis, others develop problems:
    -   ☝ ThePaleoMom Adverse Reactions to Ketogenic Diets: Caution Advised

---

Design a Ketogenic Diet: It takes *significant* effort to build a nutritionally-complete ketogenic diet. Research Wahls Paleo Plus™ in 📖 *The Wahls Protocol*, by Terry Wahls, MD. She sets strict vegetable requirements to provide the most nutrients within a low carbohydrate load (and she successfully reversed her MS with this diet).

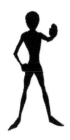

† Precautionary Considerations for Sustained Ketosis
The following are cases when it's best to avoid *sustained* ketosis. Accomplish this by increasing consumption of Paleo-friendly carbohydrates. As always, consult your physician.

1. **Type I Diabetes**
2. **Infertility**
3. **Pregnancy**
4. **High-Intensity Athletes** (example: marathoners or bodybuilders)

⤷ DrJockers When NOT To Be on a Ketogenic Diet

Keto*acidosis* – *An extreme, abnormal, uncontrolled and dangerous condition*

- Most commonly occurs in Type I diabetics due to the inability to produce insulin
- Since a Type I diabetic cannot metabolize glucose in the blood, the body naturally shifts to breaking down fat for energy, producing ketones
- In non-diabetics, insulin regulates both ketone and glucose metabolism (insulin can push ketones from the blood into cells); however, because insulin is absent in Type I diabetics, ketones accumulate uncontrolled in the blood and severely drop pH levels to a dangerously acidic state which *can be fatal!*

Paleo Advantage: At 100-150g of carbs per day from veggies and fruit, full blown ketosis won't be engaged, but neither will insulin surge nor fat be stored. Paleo is a healthy metabolic state that can be maintained indefinitely.

The majority of human evolution occurred in the backdrop of low carbohydrate intake.
~Jeff Volek PhD and Stephen Phinney MD, PhD, The Art & Science of Low Carbohydrate Living

Section II: One Final Temptation?

Last chance...do you have any last minute urges...a temptation you need to fill? Go ahead and get it out of the way. But finish before midnight, Cinderella.

Rachel's Paleo Eve: On the night before my first Paleo-style elimination diet, my friends and I had a Paleo condiment-making party...aren't we cool? We wrapped up at 11:45pm and cracked open a celebratory beer. I never would have guessed that my nightly beer habit (ahem, any good Wisconsinite can hold her own) would dwindle down to only one a rare occasion. The best part is that beer used to be a temptation and now I don't even miss it!

The only way to get rid of temptation is to yield to it... I can resist everything but temptation.
~Oscar Wilde

What were your favorite Paleo food choices from today?

Meals: _____

Snacks: _____

Beverages: _____

Did you give into a temptation?   Yes   No   If so, answer the following:

Temptation food (optional): _____

How did it taste? _____

How did it make you feel? _____

Do you think this was a proper send off for that item? Why or why not? _____

_____

Section III: Paleo Eating Quiz

Part I – Quick Eats (*Suggested answers below*)

1. Write down three recipes or snacks that you can quickly prepare:

   a. _____

   b. _____

   c. _____

2. Write down three foods that are ready to grab-and-go from your kitchen right now:

   a. _____

   b. _____

   c. _____

3. Write down three appropriate foods you could purchase in a gas station/convenience store:

   a. _____

   b. _____

   c. _____

Part II - Restaurant and Social Situation Plan*

1. Breakfast dish to order:

   _____

2. Lunch dish to order:

   _____

3. Salad bar or hot bar items to eat:

   _____

4. Beverage to drink for breakfast or lunch:

   _____

5. Dinner entrée to order:

   _____

6. Looks-like-an-alcoholic-drink-but-isn't drink to order:

   _____

7. Plan to ensure you can eat at a party:

   _____

8. Strategies you can use to navigate a dinner invitation at a friend's house:

   _____

9. Phrases you can say when others question your food choices during the next month:

   _____

   *Part I Suggested Answers – Just to jog your memory:
   1. Fresh or frozen burger, can of sardines, coconut flakes, whole carrot or bell pepper
   2. Fresh cut veggies, approved lunch meat, olives, guacamole, seaweed sheets

3. The convenience store is not too convenient for Paleo eaters, potential answers:
   - ✓ Hard-boiled eggs
   - ✓ Baby carrots
   - ✓ Pistachios
   - ✓ Sparkling water
   - ✓ Fresh fruit (might be high-sugar fruit)
   - ✓ Tuna packed in water
   - ✓ Dry-roasted nuts
   - ✓ Dry-roasted sunflower seeds

*Part II Suggested Answers:
1. Poached eggs with sautéed veggies (remember omelet mix sometimes has flour or milk)
2. Grilled salmon on top of greens
3. Steamed veggies, roasted meats, greens, hard-boiled eggs, olive oil and vinegar
4. Coffee, tea, iced tea (unsweetened)
5. Grilled steak with steamed veggies
6. Soda water with lime (also known as seltzer or sparkling water)
7. Bring your own meal, eat ahead of time, fill up on the protein and vegetables
8. Offer to make it a potluck, bring a dish to pass, suggest grilling
9. I'm working around some food sensitivities; I'm eating only anti-inflammatory foods this month; I suspect my health will improve if I skip the chips for a few weeks; I'm giving my body a break from processed foods so it can rest and reset; I'm in the middle of a food experiment

Section IV: If Cravings Hit…

It is natural to assume a craving will hit in the next month…they can be physical, mental and/or even emotional (ever cry into a pint of ice cream?). Like anything else, having a plan to deal with cravings is essential. What strategies already work for you when cravings arise?

1. _____
2. _____
3. _____

Cravings easily persuade our actions especially if we're not prepared. However, many cravings are not truly physical in nature and are relatively short-lived. Distracting yourself for 5-10 minutes with something you enjoy is an effective strategy. Name three of your favorite activities:

1. _____
2. _____
3. _____

Can any of these activities successfully create a diversion for you when cravings hit?   Yes   No

Eventually both the craving frequency and duration subsides. Here are a few more active suggestions. Check the ideas that may work for you:

- ☐ Go to the gym
- ☐ Take a walk
- ☐ Play some upbeat music
- ☐ Try some stretching
- ☐ Make some turmeric tea
- ☐ Dig into your fresh cut veggies
- ☐ Enjoy a mug of bone broth
- ☐ Read a book or some jokes
- ☐ Do some jumping jacks
- ☐ Play a game
- ☐ Find some online entertainment
- ☐ Keep postcards handy, write a quick note to a friend/relative
- ☐ Dab peppermint oil under your tongue
- ☐ Call a friend you haven't talked to in a while
- ☐ Do 5 minutes of deep breathing
- ☐ Eat some fat like guacamole, olives, coconut oil on a spoon, bacon, coconut or nut butter
- ☐ Eat some protein like jerky, deviled eggs, tuna salad, a steak, a burger or nuts (one handful)
- ☐ Brush your teeth

Carb Craving Supplements*

For those who suspect carbohydrate cravings will be a big issue (soda drinkers, grain bingers, chip chompers), it is possible to fend off cravings by taking a supplement. Again, this is not necessary, it's just a suggestion to support your transition to Paleo-eating. Shop for supplements at a trusted vendor. Browse our top picks or purchase directly at ⌐ PureRXO.com/Paleovation.

Carb Craving Supplement* Options	
✓ L-Glutamine	✓ Gymnema
✓ 5-HTP	✓ Omega-3's
✓ L-Tryptophan	✓ CarbCrave Complex†
	✓ MCT oil‡

* Before your purchase, read all supplement warnings for prescription drug
  interactions and consult a medical provider for any contraindications.
† Formulated by Pure Encapsulations as a comprehensive supplement
‡ Not available at PureRXO. Bulletproof® is a popular choice.

More Info (remember, direct links to all recommended reading are available at ⌐ Paleovation):

- ⌐ PrimalBody-PrimalMind Taming the Carb Craving Monster
- ⌐ BenGreenfieldFitness 12 Dietary Supplements That Can Massively Control Your Most Intense Carbohydrate Cravings

Section V: How to Handle a Grouchy Day

Grouchiness is common while acclimating to Paleo eating... beware that your environment may appear 100 times more annoying than usual. No worries, just set yourself up for success:

- ☐ Warn your colleagues
- ☐ Plan some nap time
- ☐ Find someone to watch your kids
- ☐ Practice deep breathing exercises
- ☐ Listen to a podcast
- ☐ Connect to nature
- ☐ Scream in a pillow
- ☐ Have a good book nearby
- ☐ Plan in some relaxing time
- ☐ Keep busy with an activity you love
- ☐ Play some music and dance
- ☐ Do something mindless (waste time on BuzzFeed)
- ☐ Do something mindful (play Scrabble or Words with Friends)
- ☐ Just mope and grouch...sometimes it feels so good!

To-Do List:

☐ **So, that's it for prep...double check your Master Preparation List and you're ready to go!**

How Are You Feeling?

- ☐ Nervous
- ☐ Sad
- ☐ Overwhelmed
- ☐ Excited
- ☐ Hungry
- ☐ Ready to go
- ☐ Uncertain
- ☐ What's the big deal?
- ☐ Bloated
- ☐ Comfortable/Prepared
- ☐ Scared
- ☐ Calm and collected

Coming Up Soon:

- Rejuvenated Health! You are now ready to take care of you. Relax, take a deep breath.

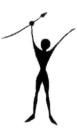

Day 1

Today's Topics:

1. Paleo-Wise: Fats Part I – Fat Fraud
2. Building a Paleo Meal: *Vegetables + Protein + Fat*
3. Tomorrow's Meal Plan

Fast Fare – Fridge Staples
♥ Baby greens sautéed in olive oil
♥ Lunchmeat wrapped around a pickle
♥ Guacamole and baby carrots

Section I – Paleo-Wise: Fats Part I – Fat Fraud

The low-fat campaign has been based on little scientific evidence and may have caused unintended health consequences. ~Frank Hu, professor of nutrition, Harvard School of Public Health

Big Fat Lies

The only thing clear about fat in the diet is that it's clearly confusing!

Decades of widely-published, inaccurate or conflicting information about dietary fat has led to mass confusion and many **blatant fat falsehoods**:

1. Eating fat makes us fat
2. Saturated fat and cholesterol cause heart disease
3. Butter, eggs, lard and red meat are unhealthy
4. Replacing saturated animal fats with unsaturated plant oils promotes health
5. Olive oil is the only healthy fat
6. Low-fat diets improve health

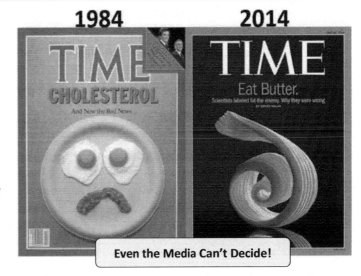

Even the Media Can't Decide!

Though conventional wisdom frequently repeats these claims, all the above misconceptions about fats have been proven false! Ironically, the promoted 'healthful' low-fat diet is a *major* culprit of the current heart disease, obesity and diabetes epidemics.

Lower Fat = Lower Health

Natural dietary fat has been blamed for health complications even though America's obesity and heart disease epidemics have skyrocketed in the face of *lower* fat intake. The problem is that the wrong food group has been attacked: when a diet is low in fat, it must be high in sugar and starch.

The low-fat nutrition advice since the 1970's has essentially been an uncontrolled, high-carb experiment on the entire population. The tragic results are evident: increased obesity, diabetes, heart disease and metabolic syndrome. It may be hard to believe, but dietary fat is not the problem. Genuine health is achieved by *seeking* healthy fats and reducing harmful sugar/starches. There's no valid evidence to justify clinging to a low-fat diet.

The Real Problem: We're eating too much sugar/starch and too little natural, healthy fat!
The Real Solution: Release the fear of fat, abandon the low-fat diet and eat traditional fats as nature intended.

Fear Sugar and Industrialized Crop Oils; Embrace Natural Fats

Over the past 100 years, fat intake has transitioned from natural, animal-based fats to unnatural, *chemically-altered* plant-based fats (such as margarine, shortening, soybean, safflower, corn, and canola oils). Not only have those industrial-manipulated fats been *disastrous* for health, but their health consequences have unfairly been projected to *all* fats, including natural, traditional fats. Science has conclusively proven the following about fats:

1. The *right fats are essential* for proper body function
2. There is NO link between saturated fat intake and risk of heart disease (Heart Disease topic on Day 18)

"Fat on the Lips" Does NOT Become "Fat on the Hips"

There is no link between the fat eaten in food and the fat accumulating around the belly. Excess body fat is the result of hormonal imbalances, especially insulin (from eating sugar) and cortisol (from stressors, *including* excess dietary sugar!). Both of those hormones induce fat-storing metabolism (more about Insulin in Prep F and Cortisol on Days 11 and 12). The correct mantra is, "*Sugar* on the lips is fat on the hips."

What Fueled the Low-Fat Obsession?

1. **Human Gullibility**
   a. Our aversion to body fat made it easy to falsely associate fat in food with fat in the belly.
   b. "Eating fat makes you fat" *sounded* true.
   c. Catchy *false* mantras convinced us that "fat on the lips is fat on the hips."
   d. Low-fat (high-carb) products justified and stimulated our sugar cravings – foods such as fat-free cookies and reduced-fat ice cream were hyped as healthy and eaten guiltlessly and abundantly.

2. **Deceptive Studies**
   a. Studies were performed using hydrogenated oils (unnatural trans fats), then the negative results were wrongly blamed on saturated fat and cholesterol.
   b. The 'Seven Countries Study' concluded that high-fat diets were unhealthy, but *rejected conflicting data from 15 countries* – there were 22 countries in the initial data set!
   c. Multiple studies determined high-fat diets caused disease symptoms but failed to disclose that the diets were *also high in sugar and starch,* the real culprit of those symptoms.

   > **Paleo Advantage:** Every clinical trial following an anti-inflammatory Paleo protocol (high in natural fat *and* low in sugar/starch) has shown increased weight loss and better health. Contrary to expectations, the *Framingham Study* (40 years of research) showed those who *ate the most* cholesterol, saturated fat and calories *weighed the least* and were the *most physically active*!

3. **Politics / Economics**
   a. **Inaccurate Food Pyramid:** In 1992, the USDA (US Dept. of *Agriculture*) promoted a grain-based, low-fat diet with a graphic food pyramid influenced by food industry lobbyists.
      i. Recommendations were based on outdated, misleading studies (see #2 above)
      ii. Simple common sense would challenge the endorsement of 6-11 servings of grains per day...seriously? How does that fit into just three meals plus snacks?! That left very little room in the diet for other food groups without overeating (which is exactly what happened).
   b. **Food Subsidies:** Food manufacturers capitalized on abundant low-cost, high-carbohydrate ingredients made possible, in part, by farm subsidies.

4. **Calorie Confusion**
   a. The false "calories in = calories out" hype demonized the higher caloric value of fat
   b. Gram for gram, sugar has lower calories than fat – but its hormonal consequences trigger both overeating and fat accumulation (eating fat doesn't do that!)

Calories are Not Created Equal	
250 Calories	**Distribution of Nutrients**
1 small 3oz bagel	• The starch is broken down into glucose which triggers insulin and sends the body into 'storage mode' • Excess glucose is converted into fat while existing fat stores are preserved
1 medium 5oz salmon filet	• The proteins are broken down to amino acid building blocks to grow and maintain muscles, bones and digestive enzymes • The healthy fats are used for cell structure and brain function • Vitamins and minerals are utilized throughout the body

> **Paleo Advantage**: Metabolism changes when sugars and starches are limited, and healthy fats are consumed:
> 1. **Fat-Adaptation** – Efficiently burn fat for fuel on a regular basis
> 2. **Calorie Liberated** – Maintain a slimmer physique despite consuming more total calories (from fats, proteins and vegetables and lower sugar/starchy carbs), *no more calorie counting*!

Importance of Fat

Our bodies *need* fat – and not just the obvious places like padding on the buttocks, feet and hands. Fats make up a large percentage of the body mass, even on lean people where it's not visually evident. Fat plays a critical role in cell structure, metabolism, hormonal balance, digestion and even cognition (the brain is mostly fat!).

Health problems emerge when healthy, natural fats are replaced with chemically-extracted, manufactured fats. Notice how low-fat, high-carb diets can compromise the following fat-based structures and functions:

Fat Structures and Functions	Low Fat Health Complications
Brain – 60% of the brain is fat and cholesterol	Alzheimer's, dementia, mood disorders and general 'brain fog'
Nerve Function – myelin insulation around nerves is made of fat, increasing transmission efficiency	Poor coordination, slow reflexes Fast Fact: myelin is damaged in Multiple Sclerosis
Steroid Hormones – estrogen, progesterone, testosterone and cortisol are made from fats	Infertility, low testosterone, PMS, menstrual and menopause symptoms, hormonal imbalance
Cell Walls/Membranes – fats provide foundational cell structure throughout the body	Leaky gut, fatigue, allergies, migraines, bruising, increased susceptibility to free radical damage
Healthy Skin – essential oils make skin waterproof, elastic and antimicrobial	Skin cancer, wrinkles, blemishes, acne, rashes, immune stress
Vitamin Absorption – fats are necessary for transport and absorption of fat-soluble vitamins	Deficiencies especially in vitamins D and K2 (more on Days 7 and 16) but also vitamins A and E
Healthy Digestion – bile in the gall bladder is made from fat and is required to digest other fats	Gall bladder dysfunction or removal, digestion disorders
Bone Health – fats are necessary to incorporate calcium into the bones (more on Day 16)	Prevalence of osteoporosis, osteopenia, degenerative discs and worn out joints

Examples of Healthy, High-Fat Lifestyles

There are many cultures that consume more fat than the U.S. population, yet still have lower rates of obesity and cardiovascular disease. These examples are often disregarded as paradoxes:
1. **Mediterranean**: Low rates of heart disease even though a larger percentage of calories are from fat
2. **European**: The countries that consume the most saturated fats have the lowest death rates from cardiovascular disease (especially France, Switzerland, Holland and Iceland)
3. **France**: Lowest rates of heart disease deaths in Europe even though the diet is loaded in saturated fats like butter, eggs, cream, cheese, liver, meats and foie gras
4. **Oldest American**: Gertrude Baines lived to age 115 and often ate bacon, fried chicken and real ice cream!

> *From lowering bad cholesterol and helping shed excess weight, to giving you shiny hair and healthy nails, your body will reap the benefits of healthy fats.* ~Josh Axe, DC, author of Eat Dirt

Add *More* Healthy Fats to your Diet

In current fat-phobic modern cultures, the concept of increasing fat consumption is completely foreign and creates anxiety. However, knowledge is power – understanding what types of healthy fats to include, why to include them and where to find them is critical for good health. Upcoming Paleo-Wise topics on Days 2, 3 and 4 will elaborate on all the 'big fat details.' For now, start adding traditional Paleo fats (listed in the chart[†] on the next page) to *every* meal.

    📖 *The Big Fat Surprise,* by Nina Teicholz
    📖 *Primal Fat Burner,* by Nora Gedgaudas

Section II: Building a Paleo Meal

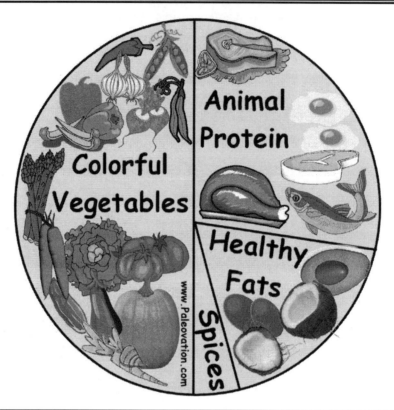

Veggies	Protein	†Healthy Fats	Seasonings*
Green	Beef / Bison	Coconut / Coconut Oil	Italian
Yellow / Orange	Pork	Olives / Olive Oil	Mexican
Red	Poultry / Eggs	Avocado / Avocado Oil	Curry
Blue / Purple / Black	Fish	Grass-fed Butter / Ghee	Asian
White / Tan	Seafood / Shellfish	Pastured Lard	Salt and Pepper
	Wild Game	Pastured Tallow	Herb de Provence
	Lamb / Goat	Duck Fat	Lemon Pepper
	Organ Meats	Drippings	Garlic and Herb

*Spice Guide on Day 2

Meal-Building Parameters

A well-built Paleo meal contains lots of veggies, a moderate portion of protein and a dollop of healthy fat. For the first few weeks of the program, build your meals around the following recommendations:

1. **Abundance of Vegetables** – Vegetables provide the vitamins, minerals, antioxidants and fiber your body needs to function and digest properly. Each color group includes different nutrients so select a variety of colors throughout the day (see chart on the next page).
    a. Consume Vegetables at Every Meal
    b. Ensure Half of Your Plate (or *more*) is Comprised of Vegetables
    c. Incorporate Green Vegetables Daily
    d. Include a Wide Variety of Colors – eat the full rainbow over the course of a week (or even daily!)
    e. Eat a Rich Assortment of Vegetables (rather than the same five or six favorites)

Vegetables by Color					
Red	**Yellow/Orange**	**White/Tan**	**Green**	**More Greens**	**Purple/Black**
Radishes	Yellow Beets	Cauliflower	Endive	Artichokes	Black Olives
Red Lettuce	Butternut	Celeriac	Asparagus	Turnip Greens	Purple Asparagus
Radicchio	Carrots	Garlic	Bok Choy	Mustard Greens	Purple Cabbage
Red Onion	Spaghetti Squash	Ginger	Arugula	Broccoli / Rabe	Purple Carrots
Rhubarb	Pumpkin	Sunchokes	Beet Greens	Brussels Sprouts	Purple Kale
Tomatoes‡	Rutabaga	Jicama	Leeks	Chinese Cabbage	Purple Endive
Red Peppers‡	Summer Squash	Kohlrabi	Lettuce	Green Beans	Taro
Chili Pepper‡	Sweet Potatoes	Mushrooms	Fennel	Green Cabbage	Purple Basil
Red Potato‡	Turmeric	Onions	Okra	Sugar Snap Peas	Black Salsify
(with skin)	Yellow Beans	Parsnip	Celery	Chayote Squash	Beets
	Winter Squash	Shallot	Snow Peas	Romanesco	Purple Cauliflower
	Yellow Tomato‡	Turnip	Cucumbers	Green Olives	Purple Tomatoes‡
	Yellow Peppers‡	Potatoes‡	Kale	Green Onions	Eggplant‡
	Orange Peppers‡		Herbs	Collard Greens	Purple Potatoes‡
	Chili Peppers‡		Spinach	Sea Vegetables	Purple Peppers‡
			Watercress	Green Peppers‡	
			Zucchini	Green Tomato‡	
			Avocado	Jalapeño Chilies‡	
			Chives	Tomatillo‡	

‡ *Nightshade vegetable – Remove if following the autoimmune protocol (AIP)*

2. **Moderate Protein**

Paleo proteins center on animal products with occasional small servings of nuts and seeds. Proteins comprise a reasonable portion of the diet, but not excessive (more about Protein on Day 6).

   a. Eat 3-8 oz per serving (1-3 deck-of-cards-sized portions), let hunger and satiety be your guide
   b. Use a wide rotation of animal proteins, ideally a different protein source every meal
   c. If the protein is naturally lean, add extra healthy fats

3. **Healthy Fat**

We have only scratched the surface of the dietary fat topic. Over the next few days, Paleo-Wise information details the differences between healthy and dangerous fats. For now, know that Paleo fats are the original unadulterated fats nature provided: Grass-fed butter/ghee, animal fats from those raised on a pasture (lard, tallow, duck fat, drippings, fatty cuts like bacon or sausage), coconut products, avocado products and olive products.

   a. A fat portion ranges from 1-3 Tbsp per meal (YES!!).
   b. Sometimes the food providing the healthy fat straddles two categories (olives can be recorded as both a vegetable and a fat; salmon is both protein and fat…more examples in the next chart).
   c. The quality of fat within fatty meats depends on the source:
      i. If the protein portion is a fatty cut of meat from *pastured* animals (free-range, grass-fed or wild caught), the fat is anti-inflammatory and satisfies the healthy fat requirement.
      ii. If the protein portion is from commercially-raised, factory-farmed animals, the fat is inflammatory. Drain and discard that fat and replace with a healthy fat.

Balance Foods Throughout the Day: As you acclimate to Paleo-eating, it may take a while to establish solid meal-building. It's okay if your initial meals are not 'perfect' – aim to cover missed servings by the end of the day. Just keep practicing – think "veggie, protein, fat" when building each meal until it becomes second nature.

The best angle from which to approach any problem is the try-angle. ~ Unknown

Charting Your Meals

The following charts are designed to assist in developing well-balanced Paleo meals. The two examples illustrate the flexibility of the Paleo Lifestyle and meal-planning – one portrays a *well-planned* Paleo day and the other a *'grab-&-go'* Paleo day. Read our evaluation at the bottom of each example. The blank chart afterward is for *your* Paleo meals today.

1. Describe the Paleo meal in the far-left column
2. Put an X next to the vegetable colors that were eaten during that meal
3. Fill in the protein and fats columns
4. Evaluate for completeness: The Veggie, Protein and Healthy Fat columns should have at least one item for each meal. Assess each column for variety and completeness.

Example 1: Well-Planned Paleo Day			
Meal	**Veggies**	**Protein**	**Healthy Fats**
Breakfast 3-egg omelet cooked in grass-fed butter w/sausage, spinach, black olives, onion, multicolored peppers and salsa	X Green X Yellow/Orange X Red X Blue/Purple/Black X White/Tan	Eggs Sausage	Grass-fed butter Olives Sausage (from pastured animals)
Lunch Burger on salad greens, onion, tomato, pickle and guacamole Dress w/olive oil and lemon	X Green Yellow/Orange X Red Blue/Purple/Black X White/Tan	Hamburger	Guacamole Olive oil Burger (from pastured animas)
Dinner Chicken Coconut Curry with Thai and Japanese eggplants, onion, carrots, zucchini and yellow squash Cauliflower rice	X Green X Yellow/Orange Red X Blue/Purple/Black X White/Tan	Chicken	Coconut milk Olive oil on cauli-rice
Snack Paleo almond meal and carrot muffin with melted grass-fed butter	Green ? Yellow/Orange Red Blue/Purple/Black White/Tan	Almond meal	Almond meal Coconut oil in the recipe Grass-fed butter

Evaluating Example 1:

✓ Nice variety of vegetables, included the full rainbow within one day.
✓ Good variety in proteins with a different protein source every meal (because fish or seafood wasn't included on this day, it would be ideal to include that protein source the following day).
✓ Wide selection of fats, especially if using fats from pasture-raised animals.

Today is your day to start fresh. To eat right. To train hard. To live healthy. To be proud.
~Bonnie Pfiester, fitness expert

Example 2: Grab-and-Go Paleo Day			
Meal	**Veggies**	**Protein**	**Healthy Fats**

Breakfast
Hard-boiled eggs
  dipped in guacamole
Carrot sticks
Red pepper slices
	X Green
	X Yellow/Orange
	X Red
	  Blue/Purple/Black
	  White/Tan
		Eggs	Guacamole

Lunch*
Hot bar at a grocer:
Salad w/greens and
  multi-colored veggies
  and bacon bits
Roasted chicken and
  baby red potatoes
	X Green
	X Yellow/Orange
	X Red
	  Blue/Purple/Black
	X White/Tan
		Bacon bits
		Chicken
			Bacon bits (only if
			  pasture-raised)
			Olive oil on salad

Dinner†
Frozen turkey burger
Frozen veggie mix
All fried in coconut oil
	X Green
	X Yellow/Orange
	X Red
	  Blue/Purple/Black
	  White/Tan
		Turkey	Coconut oil

Snack
Blackberries
Handful of pistachios
Coconut flakes
	Green
	  Yellow/Orange
	  Red
	X Blue/Purple/Black
	  White/Tan
		Pistachios	Pistachios
			Coconut flakes

Evaluating Example 2:

✓ Decent variety in vegetables and covered the full rainbow in one day.

✓ Protein variety satisfactory but not great, heavy on poultry. For balance, aim to include alternative proteins the following day such as seafood, pork or red meats.

* Lunch: This meal is very lean. Add olives to the salad, dress with 2-3 Tbsp of olive oil. It's hard to find grass-fed butter for potatoes; carry some with you or use olive oil again.

† Dinner: This meal is also fairly lean. Add more coconut oil, top the burger with avocado slices and melt some grass-fed butter on it.

✓ Convenience foods tend to be lean (byproduct of society's fear of fat). Carry some healthy fat with you like coconut milk for coffee, homemade salad dressing (commercial dressings are made with inflammatory fats), nut butter pouches or even a serving of grass-fed butter.

God grant me the serenity to accept the people I cannot change, the courage to change the one I can, and the wisdom to know it's me. ~ Unknown

Fill in the Chart: Today's Meals

Record your menu for today. Do not worry about any gaps, just note how well you're doing. This template will be included daily for the first week to encourage deliberate meal-building.

Note: A downloadable/printable copy is at 🖰 Paleovation

My Paleo Meals: Day 1			
Meal	**Veggies**	**Protein**	**Healthy Fats**
Breakfast	Green Yellow/Orange Red Blue/Purple/Black White/Tan		
Lunch	Green Yellow/Orange Red Blue/Purple/Black White/Tan		
Dinner	Green Yellow/Orange Red Blue/Purple/Black White/Tan		
Snack	Green Yellow/Orange Red Blue/Purple/Black White/Tan		

Staying Accountable

For those who need motivation to stick to their Paleo plan, we suggest keeping a food journal (extra blank meal charts can be copied from the Resource Section, or 🖰 MyFitnessPal is an electronic option). Consider having someone else review it every day or two. Remember this is not about cutting calories, it's about building nourishing and satisfying meals – portion sizes are to your satisfaction.

Checkmark the meal-building principles you are following well. Circle or highlight the areas for improvement.

- ☐ Eating lots of veggies
- ☐ Eating a colorful range of veggies
- ☐ Eating protein at every meal
- ☐ Eating a wide variety of proteins
- ☐ Eating healthy fats at every meal
- ☐ Adding traditional fats to a naturally lean meal

What is your plan to address any shortcomings and/or build well-balanced Paleo meals tomorrow?

_____

What was your favorite food from today? _____

Section III: Tomorrow's Meal Plan

Do you have meals on hand for tomorrow? At a minimum, select your breakfast menu before you fall asleep tonight – this guarantees you successfully start Day 2 with a Paleo meal. List some ideas here:

1. Breakfast: _____

2. Lunch: _____

3. Dinner: _____

4. Snack: _____

20-Minute Recipe Ideas

The modern 'meal-out-of-a-box' lifestyle creates a dependence upon quickly-prepared meals that don't need much mental energy or physical effort. Many Paleo newcomers are reluctant to start cooking from scratch; but transitioning to Paleo doesn't require slaving in the kitchen or agonizing over extravagant menus. In fact, an old favorite recipe can often be modified to fit the Paleo Template.

1. Include the best quality fat and protein your budget allows
2. Eliminate grain and dairy ingredients – sometimes use a substitution, other times just omit

There is no reason to fret over fancy meals; note how the following fast meal ideas can accommodate Paleo guidelines. Surprisingly, even omitting a key ingredient like breadcrumbs may be unnoticeable in the final meal.

Tweaking a 20-Minute Recipe	
Fast Meal Idea	**Substitutions* or Omissions**
Stir Fry	Rice → substitute cauliflower rice Soy sauce → *omit,* optional to substitute coconut aminos
Omelet	Cheese → *omit* Milk in omelet mix → *omit,* optional to use coconut or almond milk
Taco Salad	Shell / cheese / refried beans → *omit* Sour cream → *omit,* optional to use extra guacamole or salsa
Tuna Salad Sandwich	Mayo → substitute olive oil, guacamole, chopped egg, mustard, mashed sweet potato Bread → substitute cucumber boat, bell pepper half, lettuce leaf
Sausage and Sauerkraut	Bun → *omit*
Salmon Cakes	Bread crumbs → *omit,* optional to substitute crushed pork rinds
Pasta and Sauce	Pasta → substitute spiralized vegetables (or strips cut with a peeler) Cheese sauce → substitute marinara, garlic-and-herb sauce Parmesan → *omit,* optional to substitute Rawmesan®

*An extensive list of Paleo-friendly substitutions is in Day 6

Heating leftovers is one of the fastest solutions for a satisfying meal. What other ideas work for you?

1. **Use a Planned-Over** – Use prepared portions from a batch-cooking recipe during the prep
2. **Fill a Crockpot Tonight** – It's easy to fill a slow cooker with chicken or beef and veggies
3. **Search Online for "Fast Paleo Recipes"** (remember, direct links available at ⌐ Paleovation)
    - ⌐ PaleoLeap 10 Easy Paleo Recipes for Beginners
    - ⌐ PaleoGrubs 37 Super Easy Paleo Recipes (Even a Caveman Can Make)
    - ⌐ StupidEasyPaleo Recipe Index
4. **Other Ideas from the Resource Section** – Some are fast to make, others provide lots of leftovers:
    - ☐ Turkey Chili   ☐ Hamburgers
    - ☐ Fish Cakes / Casserole   ☐ Coconut Curry

Day 1 marks an exciting point in re-establishing your health. Congratulate yourself on a day well done and build upon today's success. How are you feeling after Day 1 is done? Check all that apply.

☐ Excited	☐ Sad	☐ Not so great
☐ I got this!	☐ Thinking about food	☐ Scared
☐ Tired	☐ Happy	☐ Uncertain
☐ Hungry	☐ Irritable	☐ Worn out

Care to expand? _____

_____

_____

To-Do List:

- ☐ Bone Broth – have you started your first batch? Finish up by Day 3.
- ☐ (Optional) If you can't or just don't want to make bone broth, then you need to purchase it from a reputable source. Local health food grocers often carry *true* bone broth in the freezer section (read the label to make sure it was cooked an extended period of time, roughly 24 hours). Popular online sources:
    - GrassLandBeef – *US Wellness Meats* sells high quality broths and enhanced gelatin broths from a variety of animal sources
    - KettleAndFire – *Kettle and Fire* produces grass-fed beef and free-range chicken broth
- ☐ Low-Carb Flu Remedy – symptoms may be approaching. Do you want to line up a strategy? See suggestions in Prep E.
- Ensure you have quick meal ingredients on hand all week:
    - ☐ Restock fresh veggies
    - ☐ As you sample your foundation recipes, restock ingredients if you enjoyed the meal and plan to make it again. If not, find another foundation meal to replace that recipe.

Coming Up Soon:

- Tomorrow's Paleo-Wise extends the topic of fats with desirable properties of naturally-saturated fats
- Paleo snack ideas and spice recommendations

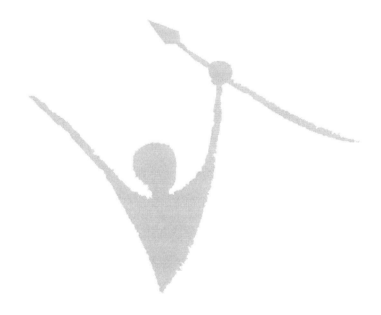

Day 2

Today's Topics:
1. Paleo-Wise: Fats Part II – Saturated & Mono-Unsaturated Fats
2. Meal Building = Vegetables + Protein + Fat
3. Paleo-Friendly Snacks
4. Seasoning, Herb and Spice Guide
5. Plan Low-Carb Flu Relief Strategies

Fast Fare – Frozen Foods
♥ Frozen stir fry veggie mix
♥ Frozen peeled shrimp
♥ Frozen cauliflower rice

Section I – Paleo-Wise: Fats Part II – Saturated and Mono-unsaturated Fats

The idea that saturated fats cause heart disease is completely wrong, but the statement has been 'published' so many times over the last three or more decades that it is very difficult to convince people otherwise.
~Mary Enig, PhD, Nourishing Traditions, cofounder of Weston A. Price Foundation

A. Saturated Fat: Bad Science, Not Bad Fat

Saturated fats have been falsely blamed for many modern ailments, but blanket accusations aren't a fair representation of any subject, including fat. The truth is, the entire lipid *hypothesis* (the *theory* that fat you eat is the same fat that clogs arteries) was built on faulty science.

Natural Saturated Fat – A Victim of Bullying

There is a BIG difference between *naturally-sourced* saturated fats and *chemically-altered* varieties. Natural saturated fats are *essential*. They are *benign, healthy* and *vital* for body structure and function!
1. No studies can confirm that high saturated fat intake *causes* cardiovascular disease. Many studies making such claims did not control for sugar/starch (the real culprit of arterial stress and systemic inflammation) or were tainted with other contributors (like trans fats).
2. The truely problematic fats are oxidized PUFA fats (detailed on Day 3) and trans fats (Day 4).

Properties of Saturated Fat

To understand why natural saturated fats are healthy and unique, we must briefly mention their molecular structure. The backbone of every fat molecule is a chain of carbon atoms. Saturated fats are distinct because their carbon chain is absolutely straight, with no bends or kinks. This is significant for two reasons:
1. Any bend or kink in a fat's carbon chain is susceptible to structural damage caused by oxygen or heat. Because saturated fats are straight, there is little chance of oxidative damage (going rancid).
2. Straight molecules can pack tightly together, therefore saturated fats are *solid at room temperature*.

Desirable Properties of Saturated Fat	
➤ Close-fitting molecules are remarkably stable ➤ Long shelf life	➤ Highly resistant to oxidation from air, light or heat exposure – saturated fats don't go rancid easily ➤ Stable at high heat – perfect for cooking, frying and baking

Vibrant Health Depends on *Natural* Saturated Fat

Saturated fat's stability and resistance to oxidation applies inside our bodies too – it won't break down to generate free radicals! Eating natural saturated fat builds a strong, highly-functional body:
- ✓ Supports brain function – enhances nerve transmission
- ✓ Increases nutrient absorption – transports fat soluble vitamins: A, D, E, K
- ✓ Slows aging, less wrinkles! – makes up 50% of cell membranes, improving cell structure and integrity
- ✓ Supports strong bones – assists with transporting calcium into bone
- ✓ Provides padding on high-impact structures – palms, bottom of feet, butt bones
- ✓ Protects liver from damage by chemicals (i.e. medications, alcohol, food additives, environmental toxins)

| Natural Saturated Fats (Eat These!) ||
Tropical Oils	Animal Fats (from Grass-Fed/Pastured Animals)
Coconut Oil – *highly* beneficial (details below) **Palm Oil** – from the fruit of the palm tree, high in antioxidants (which give it a red/orange color)	**Butter** – highly beneficial (more info below) **Lard** – pig/pork fat **Tallow** – beef or mutton fat

The best beauty products are made with natural saturated fats. Would you condition your hair or moisturize your skin with low-fat salad dressing? If I can't put it on my skin, I won't put it in my mouth.
~ Catherine Shanahan, MD, Deep Nutrition

Melt in the Mouth: Because saturated fats are solid at room temperature, it's assumed they are also solid in our arteries. *Not true!* Natural saturated fats like coconut oil, butter and lard have low melting points and are liquids at body temperature (98.6°F). However, chemically-saturated fats, including hydrogenated fats such as shortening or margarine, are designed to stay solid up to 119°F...way above body temp! Yikes!

Length of the Fat Chain – Size Matters

Another factor that influences the properties and function of saturated fat is the molecular length: short, medium or long chains. This length determines how the fat is digested and used within the body. Most natural saturated fats from meat, milk, eggs and nuts/seeds are long-chain varieties. Long chains require assistance to digest, enlisting bile from the gall bladder and digestive enzymes. However, the less common medium- and short-chain fats digest much easier, giving them unique nutritional advantages that are worth seeking out.

Coconut is King!

Coconut is a highly nutritious *natural* saturated fat, rich in fiber, vitamins and minerals. Furthermore, coconut is classified as a "functional food" because it provides health benefits beyond its nutritional content, including noteworthy healing properties. Formerly touted as unhealthy because of its high saturated fat content, coconut oil has now been scientifically vindicated and its unique health-giving qualities are praised.

Fast Fact: The coconut palm is so highly valued by Pacific and Asian cultures as both a source of food and medicine that it is called *"The Tree of Life."*

MCT Oil – "Miracle Coconut Trademark"

The saturated fat in coconut oil is unique because it's predominately *medium-chain triglycerides* or MCT (about 65%). Due to the shorter length, MCTs are easier to digest than long-chain fats, bypassing the need for digestive assistance from the gall bladder. MCTs immediately break down into *ketones* which are directly absorbed into the blood. Ketones are an alternate, and arguably preferable, energy source to glucose. However, unlike glucose, excess ketones are excreted in the urine and are *not stored as fat*!

Benefits of MCTs *and* Coconut Oil:

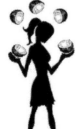

- ➤ **Quick Energy** – MCTs are easily absorbed and quickly metabolized into ketones
    - The body immediately burns MCTs as fuel rather than store them as fat
    - MCTs do not require bile from gall bladder to be digested
        - ✓ Transported directly to the liver where they're converted to ketones
        - ✓ Perfect for those with gall bladder dysfunction or fat absorption issues
    - MCTs provide energy *without* negative blood sugar and insulin impact
- ➤ **MCTs Promote Weight Loss**
    - Encourage fat-burning metabolism and preserve muscle mass
    - Jumpstart metabolism conversion from "sugar-burner" to "fat-adapted"
    - Not stored as fat – any excess is excreted in the urine!
    - Naturally suppress appetite
    - Increase metabolism by boosting thyroid function
    - Reduce insulin production (insulin is the 'storage' hormone)

> **Brain Health** – The brain prefers to use ketones from MCTs over glucose for energy!
> **Digestive Health** – Coconut oil, as a whole, is soothing to the intestines.
>   - Improves gut flora balance (reduces pathogens and boosts beneficial flora)
>   - Helps heal leaky gut
>   - Relieves bloating, constipation
> **Antioxidant and Anti-Inflammatory Properties Abound in Coconut Oil**
> **Coconut Oil for Topical Skin Therapy and Wound Healing**
>   - Therapeutic for acne, eczema, psoriasis, dry skin
>   - First Aid for scrapes, sunburn and rashes
> **Medicinal/Healing: Anti-Viral, Anti-Bacterial, Anti-Fungal and Anti-Parasitic:**

Coconut Oil as Medicine: Effective in Killing or Expelling the Following			
Viruses	**Bacteria that Cause:**	**Fungi and Yeast**	**Parasites**
Influenza	Acne	Candidiasis	Tapeworms
Herpes	Urinary Tract Infections	Ringworm	Lice
Measles	Gum Disease / Cavities	Thrush	Giardia
Hepatitis C	Pneumonia	Athletes Foot	
AIDS	Throat Infections	Diaper Rash	

Try these: Coconut oil is well-suited for personal care and cosmetic uses – skin moisturizer, hair conditioner, toothpaste, mouthwash (oil pulling), deodorant, cold sore ointment, cough suppressant, sore throat soother, sunscreen (roughly SPF7), personal lubricant (though not compatible with latex condoms) and more, wow!

Most Potent MCT

Like other fats, MCTs have different molecular lengths and are identified by the number of carbon molecules in the fat chain. Two varieties of MCT particularly prompt the body to burn fat to use as fuel, the most potent of which is the 8-carbon variety, caprylic acid (C8). The next most favorable MCT is 10-carbon capric acid (C10).

The primary MCT in coconut oil is 12-carbon lauric acid (about 50%). Though lauric acid is a uniquely useful, healthy saturated fat, it doesn't provide the same potency of fat-burning advantages as the shorter C8 and C10 varieties. Concentrated MCT oils specifically comprised of C8 and C10 MCTs are pricy but may be worth seeking.

- HealthLine MCT Oil 101 – A Review of Medium-Chain Triglycerides
- Bulletproof What is MCT Oil Really?

Butter – Source Matters!

Butter is a phenomenal, natural saturated fat, *but only when it is from the right source*. The quality and nutritional caliber of butter varies greatly depending on how the animal was raised. Before expanding on benefits of butter, we need to identify the ideal butter and clarify some animal husbandry terms:

> **Grass-Fed or Pastured** – Cattle are fed their natural diet of grass or raised on a foraging pasture.
> **Organic** – Cattle have access to a pasture but the feed can be supplemented with organic grain/soy (practices vary farm to farm). Because grains and legumes are not their natural diet, an inflammatory reaction is triggered. Consequently, the resulting fat in butter and beef products from these cattle can be pro-inflammatory, albeit with less toxin residue than conventional.
> **Conventional (what most people buy)** – Cattle are raised on feed lots (referred to as CAFOs, Concentrated Animal Feeding Operations). Animals are fed an unnatural diet of chemically-tainted grains, soy and fillers, treated with antibiotics and growth hormones. They are kept in confined, often unsanitary, conditions. Fatty products from these CAFO sources are pro-inflammatory and often have digestion-disrupting antibiotic, hormonal and chemical residues.

Best Beef, Best Butter: A *grass-fed AND organic* beef/butter product is the best of both worlds: from cattle fed their natural diet AND with no antibiotics, hormones or chemical residues.

"Butterful" *Grass-Fed* Butter!

> *You are what you eat eats.* ~ Michael Pollan, In Defense of Food

Grass-fed dairy fat (found in butter, clarified butter or ghee) contains vital nutrients including fat soluble vitamins and even the same anti-inflammatory fats touted in fish oil! And the taste is amazing! Here are the benefits of grass-fed, pasture-raised butter:

- ➤ Provides essential fat soluble vitamins A, D, K2 and E along with natural cofactors for easier absorption
    - The form of vitamin A in butter is the most easily metabolized
    - One of the few sources of vitamin K2, critical for bone health (read Bone Health on Day 16)
- ➤ Includes anti-inflammatory EPA & DHA, the same essential fats as fish oil (although a lesser percentage)
- ➤ Constructed of short-chain fatty acids, similar benefits to MCTs noted above
    - Quick energy source – acts as fuel for intestinal cells and good gut flora
    - Improves digestion – easy to digest, does not require bile and is quickly absorbed for energy
- ➤ Anti-microbial, anti-tumor
- ➤ Contains trace minerals
- ➤ Source of Conjugated Linoleic Acid, CLA (more about CLA on Day 4)
    - Shown to aid in weight loss and weight management
    - Helps the body build muscle rather than store fat
    - Protects against cancer

Double Up: You can simultaneously reap the benefits of MCT oil *and* grass-fed butter by whipping them both into your coffee or tea! Learn the science behind Bulletproof® Coffee and the technique here:
⏻ Bulletproof How to Make Your Coffee Bulletproof and Your Morning Too

---

B. Mono-Unsaturated Fats

The two most recognizable mono-unsaturated fats are olive oil and avocado oil. These fats are accurately referred to as *heart-healthy good fats* and embraced for their multitude of health benefits:

- ✓ Improve insulin sensitivity
- ✓ Support cellular structure – anti-wrinkles!
- ✓ Protect the heart by lowering blood pressure, improving cholesterol profile and lipid panels, and decreasing risk of cardiovascular disease

Fats Are Not Created Equal

To understand the qualities of mono-unsaturated fats, a little more chemistry is necessary to explain the technical terms (often found on food labels). Identifying them here will help with differentiating between healthy and unhealthy fats.

Saturated

The Backbone Structure of Fat

As mentioned previously, fat molecules have of a backbone carbon chain. Each carbon atom can hold several hydrogen atoms. The amount of *hydrogens* the fat contains largely determines its properties.

Mono-Unsaturated

- ➤ **Saturated Fat** – The carbon chain is completely filled, or *saturated*, with hydrogen atoms (and the chain is straight).
- ➤ **Mono-Unsaturated Fat** – The carbon chain is missing hydrogens at just *one* (*mono*) juncture. Note that this hydrogen gap causes the chain to kink and creates a point of structural vulnerability.

Hydrogenated Oil (a Common Term on Food Labels)

The term *hydrogenated* refers to the chemical process of adding hydrogens to an unsaturated (kinked) fat chain to make it more saturated (straight). This physically transforms liquid oil into a more solid fat, enhancing stability (shelf life) and creaminess. However, the resulting foreign fat is severely destructive and a primary trigger for inflammation. Products typically containing artificially *hydrogenated* fats include margarine, shortening, baked goods and peanut butter. Read labels and avoid hydrogenated oils (more about Trans Fats on Day 4).

Fat Fact: If you wanted to make solid hydrogenated fats like margarine or vegetable shortening, you would need a chemistry lab! However, if so inclined, it is possible to make natural saturated fats like coconut oil, butter, lard and tallow right in your own kitchen.

Mono-Unsaturated Oxidation Vulnerability

Structurally, mono-unsaturated fats have one area of the carbon chain that is missing hydrogens. This kink in the chain is susceptible to damage from air, light or heat exposure. The decay process of *oxidation* begins at these gaps and produces toxic compounds and destructive free radicals (oxidation is why an apple turns brown when exposed to air). Mono-unsaturated fats do not have the resilient structure of saturated fats, but luckily, their vulnerability is limited to just one gap, so they're relatively stable especially when found in whole food form.

In their original state within seeds and nuts, unsaturated fats are naturally protected from oxidation by the nut meat and shells. However, once the oil is removed, it becomes vulnerable. To protect these fats from air, light and heat, purchase mono-unsaturated oils in smaller quantities, select dark-colored bottles and store at cool temperatures.

Liquid Fat

Straight saturated fats pack tightly, making them solid at room temperature. The unsaturated area in a fat chain creates a slight kink which doesn't allow the molecules to pack as tightly together. Therefore, mono-unsaturated fats are less dense, making them liquid at room temperature (but generally thicken at refrigerated temperatures).

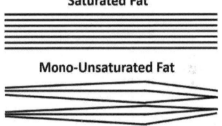

Paleo Sources of Mono-Unsaturated Fat	
Fruit and Fruit Oils	**Nuts/Seeds and Their Oils**
Olives and Extra Virgin Olive Oil from the first cold-pressing of olives **Avocados and Avocado Oil**	**Select Nuts and Nut Oil** – macadamias are best, followed by hazelnuts and cashews **Seeds** – especially sesame, pumpkin and sunflower

C. Cooking with Oils: High Heat Precautions

Applying heat to fat for cooking purposes accelerates the oxidation process, leaving toxic compounds in the oil. This is the primary reason not to reuse deep-frying oil (and good motivation to avoid fried restaurant food where unstable oils are typically reused for days).

To Prevent Fat Oxidation During Cooking:
1. Select a stable, saturated or monounsaturated fat or oil
2. Cook below the smoke point temp

Natural saturated fats generally are the most stable and include tropical oils and animal fats. Surprisingly, olive oil and avocado oil also withstand heat well due to presence of antioxidants and a substance called oleic acid.

Though smoke point is a good rough guide, oxidation can occur before the oil starts smoking, especially for highly-unstable *poly*unsaturated oils (more on those tomorrow).

- ⌂ BalancedBites FAQs What are Safe Cooking Fats & Oils
- ⌂ DrAxe Coconut Oil Uses

Stable Fats for Cooking	
Saturated Fat	**Smoke Point (°F)**
Coconut Oil / Refined	350 / 450
Butter	350
Ghee or Clarified Butter*	460
Tallow (beef fat)	400
Palm Oil	455
Lard (pork fat)	375
Duck Fat	375
Mono-Unsaturated Fat	
Avocado Oil	450
Extra Virgin Olive Oil	355

*Purified Butter: Clarified butter is made by gently melting the butter, skimming off the white protein solids and reserving the clear yellow liquid (pure butterfat). Ghee uses the same process but lets the milk solids sink to the bottom of the pan to toast before separating, imparting a nutty flavor.

Section II: Meal Building – Vegetables + Protein + Fat

Today's Meals: What does your meal plan look like today?

My Paleo Meals: Day 2			
Meal	**Veggies**	**Protein**	**Healthy Fats**
Breakfast	Green Yellow/Orange Red Blue/Purple/Black White/Tan		
Lunch	Green Yellow/Orange Red Blue/Purple/Black White/Tan		
Dinner	Green Yellow/Orange Red Blue/Purple/Black White/Tan		
Snack	Green Yellow/Orange Red Blue/Purple/Black White/Tan		

Beverages: _____

How easy is it to include all components in each meal? What works best so far?

_____

_____

Improvise Meal Components

Meal-building is not an exact science – improvising is absolutely fine. Low on fat? Add in a handful of olives or an extra pat of butter. Forgot the veggies? Grab a squeeze pouch of sweet potato, sprinkle some seaweed flakes on your lunch or keep fresh cut or roasted veggies on hand (directions to roast vegetables in Prep E).

Tomorrow's Food Plan:

If/when low-carb flu symptoms develop, bone broth is therapeutic. Having it on hand saves you from cooking when you're not feeling well. Is your bone broth started or have you purchased quality broth?   Yes   No

What meals are ready for tomorrow? If necessary, look back to yesterday's 20-minute meal ideas.

Section III: Paleo-Friendly Snacks

Quick Snacks
As you peruse snacks ideas below, note that some are too high in sugar for the Strict Paleo Protocol, save those for after this month (ex: high-sugar or *dried* fruits, honey, dates or maple syrup). Prep or purchase some snacks and divide into servings so they're ready to grab-n-go. Use zipper bags or try 4-8oz canning jars (durable, easy snack-sized way to utilize glass over plastic).

Basic ideas are provided but many more can be found with an online search for "paleo snacks." Also check Paleo shopping sites to browse new products for inspiration (remember, direct links available at ⏥ Paleovation).

☐ ThriveMarket   ☐ BarefootProvisions   ☐ OneStopPaleoShop   ☐ PaleoFoodMall   ☐ StevesPaleoGoods

Dips and Spreads
Dip or spread on veggies, deli meat, bacon, cut green apples, smoked salmon or Paleo crackers
- ➢ **Dip/Spread Ideas**
  - Guacamole (convenient single serving sizes available by Wholly Guacamole®)
  - Avocado oil mayo or coconut oil mayo (now available in retail grocers)
  - Homemade Paleo mayo (see cooking assignment #2 on Day 4)
  - Salsa
  - Paleo hummus (homemade using cauliflower, palm hearts or cashews)
  - Pureed pumpkin with cinnamon
  - Non-dairy cheese spreads (read ingredients carefully, Day 6 has Paleo-friendly suggestions)
  - Cashew or coconut milk "cheese" (Recipes online such as ⏥ TheSpunkyCoconut 5 Minute Coconut Cream Cheese Paleo Dairy-Free, note the sugar is okay, it feeds the bacteria for fermentation)
  - Chimichurri (pureed herbs and olive oil)
  - Mustard
  - Olive tapenade
  - Pesto (homemade, omit cheese)
  - Coconut butter (purchased or homemade, more info later today)
  - Liverwurst pate (sugar- and dairy-free, check ⏥ GrassLandBeef)
  - Nut butters (some available in small serving squeeze packets for grab-n-go convenience)

Veggies
- ➢ **Serving Ideas**
  - Serve with dips/spreads
  - Wrap in bacon or deli meat
  - Mason® jar salad
- ➢ **Veggie Snack Ideas**
  - Fresh cut – cut your own, buy pre-cut from a salad bar or prepackaged veggie tray
  - Cherry tomatoes
  - Sweet bell pepper (red, yellow orange) eaten whole like an apple or filled w/tuna or egg salad
  - Cucumber slices (top with a spread, salmon or tuna; cucumber sandwiches; use for dipping)
  - Pea pods, snap peas or green beans
  - Pickles (available prepackaged in a pouch)
  - Dehydrated veggie chips (purchased or homemade oven-dried kale, zucchini, sweet potato)
  - Marinated mushrooms
  - Artichoke hearts (frozen or packed in water or olive oil)
  - Sauerkraut (raw cultured preferred, in the refrigerator section)
  - Sweet potato fries/chips (purchased or homemade; cooked in lard, coconut or palm oil)
  - Roasted veggies (made ahead)
  - Olives

Eggs

- ➢ **Serving Ideas (all make ahead)**
    - Hard-boiled
    - Deviled eggs
    - Egg salad - use as a dip or a spread (for shortcut, use scrambled eggs as the base)
    - Omelet muffins / mini crust-less quiche
    - Scrambled eggs

Nuts and Seeds

Nuts and seeds are limited to one handful per day:

- ➢ **Serving Ideas**
    - Mix with berries, coconut flakes, bacon bits, cocoa nibs
    - Paleo trail mix (nuts, seeds, coconut flakes)
    - Paleo granola (purchased or homemade, cooking assignment #4 on Day 11)
    - Top with coconut milk or almond milk
    - Spiced nuts/seeds
- ➢ **Nut and Seed Ideas**
    - Macadamias
    - Almonds
    - Walnuts
    - Pecans
    - Cashews
    - Pistachios
    - Pine nuts
    - Brazil nuts
    - Hazelnuts/filberts
    - Chestnuts
    - Pumpkin seeds
    - Sunflower seeds
    - Flax seeds
    - Hemp seeds
    - Sesame seeds

Seafood

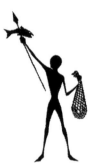

- ➢ **Serving Ideas**
    - Mix with Paleo mayo (Day 4), mustard, guacamole or salsa
    - Make a seafood salad and use as a dip or a spread
    - Serve with olives or capers
- ➢ **Seafood Ideas**
    - Tin of tuna, sardines, baby shrimp, oysters or salmon
    - Smoked salmon or lox (spread with a Paleo dip)
    - Salmon jerky – difficult to find sugar-free (cooking assignment #4 on Day 11)
    - Shrimp cocktail (watch for sugar in cocktail sauce)

Meats

- ➢ **Serving Ideas**
    - Use bacon or deli meats as a wrap for veggies, olives, pickles or spreads
    - Use crispy bacon or fried salami as a cracker substitute
- ➢ **Meat Snack Ideas**
    - Bacon
    - Meatballs
    - Jerky
    - Deli meat (make roll-ups)
    - Salami
    - Hot dogs (grass-fed, no filler)
    - Paleo chicken tenders (homemade)
    - Chicken drumsticks or wings (make ahead)
    - Pork rinds (in chip section at grocers or convenience stores)
    - Leftovers – roasted beef or chicken
    - Grass-fed meat sticks (homemade or purchased)

Chips/Crackers (homemade or read labels to avoid industrial oils)

- Kale chips
- Pork rinds
- Dehydrated veggies
- Go Raw® Flax Snacks
- Seaweed sheets for sushi
- Some seaweed snacks
- Sweet potato chips
- Paleo crackers (try Jilz® brand or homemade

Berries/Fruit

Low-sugar fruits are limited to one daily serving:

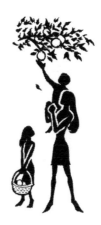

- ➢ **Serving Ideas**
    - Raw, frozen, freeze dried, dehydrated
    - Mix with nuts, coconut, cocoa nibs
    - Top with coconut milk or coconut cream
- ➢ **Berries/Fruit Ideas**
    - Blueberries
    - Raspberries
    - Strawberries
    - Blackberries
    - Green apples, wrapped in bacon or use for dipping
    - Grapefruit half

Fats

- Olives (available prepackaged in a pouch)
- Coconut (fresh, flakes or creamed)
- Avocado
- Paleo meltaways or "fat bombs" (many recipes available online, more info in Day 3)

Miscellaneous

- Bone broth in a mug

Sweets and Treats

Be careful because many Paleo treats are too high in sugar for the Strict Paleo Protocol, search online for 21-day sugar detox recipes "21DSD treats" such as ◌ BalancedBites Lemon Vanilla Meltaways

- Dark chocolate – 85% or higher (look for brands without soy lecithin)
- Strawberries (or bacon) dipped in dark chocolate
- Berries in creamed coconut
- Paleo meltaways or "fat bombs"

Energy/Protein Bars

Disclaimer: Ideally a protein bar would have little sugar, but some are fruit-based and have a high carbohydrate load. If we had to make a rule, it would be to keep the sugars <2 g per bar. However, if you find a bar with <9g sugar per bar, it could be an *occasional* treat. Any bar more than 9g should be avoided while eating a Strict Paleo Protocol. The following brands have Paleo-friendly bars, but read labels carefully – not all are low sugar:

- Tanka®
- Larabar®
- Epic®
- Exo®
- Granilla®
- Rx® bar
- Wild Zora®
- Bearded Brothers®
- Chomps® Snack Sticks
- Bulletproof® Collagen Bar

What snacks are ready for tomorrow?

_____

_____

Section IV: Seasoning, Herb and Spice Guide

- ➢ **Herbs** – from leafy and green plant parts; examples: basil, oregano, rosemary, thyme, mint, parley, dill.
- ➢ **Spices** – from non-green plant parts like roots, stems, bark, seeds and bulb; examples: ginger, cinnamon, cumin, saffron, fennel, licorice.

The Nose Knows: Spice blending does not need to be intimidating. Open spice containers and sniff their combined aromas. If they smell good together, they will taste good together!

Tip: If you are still unsure, the internet also knows – search "Paleo + [your spices]" for recipe options
For example, "Paleo Dill Cinnamon" locates ◌ PaleOMG Bacon Lime Sweet Potato Salad!

> *Ounce for ounce, herbs and spices have more antioxidants than any other food group.*
> ~Michael Greger, MD, How Not to Die

Seasoning Guide‡		
Spices	**Herbs**	**Spice Blending†**
Allspice	Basil*	
Anise	Chamomile*	***Italian Herbs*** – oregano, basil, rosemary, thyme,
Bay Leaf	Chervil	marjoram
Black Pepper*	Chives*	
Caraway	Cilantro*	***Italian Sausage/Pizza*** – salt, pepper, fennel/anise, +
Cardamom*	Dill Weed	Italian herbs
Cayenne Pepper*	Dill Seed	
Celery Seed	Lavender	***Chili Seasoning*** – chili powder, cumin, garlic, oregano,
Chili Pepper	Lemon Balm	onion, paprika
Cinnamon*	Lemongrass	
Clove*	Marjoram	***Curry Powder*** – turmeric, coriander, cumin, ginger,
Cocoa Powder	Mint	nutmeg, cinnamon, garlic, clove, pepper
Coriander	Oregano	
Cumin	Parsley*	***Herbes de Provence*** – thyme, rosemary, basil, oregano,
Fennel	Rosemary*	dill, tarragon, fennel
Garlic Powder*	Sage	
Garlic*	Savory	***Mexican*** – paprika, salt, onion, garlic, cumin, oregano,
Ginger*	Tarragon	pepper, cocoa
Horseradish	Thyme	
Lemon Zest		***Asian 5 Spice*** – ginger, nutmeg, cinnamon, anise, clove,
Mace		pepper
Mustard		
Nutmeg*		***Lemon Pepper*** – pepper, lemon zest, salt
Onion Powder		
Paprika		***Garlic & Herb*** – garlic, basil, parsley, oregano
Poppy Seed		
Saffron		
Shallots		
Star Anise		
Turmeric*		
Vanilla Bean (not extract)		

*Anti-inflammatory properties, especially turmeric and ginger

‡ Auto-Immune Protocol: the AIP Guide in the Resource Section identifies problematic nightshade- and seed-based spices

† For spice blending recipes check ⌕ WellnessMama 14 Homemade Spice Blends

Section V: Low-Carb Flu Relief Strategy

It may be a day or two before the low-carb flu sets in. Re-read the low-carb flu information in Prep E. Select two strategies you can implement right now for low-carb flu:

1. _____

2. _____

Select two more strategies that you could arrange with a touch more effort:

1. _____

2. _____

How Did Day 2 Go?
Check all that apply:

☐ Rather smoothly	☐ Thinking about food, a LOT	☐ Tired
☐ Cravings galore!	☐ Way different than Day 1	☐ Hungry
☐ Low energy	☐ Piece of cake	☐ Headaches
☐ Snacks were well-planned	☐ Not so great	☐ Satisfied
☐ Up and down	☐ Need more leftovers	☐ I'm out of veggies!

Other thoughts:

_____

_____

Day 2 Review:

1. Do you think your food choices are providing your body the nutrients it needs?   Yes   No
2. Do you feel you are on the right path, food-wise?   Yes   No
3. Are you getting enough variety in your foods?   Yes   No
4. How do you feel about your food choices so far?

   _____

5. Any concerns you have about the foods you are consuming?

   _____

6. Any concerns about the foods you are *not* consuming?

   _____

7. How can you make Day 3 go better than today?

   _____

   _____

To-Do List:
☐ Bone broth will be done (or purchased) by tomorrow – check off when yours is cooked, strained and stored
☐ Prepare a low-carb flu relief strategy
   ✓ Give yourself permission to rest, an earlier bedtime is completely acceptable during the Paleo Transition
☐ Continually restock fresh veggies so you have plenty on hand all week for meals and snacks
☐ Prepare for Cooking Assignment #2: Paleo Mayo (instructions on Day 4) – you will need:
   ✓ Blend of oils/fats such as olive, avocado, macadamia, coconut, ghee or reserved bacon drippings
   ✓ 1-2 high-quality pasture-raised eggs*, lemon juice/vinegar and mustard
   ✓ Tools: a blender (regular or immersion), food processor, stand mixer or large whisk + muscles
      * Egg-free versions use canned coconut milk + bacon drippings or olive oil + coconut butter‡

> ‡ **Make Your Own Coconut Butter:** No need to break the budget – blend dried coconut flakes into a paste in a food processor. It takes 15-20 min and ☝ MarksDailyApple *10 Tips for Making the Best Coconut Butter Ever* has a helpful picture blog on the process. Tip: dog-ear this page if you think you'll need this article in the future.

Coming Up Soon:
- Polyunsaturated Fats like canola oil, corn oil or 'vegetable' oil are the next topic
- Optional Paleo Crutches for those struggling with full compliance

Day 3

You will never change your life until you change something you do daily. The secret of your success is found in your daily routine. ~John C. Maxwell, The 15 Invaluable Laws of Growth

Today's Topics:

1. Paleo-Wise: Fats Part III – Polyunsaturated Fats
2. Prep Low-Carb Flu Relief Strategies
3. Curb Hunger by Adjusting Fat and Protein Levels
4. Paleo Crutches
5. Find Some Humor, Somewhere

Fast Fare – Freezer / Fridge / Pantry
♥ Fish filet sautéed in butter w/lemon
♥ Coleslaw mix with olive oil & vinegar
♥ Microwaved sweet potato (pricked)

How does today's meal plan look?

My Paleo Meals: Day 3			
Meal	**Veggies**	**Protein**	**Healthy Fats**
Breakfast	Green Yellow/Orange Red Blue/Purple/Black White/Tan		
Lunch	Green Yellow/Orange Red Blue/Purple/Black White/Tan		
Dinner	Green Yellow/Orange Red Blue/Purple/Black White/Tan		
Snack	Green Yellow/Orange Red Blue/Purple/Black White/Tan		

Have you been satisfied between meals?   Yes   No

What has helped you to feel comfortably full (more strategies listed below in Section III)?

_____

Is there a certain color(s) of vegetables you need to add to your grocery list?   Yes   No

If yes, write down the color and the specific vegetables you'll buy (Day 1 has the Veggie Guide):

_____

Section I – Paleo-Wise: Fats Part III – Polyunsaturated Fats (PUFAs)
Including Essential Fats, Omega-3 Fats, Fish Oils and Omega-6 Fats

Today's opening quote references that personal change can happen daily; yet on a large scale, change is slow. Despite knowing the health repercussions of polyunsaturated oils *decades* ago (exactly when saturated fats were demonized and PUFAs were encouraged as a replacement), many still consider them 'heart-healthy' and the misinformation of saturated fat persists. The shift to healthier oils is definitely a slow change:

> *Excess consumption of polyunsaturated oils has been shown to contribute to a large number of disease conditions including increased cancer and heart disease; immune system dysfunction; damage to the liver, reproductive organs and lungs; digestive disorders; depressed learning ability; impaired growth; and weight gain.* ~Sally Fallon and Mary Enig, PhD, <u>Nourishing Traditions</u>. Referenced research was published from 1973- 1994.

Consistent with the general topic of fats, polyunsaturated fatty acids (PUFAs) are immersed in controversy and confusion, exhibiting some good and some bad characteristics. We'll start with the good.

Fish Oils: Essential EPA and DHA, the Omega-3 Fats

The most notable healthy fats in the polyunsaturated category are the *essential* fatty acids, EPA and DHA, also referred to as omega-3's or fish oils. These are *required* for body function and optimal health. Interestingly, we cannot manufacture EPA and DHA as we can other fats, so it is *essential* to attain them from the diet. Omega-3's are primarily acquired from animal products, though an algae-based source of DHA is available via supplement.

Benefits of EPA and DHA Fats

The tremendous health benefits of the omega-3 fatty acids, EPA and DHA, are well-established.

- ➢ **Potent Anti-Inflammatory**
  - Generates pain-relieving, *anti*-inflammatory compounds called resolvins
  - Decreases production of irritating, inflammatory compounds called cytokines
  - Reduces production of free radicals associated with aging and degenerative diseases
- ➢ **Brain Function**
  - Supports memory, concentration and focus; decreases symptoms of ADHD
  - Reduces risk of dementia
  - Supports mood and reduces symptoms of depression and anxiety
- ➢ **Cell Structural Support** (Anti-Wrinkle!)
  - Half the cell membranes are comprised of omega-3s (the other half is saturated fat!)
- ➢ **Eyesight**
  - DHA is a key structural component of the retina
- ➢ **Bone Structure**
  - Associated with higher bone mineral content and bone density
- ➢ **Heart Health**
  - Natural blood thinner
  - Lowers blood pressure
  - Lowers blood triglycerides
  - Maintains normal heart rate
  - Reduces arterial plaque formation

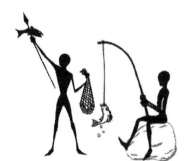

DHA, a No-Brainer: DHA stimulates growth of new brain cells, protects existing brain cells, enhances the connections between brain cells (neuroplasticity) and is anti-inflammatory (inflammation is a key factor in Alzheimer's, Parkinson's disease and in many other neurodegenerative conditions). DHA is *critical* for brain function and *must* come from the diet.

Read More about Benefits of Omega-3 Fats:
    ⁋ <u>HealthLine 17 Science-Based Benefits of Omega-3 Fatty Acids</u>

Sources of EPA and DHA

Omega-3 precursors are found in algae, seaweed and green grass. The fish and animals that eat these green foods have the necessary enzymes to convert them into EPA and DHA, which are then stored in their fat. Since humans lack this capability, the most efficient way to attain these essential omega-3's is by consuming animal fats (*but only if the animal's diet contained the required green foods as a primary component*):

1. Wild-caught *fatty* fish: salmon, mackerel, sardines, herring, halibut, cod, anchovies, etc
2. Butter from grass-fed or pastured cows
3. Pasture-raised or omega-3 enriched eggs
4. Grass-fed/pastured beef and other ruminant animals, although less than seafood sources
5. Wild game

> **Wild for Omega-3's:** Unlike wild fish that eat algae or seaweed, farm-raised fish are fed an unnatural grain-and soy-based diet deficient in the EPA/DHA precursors. Therefore, farm-fed fish *contain lower concentrations* of EPA and DHA…yet fatty farmed fish are still an adequate omega-3 source and much better than no fish at all.

Facts on Flax: Plant-Based Omega-3's

There is a third omega-3 fat called ALA, alpha-linolenic acid. This is the plant-based omega-3 found in flaxseed, chia, hemp and to a lesser extent, walnuts. Unlike animal-based EPA and DHA, our bodies can manufacture the minor amounts of ALA needed; consequently, ALA is not classified as essential.

ALA is beneficial for a variety of reasons but is *not* anti-inflammatory like EPA and DHA. Many people mistakenly consume ALA, commonly in the form of flaxseed oil, with the intention of reaping the benefits of EPA and DHA. However, humans lack the enzymes to efficiently convert ALA into EPA or DHA, with a conversion rate of less than 5%. Plant-based omega-3 can be part of a healthy diet but is *not an acceptable substitute* for EPA and DHA.

> **Best Practice for Flax:** Purchase flaxseeds whole and grind at home when ready to consume. Why? The seed's hull protects the delicate omega-3 oil from oxidation. Pre-ground flax meal or cooked flax products (muffins) are oxidized, negating the nutritional benefits. For flaxseed oil, select refrigerated brands in a dark bottle.

PUFAs: Perishable Liquid Fats

All polyunsaturated fatty acids (PUFAs), whether 'good' such as fish oils or 'bad' such as industrial oils (we'll get to those in a moment) are far more unstable than the mono-unsaturated or saturated fats. Polyunsaturated fats have several gaps in the carbon chain where hydrogens are missing (*poly* = many). As mentioned in yesterday's reading, these junctures create a vulnerable kink in the fat structure where exposure to light, heat or oxygen will rapidly stimulate oxidation (rancidity) and free radical production.

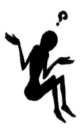

Refrigeration Test – A Benchmark for Identifying Inflammatory PUFAs

Due to multiple kinks in PUFA carbon chains, molecules pack very loosely and will remain liquid even at *refrigerated temperatures*. In fact, this is a major identifying factor for inflammatory PUFAs – *most* oils that stay liquid in the refrigerator are vulnerable to oxidation and are a potential concern. The refrigeration *clue* is a starting point for recognizing quality oils, but there are exceptions – healthy avocado oil will remain liquid with refrigeration.

Furthermore, although *most* inflammatory PUFA fats are liquid at refrigerated temperatures, food manufacturers may use a blend of oils either to cut costs or to imitate qualities of healthier oils. It is advisable to read labels of any refrigerated liquid fats (salad dressing may not be as healthy as you think!). As mentioned yesterday, *most* quality olive oils will thicken or even solidify in the refrigerator, yet some may not due to the variety of the olive or the season of harvest. Because quality fats are crucial for quality health, it's recommended to research your oil and locate an olive oil company you trust.

Read More about Olive Oil:
- ⌐ DrChristianson How Do You Know if your Olive Oil is Real?
- ⌐ OliveOilTimes Olive Oil Fridge Test Don't Count On It

Essential Omega-6 Fat Sources

Omega-6 oils are the other *essential* polyunsaturated fat. Omega-6's are required in *small* amounts and beneficial when consumed from whole-food, anti-inflammatory sources:

> ➢ Nuts and seeds, avocado, grass-fed or pasture-raised meat, game, pork, poultry and eggs

These oils are a chief source of controversy in the topic of essential fats, primarily because their health-boosting properties are *conditional*. When consumed in high proportions, omega-6's switch from being beneficial to extremely detrimental. *Excess* omega-6 PUFAs are *highly* inflammatory and contribute to chronic disease.

When Omega-6 Oils Become Inflammatory

Inflammatory Omega-6 Oils
💧 Soybean
💧 Canola
💧 Corn
💧 Peanut
💧 Safflower
💧 Cottonseed
💧 Sunflower
💧 Grapeseed
💧 Vegetable

Although the human body needs both omega-3 and omega-6 fats, the *proper balance* is a critical tipping point between maximizing health versus triggering disease. In high amounts, omega-6 fats convert to *pro-inflammatory* compounds, counteracting and suppressing the anti-inflammatory benefits of omega-3 fats.

With industrial processing, an influx of unnatural omega-6 fats has flooded the food supply. Manufacturers extract these fats from naturally-protective seed hulls using chemical solvents to isolate the oil; then they refine, bleach, degum and deodorize it. Nutrients are stripped out – residues are inevitable in the final product. During processing, these oils are repeatedly exposed to air, light and heat causing oxidization and rancidity.

The modern diet is *loaded* with these inflammatory oils, present in most packaged or prepared foods (read labels!). The primary problematic oils are listed in the table.

> **Fat Fact:** "Going rancid" is an oxidation process that generates toxic free radicals which attack the body, damage the liver, trigger inflammation, interrupt digestion and contribute to chronic disease.

> *What was healthy in the seed is not healthy in the bottle!*
> ~Cate Shanahan, MD, Deep Nutrition

Analogy: Not Too Hot, Not Too Cold

To better comprehend omega balance, think of omega-6's as being a hot (inflammatory) water tap and omega-3's being the cold (anti-inflammatory). A comfortable temperature range is created by regulating hot and cold.

Unfortunately, the westernized diet fuels omega imbalance due to an overabundance of chemically-extracted seed oils and a deficit of wild-caught fish and naturally-raised animal products. This is like turning the hot (inflammatory) tap on full force while leaving the cold (anti-inflammatory) tap dribbling.

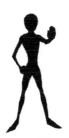

PUFA Vegetable Oils Are Highly Unstable

Industrially-extracted PUFA oils are *so* unstable that even indirect light and room temperatures will damage them, yet they are commonly sold in clear bottles, unrefrigerated! Do not buy them – they are already rancid on the store shelf. Why don't they smell rancid? They have been deodorized.

PUFA oils are falsely labeled as 'vegetable' oil to enhance health appeal. Do not be fooled. They are not safe for cooking or deep frying. When heated, PUFAs create toxic byproducts such as formaldehyde and trans fat!

> **Point to Ponder:** Although PUFAs are often called 'vegetable' oils, these fats are from seeds, legumes or grains, *not* vegetables! It is ludicrous to imagine fats extracted from true vegetables like cauliflower, kale or carrot oils.

> *The final chemical product of vegetable oil quickly goes rancid with its short shelf-life, is defenseless against free-radical attack, is stripped of its healthy antioxidants, and often contains cancerous chemicals and compounds.*
> ~Colin E. Champ, MD, author of Misguided Medicine

Deep-Fried Nightmare

Restaurants typically use cheap, inflammatory omega-6 oils in deep fryers. To make matters worse, instead of refilling fryers with fresh oil, they may just top it off every few days, or weeks, before replacing the entire batch. Repeatedly heating these oils magnifies the negative consequences to the oil and ultimately, to our health.

Read More about Dangers of Heating PUFAs
- ⁰ ChrisKresser An Update on Omega-6 PUFAs
- ⁰ WestonAPrice The Big Fat Surprise: Toxic Heated Oils

Damaged Oil = Damaged Body

Omega-3 and omega-6 fats compete with each other for placement within the body. They are incorporated as building blocks into all cell membranes including skin, organ linings, blood vessels, nerves and brain tissue.

In absence of sufficient anti-inflammatory omega-3 fats, overabundant *and often damaged* omega-6 fats must be allocated to build body structures. This causes weakness and instability of every cell in the body! Impaired cells easily succumb to inflammatory free radicals which create additional destruction and health compromise.

> **Analogy:** Over-consuming processed, omega-6 vegetable oils means the body must build tissues with damaged fats. This is like building a house with termite-ridden wood! Consequences are inevitable.

Balancing Act, Omega-6 and Omega-3

To be clear, small amounts of omega-6 fats *from natural sources* are essential and healthy. The critical part is to balance their consumption with appropriate amounts of omega-3 fats. To minimize the inflammatory effects of too much omega-6, their consumption should be *no more than* 4 times the amount of omega-3. This is achieved by regularly eating fatty fish *and* limiting omega-6 to whole food sources like nuts, seeds and meats.

Modern agricultural practices and food processing have created an exponential shift in liquid fat consumption. It is not uncommon in a contemporary diet to consume 30-50 times more omega-6 than omega-3!

> *Soybean oil alone is now so ubiquitous in fast foods and processed foods that an astounding 20 percent of the calories in the American diet are estimated to come from this single source.* ~Andrew Weil, MD, Healthy Aging

> **Point to Ponder:** Today's *conventional* beef is high in inflammatory omega-6 fat due to cheap grain and soy feed. Interestingly, cattle fed an unnatural grain/soy diet sustain the same consequence as humans: inflammation and accumulation of fat! Just a few generations ago, pasture-raised, grass-fed beef was the only meat available (higher in healthy omega-3's) and industrial oil processing had not yet been invented (lower omega-6 exposure). With those two factors alone, our great-grandparents easily consumed an appropriate balance of omega-6 and omega-3 fats.

Paleo Naturally Balances Omega-3 and Omega-6 Fats

Merely increasing intake of omega-3 is not enough to offset the extremely high omega-6 consumption typical in modern diets. It is absolutely crucial to decrease intake of omega-6 fats. The Paleo Diet naturally accommodates this by eliminating inflammatory omega-6 sources from grains and legumes (and their oils), while simultaneously increasing omega-3 consumption via fish, seafood, pastured animal products or omega-3 enriched eggs.

A simple strategy to ensure sufficient omega-3 intake is to eat *fatty* fish at least twice a week. Fresh, canned, pickled, smoked or frozen/previously-frozen are all acceptable.

- ➤ Salmon (wild-caught, red or sockeye preferred)
- ➤ Mackerel
- ➤ Sardines
- ➤ Anchovies
- ➤ Whitefish
- ➤ Trout
- ➤ Tuna
- ➤ Herring

> **Salmon Omega Balance:** Wild-caught salmon is leaner than its farm-raised cousin. Though both fish have the same amount of omega-3 per serving, wild fish has *far less* omega-6, amplifying the anti-inflammatory benefits. Still, if wild-caught is not an option, farmed salmon (especially from Norway) is an excellent source of omega-3s.

Supplementing with Omega-3 Oils

Ideally, a diet rich in wild-caught, fatty fish and grass-fed or pastured animal products would negate the need to take a fish oil supplement. Realistically however, most people do not consume enough fish to support essential omega-3 needs. Additionally, some people may temporarily need extra omega-3 to unwind the damage from chronic omega-6 consumption. Individual evaluation is required regarding supplementation.

> **Fish Oil Fantasy:** Taking fish oil supplements is not a "Get-Out-of-Jail-Free" card to justify a diet loaded with omega-6 fats. Inflammatory seed oils and packaged/prepared foods need to be reduced as well.

For many individuals, a high-quality fish oil supplement is valuable. To prevent spoilage, store in a dark, cool place (or refrigerator) and do not buy in bulk. Taking up to 2000 mg of omega-3 per day from supplements* is safe according to the FDA. *Speak to a doctor if you take blood thinning medications or have a bleeding disorder.*

*Supplements must contain EPA and/or DHA (flaxseed oil is not an adequate substitute). Several high-quality products are listed at ⌐ PureRXO.com/Paleovation under "My Picks." The following omega-3 recommendations contain 1000mg of EPA/DHA per capsule (much more than grocery store brands):

- **O.N.E. Omega** by Pure Encapsulations
- **ProOmega 2000** by Nordic Naturals

Budget Concerns - Keep Calm and Paleo On

Though we emphasize the importance of sourcing animals that eat their natural diet (wild-caught, pastured, grass-fed), we do not want to discourage an individual who cannot acquire or afford those animal products. Do what is best for your budget – perhaps that means buying high-quality, grass-fed butter but lower quality conventional lean meats. Regardless, a Paleo Diet with conventionally-raised products is still a *major* improvement from a westernized diet loaded with sugar/starch. Each step is a step in the right direction.

Further Reading:
- ⌐ ThePaleoMom Can I Still Do Paleo if I Can't Afford or Source Grass-Fed Beef
- ⌐ DrCate List of Good Fats and Oils versus Bad

> *Give up grains and fried restaurant foods. Doing that pretty much gets you most of the way there.*
> ~Mark Sisson, Primal Blueprint, The Keto Reset Diet

Section II: Withdrawal Relief

By Day 3, symptoms of sugar/carb withdrawal set in. It may not escalate into full blown low-carb flu (more info in Prep E), but the following relief strategies can ease symptoms of both withdrawal and low-carb flu.

- ☐ **Sleep** (nap, early bedtime, sleep in)
- ☐ **Sweat** (sauna, steam, hot bath, hot tub, sweat lodge, Epsom Salt bath)
- ☐ **Stretch** (gentle yoga, Tai Chi, stretching)
- ☐ Push **fluids** (tea, water, lemon water, bone broth)
- ☐ **Move** the lymph (take a walk, get a massage, use a foam roller, dry brush)
- ☐ **Reduce energy** requirements (lower workout intensity, stroll, rest/relax)
- ☐ Supplement with **salt** (add extra sea salt or coconut aminos to food/drink)
- ☐ Utilize **detoxification support** details in Prep E (activated charcoal, clay, fresh herbs, supplement*)
  - *find our top 3 detox supplements at ⌐ PureRXO.com/Paleovation

Have you started to show signs of withdrawal?   Yes   No

What, if any, relief strategies have you tried? _____

Do you feel any are helping? _____

Is there anything else you plan to do to ease withdrawal symptoms?

_____

Section III: Hunger Levels

How Are Your Hunger Levels?

- ☐ Hungry all the time
- ☐ Strangely satisfied
- ☐ I need some snacks

- ☐ Lost my appetite
- ☐ Too busy to be hungry
- ☐ Thinking about food, a LOT

- ☐ Feeling pretty normal
- ☐ Missing my favorite food
- ☐ Feeling "off"

Curbing Hunger:

Protein and fat are more satisfying than carbs – adding more to each meal/snack can temper hunger levels. Which fats and proteins taste good to you right now?

_____

Select Several Strategies for Adding Fats/Proteins:

- ☐ Salads need olives, avocado and meat
- ☐ Use extra olive oil on your salad
- ☐ Add extra fats when preparing meals
- ☐ Top your eggs with guacamole
- ☐ Snack on protein like hard-boiled eggs or jerky
- ☐ Bacon, need we say more?
- ☐ Sip on canned coconut milk (may water down)
- ☐ Add coconut milk to coffee or tea

- ☐ Snack on fats like olives, guacamole, coconut oil on a spoon, nut butter or coconut butter
- ☐ Use drippings from cooking to make a sauce
- ☐ Melt grass-fed butter into your hot drinks
- ☐ Make a coconut milk-based soup or sauce
- ☐ Top a steak with a pat of grass-fed butter
- ☐ Sprinkle your entrée with coconut flakes
- ☐ Snack on a handful of nuts (one serving daily)

Section IV: Different Routes to Paleo Success

The only difference between stumbling blocks and stepping stones is the way you use them. ~American Proverb

Are you having any difficulty with cravings? Common cravings include sugar (carbs), salt and for some, alcohol. Occasionally a craving is just missing a favorite food or habitual snack like a morning latte or smoothie. Yet, other cravings can be strong enough to completely unravel personal commitment to dietary change. These strong and persistent cravings need to be approached in a rational manner.

If your cravings are intensifying to the point that you are considering quitting, it is best to consciously acknowledge them and address them directly. Do not allow food urges to interrupt your commitment to better health. Instead, incorporate some dietary hacks or crutches to stay on track toward the long-term goal.

Two options to manage cravings and keep you en-route to Paleo success:

1. **Direct Route:** Remain strict with Paleo Protocol but incorporate some Paleo-friendly hacks
2. **Roundabout Route:** Bend the rules to allow Paleo-ish exceptions (crutches) normally reserved for those in maintenance mode. Understand that this will elongate the program and cravings can linger. However, it may be worth it if your stress levels are reduced and you remain on track toward the long-term goal.

Success is the goal! There is nothing right or wrong with selecting either path. If you need assistance, we suggest trying the hacks in Route 1 before implementing the crutches listed in Route 2.

Route 1: Direct Route – Remain on the Strict Paleo Protocol

The following Paleo hacks assist in reducing cravings while the body is transitioning out of a westernized diet. These will allow you to calm symptoms while adhering to the Strict Paleo Protocol.

Craving Hacks

- ➢ Promote ketone production by consuming easily-digested fats (for more info about ketones and fat burning, see Prep G and Day 2)
  - ✓ Coconut oil (contains MCTs, medium chain triglycerides)
  - ✓ Concentrated MCT oil (more information in the saturated fats topic on Day 2)
  - ✓ Grass-fed butter, ghee or clarified butter (contains a special short chain fat, butyrate)
  - ✓ Bulletproof coffee/tea (uses MCT oil plus grass-fed butter: ⌐⊕ Bulletproof How to Make Your Coffee Bulletproof and Your Morning Too)
  - ✓ Make a "fat bomb" snack (see recipes next page)

- Supplement with L-Glutamine* to quickly stop a craving for sugar or alcohol: start with a 500 mg - 1000 mg dose (empty stomach is best), wait 10 minutes, take a second dose if necessary
  *for quality L-glutamine, go to 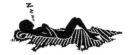 PureRXO.com/Paleovation – select 'My Picks'
- Review other carb craving strategies and articles in Prep G
- If you are craving cheese (Day 7 explains why that happens), Day 6 gives cheese alternatives in the Paleo food substitution charts
- Have a *single* serving of 85+% dark chocolate (without soy lecithin)

Food Hacks
- Cinnamon, coconut and powdered vanilla naturally have a sweet flavor; use liberally
- Try *unsweetened* fat bombs made from Paleo ingredients (note: when searching 'Paleo fat bombs' online, many recipes are sweetened with dates, maple syrup or honey – stay clear of those for now)
  - DitchTheWheat Cinnamon Bun Fat Bomb Bars
  - FreeCoconutRecipes Strawberry Coconut Bites
  - TheHealthyFoodie Almond Pistachio Fat Bombs
  - PrimalPalate Paleo Recipes Peppermint Patties 2
- Eat something that feels decadent to curb a craving – macadamia nuts or sunflower seed butter are perfect Paleo indulgences (review the Paleo Yes Foods chart in Prep B for other enticing ideas)
- For a sweet-ish side dish, caramelize vegetables in the oven such as onions, sweet potatoes, cauliflower, bell peppers, carrots, winter squash or broccoli
- Use your daily fruit serving wisely:
  - Grate a green apple into coconut or almond butters
  - Sauté fruit in grass-fed butter/ghee and add cinnamon or coconut flakes
  - Make a berry purée to sweeten a sauce, use as salad dressing or freeze in a popsicle mold

Energy Hacks
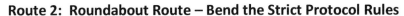
- Meditation or deep breathing exercises
- Movement: exercise, yoga, dance, Tai Chi
- Take a power nap
- Aromatherapy: Place a drop of essential oil or extract such as peppermint on your palm, cup your hands around your nose and enjoy the scent for two minutes

Route 2: Roundabout Route – Bend the Strict Protocol Rules
If you are at a point where bending the rules makes the difference between sticking to the program versus quitting, we prefer you proceed and use a Paleo crutch. Success is the goal! Although these options aren't *strict* Paleo Protocol, they are still Paleo-friendly and commonly incorporated by individuals in maintenance mode.

Do You Need a Crutch?
Our advice is to stay as close to strict Paleo as you comfortably can. In a few weeks when food reintroductions begin, your readiness is kept in perspective by considering how many crutches were used. Depending upon how far you selectively stray, your program may need to be extended by 2-4 weeks.

It does not matter how slowly you go so long as you do not stop. ~Confucius

Is a Crutch Worth It?	
Advantages	**Disadvantages**
- Satisfies short-term cravings - Remains on track to long-term goal - Avoids indulgence in less Paleo options - Prevents quitting the program altogether - Reduces stress if the Strict Paleo Protocol is overwhelming - Allows modification for personal temperament	- Postpones reaping the full health benefits of Paleo - Lengthens the time commitment before truly reaching Paleo maintenance mode - Encourages cravings/addictions to linger - Delays addressing the crutch to a future date - Can increase the time experiencing sugar/carb withdrawal symptoms

Questions to Ponder

Before you decide to read through the roundabout route's selective deviations, consider these questions:

1. Did the Paleo Hacks provide enough latitude so you can adhere to the program as is?   Yes   No
2. Have you browsed the Paleo Substitution charts on Day 6 to check alternative ingredients?   Yes   No
3. Can you commit to one more day of the Strict Paleo Protocol before you implement a crutch?   Yes   No

The goal is to make conscientious choices that impact health and wellness – Paleo-with-a-crutch satisfies that. Feel free to mix and match the following ideas, gradually tapering your craving crutches over time. Use the least amount of your selected crutch as possible to steadily reduce your brain's 'bliss point.'

1. **Fruit Options**
   - Indulge in a high sugar whole fruit such as apple, mango or peach (not canned)
   - Add a 2nd or 3rd low-sugar fruit serving
   - Use fruit as a dessert
      - Unsweetened applesauce
      - Purée frozen fruit with nut butter and coconut milk to make 'ice cream'
      - PaleoTable Chocolate Banana Pudding

2. **Sweeteners, Including Stevia or Hardwood Xylitol (not xylitol from corn)**
   These are acceptable sweeteners that will not impact blood sugar levels; however, they do continue to stimulate sweet cravings. Look for pure stevia (many brands are mixed with dextrose). Also, sugar alcohols like xylitol are linked to digestive disruption (often causing bloating) so proceed with caution.
   - Add sweetener to drinks, homemade Paleo muffins or pancakes
   - Make a *sweetened* fat bomb (remember, direct links available at Paleovation)
      - GrassFedGirl Low Carb Chocolate Coconut Fat Bombs
      - WholeNewMom No Bake Coconut Delights
      - TheNourishedCaveman Coconut Chocolate Bars Low Carb Snacks
      - OurFourForks Homemade Chocolate

3. **Alcohol, Gluten-Free**
   Alcohol is not recommended except in the worst-case scenario → you are ready to quit the program! Your liver is already being taxed with neutralizing toxins released during these dietary changes. Furthermore, alcohol can spike insulin and slow the rate that fat is mobilized for energy.

   Limit yourself to 1 drink per week. Try a smaller half-sized serving, drink earlier in the evening and only drink with a meal. Internet search "*Paleo Supplements for Alcohol Hangover*" for recommendations to assist your body with processing alcohol. These are the cleanest options (more about Alcohol Day 26):
   - Hard liquors (lowest carb options and gluten-free)
      - 100% agave tequila   • Vodka made from grape or potato   • Gin
   - Limit mixers to seltzer, sparkling water, fresh squeezed citrus juice or coconut water
   - Blend with fresh vegetables like cucumber and tomato or fats like coconut milk and avocado
   - Gluten-free beer or hard cider (<u>caution</u>: high carb; choose a dry cider)
   - Glass of wine (<u>caution</u>: high carb; organic dry white or dry sparkling wines are best tolerated)

4. **Paleo Treat**
   These choices are better than their conventional counterparts, but they still introduce sugars or starches that prolong cravings and interrupt the insulin-leptin balance. <u>Reminder</u>: it is difficult to eat too many baked sweet potatoes but quite easy to consume too many sweet potato chips. We suggest placing an individual serving on a plate to avoid overconsumption.
   - Sweet potato, plantain or taro chips fried in coconut/palm oil
   - Paleo-friendly protein / energy bar (suggestions on Day 2)
   - Paleo baked good, try cutting the sugar in half if making homemade
   - Dried fruit or homemade dessert using dried fruit such as date and nut balls

Which approach do you think will best serve your individual body and personality? (circle one)
1. The Direct Route – Strict Paleo
2. The Roundabout Route – Implement some Paleo crutches

> *The rung of a ladder was never meant to rest upon, but only to hold a man's foot long enough to enable him to put the other somewhat higher.* ~Thomas Henry Huxley, <u>Man's Place in Nature</u>

List any of the previous strategies you feel will help you stay on track:

1. _____
2. _____
3. _____
4. _____

Section V: Find Some Humor

Humor is stress-relieving and we know that drastically changing one's diet is enormously stressful. Shake off some of the seriousness and lighten up.
1. Look up award-winning comedy movies
2. Find clips of your favorite comedian: many SNL comedians range decades, George Carlin, Jim Carey, Lucille Ball, Jerry Seinfeld, Jerry Lewis, Laurel and Hardy, Johnny Carson, Jimmy Fallon, Carol Burnett, Eddie Murphy, Robin Williams...the list is endless
3. Internet search "humorous quotes" or "I need some humor"
4. Go to a comedy club
5. Visit ⌐ BuzzFeed LOL Feed
6. Watch a cartoon (South Park has one titled Gluten-Free Ebola)
7. ⌐ YouTube – JP Sears pokes fun at the Paleo crowd (Awaken with JP), Jimmy Fallon's Lip Sync Battles, Jimmy Kimmel's request to parents to eat their kids' Halloween candy, Poor lip reading voice-overs, your favorite sit-com or comedy show

Section VI: Finish Bone Broth

Time to cross Bone Broth off your list. Day 4 tends to bring on the low-carb flu and the first signs that the body is beginning to regulate hormones. You will be relieved to have broth prepared to nourish your body.
Hint: If you are ready to use your broth, Prep F and Day 5 have ideas.

To-Do List:
- ☐ Bone Broth – check off when yours is cooked, strained and stored
- ☐ Choose a detox relief strategy (listed in Section II today) that you can use tomorrow if necessary:

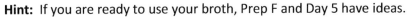

_____

- ☐ Restock fresh veggies to keep healthy snacks on hand all week

Coming Up Soon:
Prep for Cooking Assignment #2: Paleo Mayo – do you have what you need? Select the ingredients you have on hand and/or would like to use, instructions tomorrow.
- Oil choices: olive, avocado, macadamia, coconut, ghee, bacon drippings
- 1-2 high-quality eggs, lemon juice/vinegar, garlic and mustard
- For egg-free versions: canned coconut milk + bacon drippings *or* olive oil + coconut butter

Day 4

Pork chops and bacon, my two favorite animals. ~Homer Simpson

Today's Topics:

1. Paleo Meal Planning
2. Keep Calm and "Paleo On"
3. Low-Carb Flu Relief Strategies
4. Paleo-Wise: Fats Part IV – Trans Fats
5. Cooking Assignment #2: Paleo Mayo

Fast Fare – Fridge and Pantry
♥ Scrambled egg + pepperoni
♥ Marinara sauce
♥ Kale chips

Section I: Paleo Meal Planning

What is the menu today? This template will be provided for the remainder of this first week to help you build meals and monitor progress:

My Paleo Meals: Day 4			
Meal	**Veggies**	**Protein**	**Healthy Fats**
Breakfast	Green Yellow/Orange Red Blue/Purple/Black White/Tan		
Lunch	Green Yellow/Orange Red Blue/Purple/Black White/Tan		
Dinner	Green Yellow/Orange Red Blue/Purple/Black White/Tan		
Snack	Green Yellow/Orange Red Blue/Purple/Black White/Tan		

Meal-Building

Are you successfully building colorful Paleo meals?   Yes   No

What column is easiest for you get enough quantity *and* variety?   Vegetables   Protein   Fat

What parts of your meals do you need to improve?

What will you do differently so that you're prepared to build better meals tomorrow?

☐ Revisit breakfast ideas in Prep F
☐ Fresh cut veggies every meal
☐ Keep guacamole on hand
☐ Keep a bottle of coconut oil on the table
☐ Keep a bottle of olive oil on the table
☐ Buy some single serve pouches: olives, pickles, nut butter, guacamole

☐ Use canned seafood for a quick snack
☐ Check the Veggie Guide (Day 1) for colorful ideas
☐ Prepare large quantities of roasted vegetables
☐ Visit the suggested foundation meals (Resource)
☐ Decrease nut consumption
☐ Scan the 28 days of Paleo menus in Prep B
☐ Regularly rotate fish, poultry, beef, seafood and pork

Recipe Plans

Have you found any favorite or easy go-to recipes yet? Review your previous food log entries...what have you liked the best so far?

_____

_____

Meal prepping doesn't need to be time-intensive. The daily Fast Fare boxes spark ideas – here are several more:

☐ Frozen burger with tomato and greens
☐ Stir fry – use prepackaged frozen veggies or purchase pre-cut veggies from a salad bar
☐ Salad mix with canned or smoked fish
☐ Frozen cauliflower rice for fried "rice"
☐ Omelet or frittata
☐ Frozen single-serve fish filet, flash defrost by immersing packet in water before cooking
☐ Pre-made shish-kabobs at the meat counter
☐ Pre-shredded cabbage for slaw or sautéing

☐ Ground meat scrambled with lots of veggies, mix with seasoning like Italian, curry or taco
☐ Frozen sausage links
☐ Shrimp cocktail minus the sauce
☐ Hot/cold bar at a grocery store
☐ Frozen previously roasted sweet potato slices
☐ Batch cook with plenty of leftovers
☐ Sausages and kraut
☐ Bone broth soup, add sautéed veggies & meat
☐ Tin of baby shrimp mixed with guacamole

Break*fast*: Fastest Quiche Ever!

1. Grease a coffee mug with coconut oil or grass-fed butter
2. Crack in an egg, add a splash of coconut milk (optional) and seasonings
3. Add an assortment of chopped spinach, peppers, green onions and fresh herbs
4. Whisk it all up
5. Microwave for 90 seconds and invert mini-quiche onto a plate

---

The most dangerous phrase in the language is "we've always done it this way." ~ Grace Hopper

Cooking Assignments Overview

1. **Bone Broth** – Yours should be done. Use it as a cooking liquid, drink it warm out of a mug or make a creamy soup by pureeing it with cooked vegetables and coconut milk. Use your broth to nourish your body during this transition. Other ideas in Prep F and more coming up tomorrow.

2. **Paleo Mayo** – Directions later today – complete by Day 7. Ingredients should already be on hand.

3. **Substituting Veggies for Grain** – This indispensable technique provides extra vegetables while avoiding grains. Consider what grain you will substitute and purchase one of the replacement veggies by Day 7:
   a. **Rice**: cauliflower, jicama
   b. **Noodles**: consider buying a spiralizer to produce a more authentic noodle appearance/texture
      i. Sautéed: zucchini, sweet potato, yellow squash, carrots, bell peppers
      ii. Roasted: spaghetti squash
   c. **Sandwich Bun**:
      i. Latkes: sweet potato, zucchini, carrots, turnips, etc (you'll also need eggs for these)
      ii. Grilling: eggplant slices or portabella mushroom caps
      iii. Raw: lettuce leaves, cabbage leaves, bell pepper or cucumber

Section II: "Keep Calm and Paleo On"

We have repeatedly mentioned flu-like symptoms are a common side effect as the body acclimates to Paleo eating. Additionally, dietary changes of this magnitude are physically and mentally stressful. Do not be surprised by sudden emotional sensitivities including anxiety, irritability or a shortened temper. Monitor your emotional state over the next few days and know that these responses are natural and only *temporary*.

If you notice moodiness intensifying, remember that others do not know what you're going through. No one is intentionally trying to upset you. Take deep breaths, release any tension and try to stay composed. It may be a few days before your mood resets, but until then, do your best to calmly respond to outside circumstances.

- Has your mood or attitude affected interactions with others today?   Yes   No
- Stress relieving strategies such as deep breathing, meditation, muscle tensing and relaxing, or exercising can help steady an agitated mind. Do these methods work for you?   Yes   No
- Consciously pausing for 3-4 seconds when reacting to stressful situations paves the way for a calmer response. Has a technique such as this been successful for you?   Yes   No
- Any other methods that help you keep your cool? _____

Managing stress is a significant part of overall health. The Paleo hacks and crutches mentioned yesterday are viable strategies to take the edge off this dietary change. Additional stress relieving ideas are in Day 12.

Section III: Low-Carb Flu Relief Strategies

The low-carb flu manifests in many ways and usually starts around Day 4 or 5. Trust that these symptoms are temporary and will pass. How are you feeling today?

☐ Grumpy	☐ Fuzzy brain	☐ Angry
☐ Tired	☐ Exhausted	☐ Achy
☐ Nauseous	☐ Excessive cravings	☐ Dizzy
☐ Hyperactive	☐ No energy	☐ Crazy dreams
☐ Irritable	☐ Headache	☐ Worried this isn't the right
☐ I caught a cold	☐ Jitters	thing for my body
☐ Swollen glands	☐ Hungry	☐ I'm feeling pretty good

Do NOT misinterpret low-carb flu symptoms as your body rejecting the new Paleo foods. It's actually the exact opposite. These symptoms are the body's way of responding to *and* healing the damage from chronic exposure to westernized foods. They also indicate that positive physical changes are emerging in your body:

1. Toxins are being neutralized and mobilized out of your body
2. Your body is withdrawing from addictive foods (grains, cheese, sugar, alcohol)
3. Your metabolism is re-learning how to burn fat for energy instead of glucose
4. Hormonal signaling is beginning to normalize

> **Key Point:** The low-carb flu exposes the chronic damage and powerful effect that decades of westernized foods created in the body. It does not indicate anything wrong with Paleo foods. Stay strong through this transition, trust that the body is beginning to heal the damage and remember these symptoms are only temporary!

Review strategies to ease low-carb flu symptoms and/or manage cravings in Prep E, Prep G and Day 3.

1. Is there any strategy you haven't yet tried that you want to incorporate?

   _____

2. What strategy has worked for you?

   _____

3. What hasn't worked for you?

   _____

4. Are you utilizing a specific strategy today? If yes, note which one(s) and how you felt afterward:

   _____

Section IV – Paleo-Wise: Fats Part 4 – Trans Fats

What are Trans Fats?
It's generally understood that trans fats are unhealthy and are linked to heart disease, but few comprehend exactly what they are or where they lurk. Artificial trans fats were first developed in the early 1900's to create a solid fat from an inexpensive, liquid oil (originally intended for soap-making!).

The most concentrated form of trans fat is partially hydrogenated oil made from PUFA oils. For decades the food industry favored this fat because it's cheap, extends shelf-life, has higher melting points (important in the summertime) and creates flaky textures in baked goods. Additionally, because PUFAs are extracted from plants, food manufacturers deceptively boost health appeal with 'cholesterol-free' product advertisements.

Creation of Partially Hydrogenated Oil
Trans fats are created by a chemical process called *hydrogenation*. Food chemists take a highly unstable, liquid oil (like soybean or cottonseed) and alter the properties by adding and maneuvering hydrogens on the fat chain.

How to Create Partially Hydrogenated Oil
1. Begin with a cheap, unstable, liquid polyunsaturated vegetable / seed oil (PUFA)
2. Use heat and catalysts to add and rearrange hydrogen atoms on the fat chain, forcing the kinked polyunsaturated fat chain to straighten and act like a saturated fat
3. The end product mimics properties of saturated fat and extends shelf-life: more solid at room temperature, higher melting point and more stable to light, heat and air

Trans Fat is NOT Saturated Fat
Although trans fats *look and act* like saturated fats, the body *cannot assimilate* them appropriately. Trans fats neither fit nor function correctly. As our bodies attempt to incorporate trans fats into structures typically made from saturated fats (such as your brain tissue or cell membranes, more on Day 2), a host of health problems emerge. That's like the proverbial "putting a square peg in a round hole."

Trans fat is not an acceptable substitute for stable, saturated fat. The detrimental health effects that result from trans fat consumption are often incorrectly linked to naturally-saturated fats and mistakenly used to criticize healthy, stable fats like butter, pastured animal fats and coconut and palm oils.

Health Risks of Artificial Trans Fat
Industrial trans fats are *not* natural and are extremely difficult to digest. Trans fat consumption has shown to:
- Raise the risk of heart disease by elevating levels of LDL (often referred to as "bad cholesterol") and lowering levels of HDL, "good cholesterol" (read more about Cholesterol on Day 17)
- Increase triglycerides in the bloodstream
- Damage the liver
- Promote systemic inflammation
- Disrupt insulin sensitivity, raising the risk of developing type-2 diabetes
- Damage the inner lining of blood vessels and destroy blood cells
- Weaken cell membranes, allowing easier entry of toxins
- Interfere with transport of minerals and other nutrients

Although these fats extend a *food's* lifespan, artificial trans fats decrease *human* lifespan. In 2015, the FDA acknowledged their health risks and removed the GRAS status (Generally Recognized As Safe) from the main source of trans fat, *partially hydrogenated oil*. In the U.S., this specific fat is no longer allowed in food without a special permit (but is still allowed in animal feed – another reason CAFO animals products are discouraged).

You know why they call it shortening? It shortens your life. ~Mark Hyman, MD, Eat Fat, Get Thin

> **Point to Ponder:** The food industry replaced *vital* saturated fats with processed 'vegetable' oils to protect heart health. Ironically, the chemical manipulation of vegetable oils introduced trans fats into the western diet and accomplished the exact opposite.

Trans Fats Still Slip Through the FDA Ban

Because the FDA banned partially hydrogenated oil due to its trans fat content, it's increasingly rare to read the words *'partially hydrogenated'* on food packaging. Yet, trans fat is still hidden in modern prepared foods. Labeling loopholes permit manipulation of serving size and the use of alternative ingredients to avoid trans fat disclosure. Despite regulations, here are several ways artificial trans fats sneak into the food supply:

➢ **Serving Size:** Labeling laws allow up to 0.5g of trans fat *per serving* before it must be disclosed. Therefore, a manufacturer can simply reduce the serving size and still advertise "No Trans Fat."

➢ ***ALL* Highly-Processed Industrial Seed Oils:** PUFAs are extremely unstable. Heat-processing, deodorizing, degumming and other manufacturing practices create trans fats as a byproduct in any final seed oil.

➢ ***ALL* PUFA Oils Used in Cooking:** When PUFA oils are heated via cooking, trans fat are created. Therefore, they lurk in processed foods, deep-fried foods, restaurant entrees and even in our own kitchens!

➢ **Monoglycerides and Diglycerides:** Technically, the food industry only labels trans fats from *tri*glycerides. By using *mono-* and *di*-glycerides as emulsifiers, trans fats can still hide within a product. Admittedly, these contribute minimal amounts of trans fat, but demonstrates that label laws are not fully accurate.

Toxic trans fat continues to hide in plain sight! Read every label. Avoid *all* canola, soybean, corn, vegetable, safflower, sunflower, cottonseed & grapeseed oils as well as any cooked products with these oils as ingredients.

Foods that Commonly Contain Hidden Trans Fat		
Snack foods	Ice cream	Restaurant foods
Baked goods	Frosting	Margarine / shortening
Fried foods	Cheese spread	Microwave popcorn
Pre-made dough	Donuts	Nondairy creamer
Coffee creamer	Salad dressing	Peanut butter
Pie / crust	Chips	Frozen entrees / pizza
Cookies	Crackers	Chocolate-flavored candy
Shake mixes	French fries	Mayonnaise / dips

> *Remember that ALL commercial canola and soybean oils (apart from being genetically modified, which is bad enough) are partially hydrogenated as part of their deodorization process.*
> ~Nora Gedgaudas, author of Primal Body, Primal Mind

Are New Fats Better?

The food industry continues to manipulate fats to replace the now-banned partially hydrogenated oils. However, just because 'new' fats are deemed 'better' doesn't necessarily make them good for human health.

The good news is that the following fats do not contain trans fat. The bad news is they are still unnatural – they remain highly processed and hydrogen atoms are still chemically-manipulated onto the fat chain.

➢ **Fully Hydrogenated Oils** – these are made from industrial PUFA oils so genetic modification, pesticide residues and solvent residues remain concerning

➢ **Stearate or Interesterified Fat** – the manufacturing process utilizes hydrogenation, yet the final product is labeled as *interesterified, stearate* or *stearic-rich fat* instead of hydrogenated

As always, read food labels and avoid these ingredients – they cannot compete with time-honored natural fats.

> **Paleo Advantage:** Artificial trans fats do not exist in nature; it is impossible to consume them when eating whole foods.

> *Nature doesn't make bad fats, factories do!* ~Cate Shanahan, MD, author of Deep Nutrition

How to Avoid Artificial Trans Fat
- ✓ Eliminate processed foods from the diet
- ✓ Make time for home-cooked meals using fresh, whole, unadulterated ingredients
- ✓ Use a natural fat (butter, olive oil, coconut oil, avocado oil or animal fats) instead of PUFA vegetable oils
- ✓ Do not buy any products containing *partially hydrogenated* oil, monoglycerides or diglycerides
- ✓ Avoid industrial seed oils and products cooked in them (beware of prepared foods such as rotisserie chicken, hot bar items and restaurant salad dressing)
- ✓ Request that restaurant foods are prepared in butter or select steamed entrees

Natural Surpasses *Artificial* Every Time

There is one type of naturally-occurring trans fat produced in the gut of some ruminant animals during digestion, most notably cattle. This natural trans fat, conjugated linoleic acid (CLA), has a slightly different configuration than the artificial variety, so the body recognizes it as a healthy nutrient.

CLA offers remarkable benefits and is being studied in the following areas:
- ➢ **Diabetes** – Prevention and improved management of type-2 diabetes. Scientific evidence correlates higher levels of CLA with lower diabetes risk.
- ➢ **Cancer** – Blocks growth and metastatic spread of tumors.
- ➢ **Inflammation Reduction** – Interrupts omega-6 PUFA inflammatory pathways.
- ➢ **Weight-Loss** – Shown to increase lean body mass and reduce fat mass (improved body composition) because it suppresses proliferation of fat cells.
- ➢ **Heart Disease** – Epidemiological studies show CLA is beneficial or neutral regarding heart disease risk.

> **Paleo Advantage:** Artificial trans fat *increases* the risk of heart disease, cancer and obesity. The naturally-occurring trans fat, CLA, *decreases* the risks of those diseases!

CLA is primarily found in fat-rich beef, bison, goat and lamb products such as meats, butter, milk and bone marrow. CLA levels are higher in grass-fed, pastured animal products than conventional grain-fed…just another example that natural diets provide the best nutrients.

> **Beware:** CLA supplements are *not* recommended as they are often derived from PUFA oils. Consequently, CLA supplements have not been effective in clinical trials. Stick with grass-fed, pastured animal products for the best health boost!

Additional Resources:
Cate Shanahan, MD, has extensively researched the adverse effects of vegetable oils as a source of trans fat. She has coordinated the LA Lakers' nutritional program and does many interviews.
- 📖 *Deep Nutrition: Why Your Genes Need Traditional Food,* Catherine Shanahan, MD
- 🖰 DrCate Salad Dressing the Silent Killer
- 🎧 Podcasts (with transcripts)
    - 🎧 FatBurningMan Cate Shanahan: Why Kobe Bryant Drinks Bone Broth
    - 🎧 Bulletproof #376 Vegetable Oil the Silent Killer with Dr. Cate Shanahan

Section V: Cooking Assignment #2 – Mayonnaise

Until recently, all commercial mayonnaise included inflammatory PUFA oils. This meant Paleo mayo-lovers needed to make their own – and it's delicious! For those who are not willing or able to make their own, avocado oil mayo is increasingly easier to find on store shelves…but we highly encourage you to give this a try! Admittedly, the first few times takes some effort (to find a technique and recipe you like), but the process becomes much easier with a little practice and the flavor is worth the effort.

> **Retail Paleo Mayo:** Paleo-friendly mayonnaise available for purchase includes Primal Kitchen® Mayo or Chosen Foods® Avocado Mayonnaise and/or Coconut Mayonnaise.

Choose a Method and Recipe

Mayonnaise is essentially made by blending eggs and a liquid oil to create a thick, creamy sauce. Sometimes the mixture "breaks" when the egg and oil fail to emulsify, meaning they do not combine or thicken (if that happens, directions to fix your mayo are listed below). Our best success has been with a stick / immersion blender or a food processor.

No mayo recipe uses 100% extra virgin olive oil because the result tastes too bitter; however, using *part* extra virgin olive oil has a pleasant taste (if it's less than half of the total oil). Although light olive oil is often an ingredient, it may be chemically-extracted because it's not the first pressing of the oil, so not our first choice.

> **The Best Oil Choices:** avocado oil is tasteless, coconut oil for a slight coconut flavor, organically-refined coconut oil is tasteless, macadamia nut oil is a bit nutty and bacon drippings are, well, yummy! Use any combination of oils (even melted butter – clarified works best). Direct links from ⁀ᵈ Paleovation.
> - Immersion/stick blender: ⁀ᵈ TheHealthyFoodie Fail Proof Home Made Paleo Mayo
> - Hand whisk recipe and general mayo information with video: ⁀ᵈ NomNomPaleo Paleo Mayonnaise
> - Blender version with video: ⁀ᵈ MelJoulwan Homemade Paleo Olive Oil Mayo
> - Food processor version plus dip/sauce recipes: ⁀ᵈ Whole30 The Best Mayo You've Ever Made
> - Flavored and exotic versions: ⁀ᵈ PaleoGrubs 11 Homemade Mayos

Tips for Success

To improve the chances that your mayo works the first time:

Immersion Blender Method:
1. Okay to use the whole egg instead of just the yolk
2. Use a narrow container – a wide mouth canning jar works well, then store mayo in the same jar
3. Put the egg, vinegar and seasoning in the container first; pour oil on top
4. Start with the hand blender pressed to the bottom of the container; once it starts thickening, gently move up and down the mixture until mayo is blended (do not over-blend)

Food Processor, Regular Blender or Hand-Whisking Methods:
1. All ingredients must be room temperature – overnight on the counter is fine. Do NOT rush.
2. SLOWLY add oil once the base ingredients are well incorporated
   a. You cannot go too slowly
   b. Initially add the oil drop by drop until well-incorporated
   c. Eventually drizzle in a slow stream while continuing to blend
   d. If you accidentally have an "oil slick" when the stream becomes more of a pour, stop adding the oil and incorporate the slick into the mixture before resuming the slow stream
3. If you use a regular blender, let the egg and acid sit together for a minute or two before blending
4. High-powered blenders such as VitaMix® can break the mayo due to too much heat (use low speed)
5. Have an extra egg yolk at room temp in case your mayo breaks (to start fresh and re-emulsify)
6. Patience...reread all these tips again, *patience is key*

> **Kelly's Tip:** Admittedly, cooking is not my forte, but I really wanted a healthy mayo. After failing with a couple methods, I found *100% success* using the immersion blender! It's very forgiving (using avocado oil and a whole egg, even cold) and now I can whip up great-tasting healthy mayo in less than a minute.

Pasteurizing Eggs / Yolks (optional)

If using raw eggs or the risk of salmonella poisoning makes you uncomfortable, there are a few options to address those concerns and still get great mayo. Understand that the percentage of eggs containing salmonella is very low, even less in high-quality pasture-raised eggs. Furthermore, mayo recipes always contain an acid (lemon juice, vinegar) which naturally sterilizes the egg. Here's a list of best-practices or alternatives to raw eggs:
1. Buy *pasteurized* eggs (different from *pasture-raised*, these are heat-treated prior to reaching the store)
2. Buy eggs from a local source you trust – small farms have healthier living conditions than factory farms

3. Use just the yolks – salmonella tends to occur in the whites; if still concerned, hold the *yolk* in your hand and rinse it with vinegar to kill any bacteria on its surface
4. Heat or pasteurize eggs or yolks at home using one of the following methods:
   a. Plunge the whole egg in a pot of boiling water for 1 minute. Remove from water, use whole or separate if desired.
   b. Put the yolk in a glass bowl and mix with lemon juice or vinegar. Microwave for 15-20 seconds, stir, repeat once more (it is okay if the mixture rises and thickens, the goal is to keep it semi-liquid; do not let it cook through like scrambled egg).
   c. Add the yolk and lemon juice in a metal/glass bowl and place over boiling water, creating a double boiler. Stir constantly for 1 minute.
5. Use an egg-free mayo recipe (also convenient for the egg-free autoimmune protocol, AIP)
   a. Bacon dripping and coconut milk version (mustard is seed-based and should be omitted for strict AIP): ⚘ DiabeticPaleo AIP Egg-free Bacon Mayo
   b. Coconut butter* & olive oil version: ⚘ AutoimmuneWellness Sweet Potato Fries with Garlic Mayo
      *Coconut butter is sometimes called coconut crème, coconut manna or creamed coconut. Essentially it is dried coconut flakes ground into a paste. Making it in the food processor is more cost-effective than purchasing pre-made (recipe link noted on Day 2): *16oz bag of dried coconut = ~1 cup of coconut butter*

Fixing Broken Mayonnaise

Homemade mayonnaise can "break" if the egg and oil fail to blend. If that happens, here are some options:

1. **Have Another Egg at Room Temperature:** Add a touch of your broken mayonnaise to a room temp egg. Whisk/blend like crazy to get another emulsification going, then SLOWLY add the rest of your broken mixture and finally, drip in the remaining oil.
2. **Make a Mustard Sauce:** Start with 2-3 Tbsp mustard and gently whisk in the broken mixture.
3. **Use It "As Is"** – it's still healthy and yummy. Use as a salad dressing, add to guacamole for creaminess, dip veggies in it or add to a soup for a smooth texture.

Try These Recipes with Your New Mayo!	
✓ Flavored mayo dips (like onion dip)	✓ Tuna / chicken / egg salad
✓ BLT-stuffed lettuce leaves	✓ Mix into ground meats for moist burgers
✓ Creamy guacamole	✓ Ranch salad dressing
✓ Cole slaw	✓ Basting sauce for grilled foods
✓ Deviled eggs	✓ Aioli (garlic-flavored mayo sauce)
✓ Creamy base for soup	✓ Slather on a steak then grill for a crisp crust
✓ Marinate meats before cooking	✓ Mix into sautéed vegetables for a creamy sauce

To-Do List:

☐ The timeline to finish your mayo is by Day 7. Make a plan:
   I'm making my Paleo mayonnaise on _____

☐ As necessary, utilize low-carb flu relief strategies during the next few days.

- In Prep C we talked about new **healthy habits** to incorporate during the program. The first four listed below are basic strategies to complete a month of Strict Paleo Protocol. The 5th habit involves some low-level movement. Are you incorporateing some healthy habits?

   ☐ Fresh cut veggies in the fridge   ☐ Cook with coconut oil or
   ☐ Drink non-sweetened beverages   grass-fed butter/ghee
   ☐ Use veggie slices instead of breads   ☐ Take a walk daily

Coming Up Soon:

At this point, make an effort to include low-level movements each day such as a daily stroll (from the above healthy habits) or yoga, Tai Chi, Qi Gong or other gentle stretching movements. On Day 10 we'll discuss incorporating more movement and activity.

Day 5

Today's Topics:

1. Paleo-Wise: FREE Day
2. Paleo Fat Recap
3. Decoding Animal Product Labels
4. Questions for Your Animal Product Providers
5. Paleo Comfort Foods
6. Low-Carb Flu Check-In (plus Bone Broth Uses)
7. Rest (!!)

Fast Fare - Fancy
♥ Prosciutto wrapped around green apple and olives
♥ Sautéed asparagus spears and butter

My Paleo Meals: Day 5			
Meal	**Veggies**	**Protein**	**Healthy Fats**
Breakfast	Green Yellow/Orange Red Blue/Purple/Black White/Tan		
Lunch	Green Yellow/Orange Red Blue/Purple/Black White/Tan		
Dinner	Green Yellow/Orange Red Blue/Purple/Black White/Tan		
Snack	Green Yellow/Orange Red Blue/Purple/Black White/Tan		

Is this template easier to complete now that you have a few days of practice?   Yes   No

It is common to miss some of your old favorite foods, snacks or meals. Has anything been tempting you?

_____

_____

What are two strategies you use to beat cravings?

1. _____

2. _____

Section I – Paleo-Wise: FREE Day

Today is a day to physically and mentally rest. The fat information covered over the past few days is a lot to absorb, so enjoy a break from the Paleo science. Better yet, we've organized and summarized the primary fat facts into easy-to-scan tables to help you remember which fats to use and which to avoid. We've also purposely lightened other reading today – identifying quality meat products and ideas for Paleo comfort foods.

If you feel motivated, use the extra time today to re-review other Paleo-Wise topics, make your mayonnaise, try a new recipe or…just relax! Some movie and video recommendations are listed at the end of the chapter.

Section II: Paleo Fat Recap

Eliminate the fear that "eating fat makes us fat." Eating *sugar and starch* makes us fat! The following charts summarize healthy fats, tips to store them, which are best for cooking and which are best to avoid. There's an additional copy in the Resource Section (if desired, you can tear it out for quick reference).

As for butter versus margarine, I trust cows more than chemists. ~Joan Gussow, <u>This Organic Life</u>

The Bottom Line on Fats: Incorporate a wide variety of natural fats to replenish nutrients and optimize health. Avoid destructive high omega-6, chemically-manipulated fats.

Paleo-Approved Fats		
Naturally Saturated	**Mono-Unsaturated**	**Polyunsaturated (Omega 3 or 6)**
<ul><li>Coconut and coconut oil</li><li>Palm oil</li><li>Grass-fed Butter</li><li>Pasture-raised animal fats (lard, tallow, duck fat, etc)</li></ul>	<ul><li>Olives and olive oil</li><li>Avocados and avocado oil</li><li>Nuts, especially macadamias, hazelnuts and cashews (followed by almonds, pecans and pistachios)</li></ul>	3- Wild-caught fatty fish 3- Free-range or omega-3 eggs 3- Fish oil supplements 6- CLA found in pasture-raised red meat and dairy products 6- Flax, chia, hemp and walnuts

Healthy Habits for Paleo Fats	
Usage	**Details**
Fats for cooking	Use naturally saturated fats, olive oil or avocado oil
Safest processing	Choose extra virgin, virgin or organic (expeller-pressed is a distant second)
Minimalize oxidation of fragile Paleo-friendly PUFA oils	These oils include walnut oil, flaxseed oil, fish oil ✓ Select oils in dark glass or metal bottles ✓ Refrigerate nut oils and flaxseed oils ✓ Purchase in small amounts and do not store for long periods ✓ Do not heat or cook with these oils
Consume EPA & DHA	Liberally eat sardines, herring, salmon, mackerel, etc; supplement with fish oil*

*Speak to your doctor regarding dosage if you are taking blood thinners or have a bleeding disorder

Unhealthy Products	
Foods to Avoid	**Details**
Industrialized Fats	✓ Read labels to avoid hydrogenated, interesterified, mono/diglycerides ✓ All omega-6 PUFA oils such as canola, soybean, corn, vegetable, safflower, sunflower, cottonseed, etc (the deodorization process creates trans fat) ✓ All processed or restaurant foods where PUFA oils are exposed to heat *Ask for food to be cooked in butter; buy products with safe cooking fats
Avoid processed "low-fat" products	✓ Low-fat often means high sugar/starch ✓ Healthy fats are removed and replaced with sugars, chemicals, emulsifiers, etc

Section III: Decoding Animal Product Labels

Food labels are intended to *clarify* animal product quality – the healthier the animal, the healthier it is to eat. Clarification is a simple concept, but apparently it's not so simple to design exact terminology. Some labeling terms apply to animal living conditions while others describe the animal's diet. Therefore, certain terms will overlap. To add to the confusion, a few labels are non-regulated and some terms are downright deceptive (*).

A. No Label at All

Assume any unlabeled animal product means the animal lived in confined, crowded, unsanitary and stressful conditions. Antibiotics are routinely administered in factory farms to offset the chance of infectious disease. Animal feed is not a natural diet but includes cheap GMO grains/soy, animal byproducts and random fillers.

B. General Terms

1. **Organic** – Animals are fed organic, GMO-free feed (may or may not be tailored to the animal's natural diet). Antibiotics and hormones are not permitted; animal byproducts are not allowed in feed. Living conditions include clean shelter, bedding and water plus outdoor areas for exercise, sunlight and shade. Grazing animals must have access to an organic foraging pasture.
2. **Pasture-Raised*** – Animals spend most of their lives outdoors where they can forage for their own natural diet of grasses, bugs, tubers, etc. This label is loosely regulated by the USDA with no rules for pasture conditions (overcrowding, rotation schedules, green space vs bare dirt). However, if a product is *Certified Humane + Pasture-Raised*, then it indicates animals had plenty of green pasture space.
3. **Non-GMO** – This certification means animal feed does not include genetically-modified crops (which tend to have chemical residues). Any certified 100% organic product is automatically GMO-free.
4. **Certified Humane or Animal Welfare Approved** – These labels are similar in that animals are raised in clean, uncrowded environments with no crates or cages. Hormones and non-therapeutic antibiotics are prohibited. Some animals such as cattle must have access to the outdoors. Slaughter is humane.
5. **No Antibiotics** – Animals are raised without the use of antibiotics; may imply cleaner living conditions.
6. **No Hormones*** – Depends on the animal; it is illegal to administer hormones to pigs or poultry, so a 'No Hormones' label for pork, poultry or eggs means nothing because *all* pork/poultry is hormone-free. Yet, this is good news for cattle since growth hormones such as rBGH are not permitted.
7. **Naturally-Raised*** – Animals are raised without growth-promoters/hormones or unnecessary antibiotics. However, other non-natural techniques such as GMO feed or caged living conditions are not addressed.
8. **Natural*** – This term denotes that a product comes from nature, is 'minimally processed' and does not have artificial colors or preservatives. Under these 'rules,' animals raised in confinement and fed GMO crops with antibiotics and hormones are considered natural (so is high-fructose corn syrup, by the way).
9. **Nitrate-free*** – These products contain naturally-occurring nitrates in beet or celery powders versus man-made sodium nitrate curing salt. However, nitrates are not the issue, animal quality is (more on nitrates on Day 20). Consumers think they're purchasing a high-quality meat, but this label has nothing to do with animal husbandry. Choose pasture-raised and organic products first.

C. Poultry-Specific (Chicken, Turkey, Eggs, Other Birds)

The highest quality eggs have a thick shell and an orange- (or maybe even a deep orange-) colored yolk. Try your local farmer's market – very few local farmers confine poultry the way factory farms do.

1. **Omega-3 Enriched** – Birds are fed a supplement such as flaxseed so their eggs are higher in the EPA & DHA fats that humans need to consume (more on omega-3's on Day 3).
2. **Free-Range*** – Guarantees birds have access to the outdoors, but not that they ever use it.
3. **Cage-Free*** – Birds are raised in confinement but without any cages. Yes, they can move around and spread their wings, but in reality, they are raised in a large barn with thousands of de-beaked chickens.
4. **Vegetarian-Fed*** – Birds are not natural vegetarians – they are supposed to forage for worms, bugs and grubs. This label surfaced after the public learned animal byproducts are often used as fillers. Yes, this feed is higher quality, but unless poultry additionally forage for insects outdoors, it remains non-ideal.

D. Beef-Specific

1. **Grass-Fed** – This only describes the animal feed. Though it implies the animal lived on a pasture, it may only be during summer. Unless a product specifies *100%* grass-fed and grass-*finished*, the animal could be fattened up with grains and soy on a feedlot prior to slaughter (this introduces inflammatory compounds into the meat and fat, essentially nullifying the reason to purchase grass-fed products).
2. **Grass-Finished** – This desirable label describes the animal feed during the final months of life. Most conventional beef products are grain-finished on feed lots to fatten them up prior to slaughter.
3. **Angus*** – The animals exhibit a certain proportion of Angus genetics/characteristics. The meat must have uniformity in marbling and sizing of cuts. No dietary or living standards are regulated.

E. Marine-Specific

Farmed fish and shrimp are typically fed unnatural grain- and soy-based feed laced with antibiotics. Yet at the same time, wild aquatic animals may be overfished. The following sources are healthiest:

1. **Wild** – This means the aquatic animals spent their entire lifespan in the wild.
2. **Wild-Caught** – These animals may have been spawned in a hatchery before being released to the wild.
3. **Monterey Bay Aquarium Seafood Watch** – Makes recommendations for sustainably-caught wild fish.
4. **Marine Stewardship Council** – Ensures sustainability and effective management of certified fisheries.
5. **Farmed*** – Though Paleo-eaters typically condemn farmed animal products, there are a few exceptions in farmed seafood. In general, sedentary shellfish such as oysters, mussels, scallops, etc, are raised on ropes/crates in the ocean, eating their natural diet in their natural environment. Additionally, countries such as Norway, Scotland or Iceland have strict regulations on salmon husbandry, producing a healthy and sustainable farmed salmon. Search your favorites at ⌐ SeafoodWatch Seafood Recommendations.

Further Reading (Direct links from ⌐ Paleovation.

- ⌐ HumaneSociety How to Read Meat and Dairy Labels
- ⌐ CertifiedHumane Free-Range and Pasture-Raised Officially Defined by HFAC
- ⌐ NofaNY USDA Organic Livestock Requirements PDF

Section IV: Questions for Your Animal Product Providers

Unfortunately, as detailed in the above lists, label confusion does occur in the meat world: some "grass-fed" animals are fed grass in a confined facility unless it is summertime; some "pastured" animals are grain-*finished* (which fattens them up right before sale but creates inflammatory consequences).

The only way to really know how an animal is raised is to inquire directly. Farmers and butchers are eager to share information about their product quality and build relationships with customers. Even if you are not face-to-face, humane corporate farms detail husbandry practices on their websites and respond to email inquiries.

Questions for Your Farmer / Butcher / Egg Producer	
Basic Questions	**Ideal answers**
What are the animals fed?	▪ Any matter they naturally forage (plants, insects, nuts, seeds)
Is their diet supplemented with other products or feed?	▪ Perhaps vitamin/mineral supplements (ask about the source) ▪ Poultry: Non-GMO grain and seeds, garden scraps, grit such as fine gravel, clean crushed eggshells ▪ Ruminants (beef, goat, lamb, bison): Dry hay in winter ▪ Pork: Pigs are often fattened up *even* when pasture-raised – practices vary including acorns, sour milk, fermented grain
Where are the animals kept?	▪ On a green pasture with access to an open shelter ▪ Some animals: Access to woodland areas ▪ Poultry: May be in a "tractor" (moveable, protective coop)
Are there implements to support natural behaviors?	▪ Clean dry bedding, shade and sunshine access, no tethers ▪ Poultry: Perches or trees, dust wallows, no de-beaking ▪ Pork: Mud wallows, areas to root

Basic Questions	Ideal answers
Are GMOs present in the feed / field?	▪ No
Is the pasture treated with herbicide, pesticide or synthetic fertilizers?	▪ No
Do animals have clean, fresh water *both* indoors and outdoors?	▪ Yes
Do the animals receive vaccines?	▪ No
Are there antibiotics in the feed?	▪ No
Are they administered antibiotics?	▪ Only when sick, which is rare
May I visit the farm?	▪ When can you be there?

Do not be surprised if the farm does not supply *all* the ideal answers. Even at stellar farms, calves may be vaccinated for fly-borne illness, cattle or bison might receive some non-GMO grain as an incentive to move into a pen, pigs may be fed non-meat table scraps. These practices may be perfectly acceptable to you, but you won't know unless you ask. Use the website ⌁ EatWild to find a local farmer or one who will to ship to your home.

Section V: Paleo Comfort Foods

Because so many others have already completed a Paleo-style elimination, you can benefit from their experiences and ideas, especially Paleo comfort food recipes. All the following recipes have been Paleo-tized and can be found on the internet (some searches require adding the word, 'Paleo'). Additionally, there are Pinterest boards, blog posts and print cookbooks dedicated exclusively to Paleo comfort foods.

    📖 *Paleo Comfort Foods,* by Charles and Julie Mayfield

Which recipes sound good to you right now?

☐ Cauliflower grits	☐ Meatza (Paleo pizza)	☐ Sweet potato pancakes
☐ Meatloaf	☐ Chicken zoodle soup	☐ Cauliflower fried rice
☐ Stuffed peppers	☐ Bacon fat vinaigrette	☐ Cauliflower and leek soup
☐ Shepherd's pie	☐ Mashed faux-tatos	☐ Buffalo chicken egg muffin
☐ Beef stew	☐ Zucchini pasta salad	☐ Creamy butternut squash soup
☐ Paleo chili	☐ Cauliflower risotto	☐ Paleo + [insert your comfort food]

If you are interested, take a moment to look up a recipe and put the ingredients on your next shopping list.

Section VI: Low-Carb Flu Check-In and Bone Broth as a Remedy

Low-carb flu typically manifests around Day 4 or 5, often surprising those individuals who previously followed a 'heart-healthy' whole grain diet. Low-carb flu symptoms are so common that this transition has been described as *a hangover without the alcohol* (though in all truthfulness, it *IS* a hangover from pizza, pasta and pretzels!).

Each low-carb flu experience is unique, yet similar symptoms emerge repeatedly: inability to make a decision, weird donut dreams, easily offended by others' comments, headaches, no patience for traffic, surprised that weaning off the old diet is tough, secretly questioning the intelligence of colleagues (or was that out loud?)!

Mental and physical discomfort during this phase of the Paleo Transition is common and can be devastating to commitment levels. *Don't quit!* We are purposely repeating this information to help you identify emerging symptoms and act to minimize discomfort. This will help you persevere through the transition.

Please take care of yourself and understand low-carb flu is temporary and *will recede* with time. These symptoms may feel like a setback, but it truly is a step forward – a signal that your body is withdrawing from addictive foods, adjusting to the influx of fresh nutrients and finally has a proper chance to heal.

Did you try a low-carb flu relief strategy today?   Yes   No

If so, what did you try and did it help? _____

Low-Carb Flu Symptoms
Are any of these emerging for you?

- ☐ Fuzzy brain
- ☐ Exhausted
- ☐ Cravings galore!
- ☐ No energy
- ☐ Headaches
- ☐ Jitters
- ☐ Dizziness
- ☐ Cold sweats
- ☐ Nauseous

- ☐ Hyperactive
- ☐ Irritable
- ☐ I caught a cold
- ☐ Swollen glands
- ☐ Hungry
- ☐ Angry
- ☐ "Hangry" (hungry & angry)
- ☐ Crazy dreams
- ☐ Grumpy

- ☐ Worried this isn't the right thing for my body
- ☐ Body acne
- ☐ Digestive upset (diarrhea, bloating, cramps, constipation)
- ☐ Achiness
- ☐ Weak muscles
- ☐ Insomnia
- ☐ Symptom-free!!

Utilizing Bone Broth
Broth is *very* therapeutic for low-carb flu symptoms, not to mention healing and nourishing for your body and gut lining. Put your broth to good use by incorporating it all day long! Here are a few suggestions:

- ☐ Drink straight from a mug
- ☐ Stir into guacamole **or dips**
- ☐ Add a little to salad dressings
- ☐ Add to a smoothie
- ☐ Use as a base for sauce like marinara or BBQ
- ☐ In cooking, use as a liquid substitute for water, milk, bouillon or broth

- ☐ Blend into cooked vegetables for a purée – incorporate more to make a creamy soup
- ☐ Make a soup:
  - Egg drop soup
  - Chicken 'zoodle' soup
  - Paleo French onion soup
- ☐ Add a bit when reheating leftovers on the stovetop or microwave
- ☐ Use in scrambled eggs or omelets

Have you used your bone broth already?   Yes   No

What is another way you will incorporate bone broth? _____

Section VI: Rest

If you are not feeling well, please rest...take a nap, take a bath, go to bed early or just lounge on the couch. Health improvements will be appreciated sooner if you slow down now and give yourself a chance to heal. The low-carb flu is just a temporary drawback and this too will pass.

Watch a Food-Oriented Documentary
Since you are in rest mode, consider watching a food-oriented video to learn more about how industrialized food deteriorates health. This information is motivational in the midst of a major diet change. There are quite a few selections available and can be in the form of movies, TED Talks or YouTube videos. Here is just a short list (beware, some of these are B-movies but the information is terrific):

Recommended Food Documentaries			
Movies			**Not-so-Boring Taped Lecture Options**
✺ Food, Inc	✺ Ingredients	✺ Killer at Large	✺ Great Cholesterol Myth (Jonny Bowden)
✺ Fed Up	✺ Carb Loaded	✺ Hungry for Change	✺ Sugar the Bitter Truth (Robert Lustig)
✺ Fat Head	✺ King Corn	✺ Cereal Killers	✺ The Oiling of America (Sally Fallon)
✺ Origins*	✺ Food Fight	✺ That Sugar Film	✺ Minding your Mitochondria (Terry Wahls)

*Directed by Mark van Wijk

To-Do List:
- ☐ Make Paleo Mayo by Day 7
- ☐ Optional Cooking Assignment: Locate a Paleo Comfort Food recipe and prepare by Day 10

Coming Up Soon:
- ➢ Tomorrow: Proteins, budgeting quality sources and Paleo substitutes for western foods and ingredients

Day 6

Today's Topics:

1. Assess Your Need for Rest
2. Paleo-Wise: Protein
3. Budgeting and Locating Quality Protein Sources
4. Substitutes for Non-Paleo Foods

Fast Fare – On the Grill
♥ Purchased meat and veggie kebab
♥ Grilled veggie packet (salad bar veggies and grass-fed butter)

How are you eating today? Meals will be recorded with this chart through tomorrow. If you feel you've already had enough practice, skip the chart and proceed to the next section.

My Paleo Meals: Day 6			
Meal	**Veggies**	**Protein**	**Healthy Fats**
Breakfast	Green Yellow/Orange Red Blue/Purple/Black White/Tan		
Lunch	Green Yellow/Orange Red Blue/Purple/Black White/Tan		
Dinner	Green Yellow/Orange Red Blue/Purple/Black White/Tan		
Snack	Green Yellow/Orange Red Blue/Purple/Black White/Tan		

What is your favorite Paleo food you've tried so far? _____

Is it easier to incorporate vegetables every meal?   Yes   No

Is it easier to include quality fats in every meal?   Yes   No

What is working best for you?

_____

_____

Keep these tactics in mind to build upon your success.

Section I: Assess Your Need for Rest

Yesterday we mentioned that rest is an important part of the transition to a Paleo Diet. Literally, the body digests while at rest! How do you know if you need more rest? It cycles back to the symptoms of low-carb flu:

- ☐ Brain fog
- ☐ Confusion
- ☐ Nausea
- ☐ Dizziness
- ☐ Headaches
- ☐ Flu-like symptoms

- ☐ Increased allergies
- ☐ Achiness
- ☐ Low energy
- ☐ Clumsiness
- ☐ Irritable
- ☐ Swollen glands

- ☐ Tired
- ☐ Withdrawr
- ☐ Cravings
- ☐ Drowsiness
- ☐ Digestive troubles
- ☐ Something feels "off"

What other symptoms are you noticing in your body?

_____

What can you do to provide your body the rest it needs so your hormonal signaling can normalize?

- ☐ Hot bath
- ☐ Try low-carb flu relief strategies
- ☐ Try some gentle exercise
- ☐ Avoid strenuous exercise*
- ☐ Use a premade freezer meal
- ☐ Hire childcare for a day or two
- ☐ Take a nap

- ☐ Set an earlier bedtime
- ☐ Sleep in
- ☐ Take a walk (out in nature if possible)
- ☐ Eat when hungry (Paleo, of course!)
- ☐ Deep breathing
- ☐ Read a book
- ☐ Put up your feet and relax

List any other ideas:

_____

*Don't worry about a temporary break from exercise. Resting now will accelerate healing and hormonal regulation. The good news: your energy will return soon, often higher than before, allowing *increased* exercise capacity, if that's a goal.

Section II – Paleo-Wise: Protein

> *Our genetic makeup is still that of a Paleolithic hunter-gatherer, a species whose nutritional requirements are optimally adapted to wild meats, fruits and vegetables, not to cereal grains.*
> ~Loren Cordain, PhD, author of <u>The Paleo Diet</u>

Proteins – Essential Building Blocks

Proteins are the primary building blocks of all bodily tissue. In fact, the only other substance more plentiful in the body is water. If water weight is excluded, 75 percent of body weight consists of protein. Each protein is constructed from long chains of amino acids, ranging anywhere from 50 to 2,000 linked together! These chains twist and fold into complex 3D structures creating unique shapes, sizes and distinct characteristics.

Surplus protein is not stored like carbohydrate and fat. Therefore, it's *essential* to attain it regularly in the diet. If it's not available, the body will harvest missing amino acids from the breakdown of *vital* body tissues.

Essential Amino Acids

There are 20 unique amino acids that are used to build protein structures and the human body has the capability to internally manufacture about half of them. However, there are 9 amino acids that the body cannot make and, therefore, are classified as *essential* because they must be attained by dietary consumption.

> **Key Point:** There are ESSENTIAL amino acids and ESSENTIAL fatty acids, but *NO* essential carbohydrates!

Additionally, there are a handful of *conditional* amino acids which are typically made by the body, but become essential when the body is under increased stress, such as sickness, pregnancy or even eating an inflammatory diet (more about Stress and Cortisol on Days 11 and 12).

Role of Protein
The human body is made of more than 50,000 different proteins!

Structural Proteins	Functional Proteins
• Skin • Hair • Nails • Muscles • Tendons • Ligaments • Bone • Organs • Blood vessels	• ***Enzymes*** – catalysts in 4000 body reactions such as digestion • ***Neurotransmitters*** – nerve cell signaling throughout body, necessary for body function, mobility and mood stabilization • ***Antibodies*** – essential to immune function • ***Hormones*** - influencing growth, blood sugar regulation, stress management, water/fluid balance • ***Nutrient Transportation*** – LDL and HDL (lipo*proteins*) deliver fat, cholesterol, hemoglobin (for oxygen) • ***Provisional Energy*** –protein can be converted to glucose as an emergency energy supply, but is not storable • ***Satiety*** – gives a full feeling, helps prevent over-eating

Protein Deficiency

If one amino acid is deficient, then all proteins requiring that building block will be compromised. In other words, even with sufficient *total* protein intake, if the diet lacks amino acid variety, deficiency symptoms are still possible because countless required proteins cannot be properly synthesized.

It is critical to regularly consume all amino acids in sufficient proportions. This is the reason collagen protein in bone broth is so beneficial – it provides specific amino acids in sufficient supply that are not abundant in more popular muscle meats. Symptoms of protein deficiency includes:

- Lower energy levels
- Thin or fragile hair and nails
- Lower immune function
- Slow wound healing
- Weak muscles

- Weak connective tissues
- Dull skin
- Impaired digestion
- Hormonal imbalance
- Compromised brain function

- Edema/swelling
- Anemia from B12 deficiencies (B12 is found *exclusively* in animal sources and must be supplemented in a vegan diet)

Animal Protein versus Plant Protein

Though protein is available in both animal and plant sources, animal proteins have specific advantages:

1. **Concentrated** – Animal proteins have a high percentage of amino acids per serving
2. **Complete** – Animal proteins contain *all* 9 essential amino acids, though in varying proportions

The problem with trying to meet protein needs with vegan sources of protein lies in the incomplete amino acid profile and the high starch content of nearly all vegan-source protein-containing foods. ~Nora Gedgaudas

Examine the following table. When compared to animal proteins, plant-based proteins such as grains or legumes require more energy to process for a less desirable outcome, plus they add to the carb and calorie load.

Animal versus Plant Protein		
Trait	**Animal Protein**	**Plant Protein**
Anti-Nutrient and Toxin Levels	No anti-nutrients or toxins	Anti-nutrients and plant toxins interfere with digestion and absorption. In some cases, such as gluten, the plant protein *is* the toxin.
Amino Acid Profile	**Complete protein** – virtually any kind of animal product (meat, fish, eggs) *contains all 9 essential amino acids.*	**Incomplete protein** – some essential amino acids are in low percentages or completely missing. Various plants must be combined to attain full amino acid profile.
Bone Mineral Density	Associated with higher mineral density for strong bones	Associated with lower bone mineral density (osteopenia, osteoporosis)

Trait	Animal Protein	Plant Protein
Digestibility and Absorbability	Easier to digest; high bioavailability	More difficult to digest and energy consuming to break down. May absorb as little as 50% of protein consumed.
Protein Efficiency	Efficient source of protein; less calories consumed for adequate amino acid nutrition.	Plant proteins such as beans, tofu and grains significantly increase calorie and carbohydrate consumption to obtain adequate protein supply.

Animal Gratitude: A Long-Standing Tradition

Some individuals struggle with the idea of consuming animal products. However, the reality is that humans *are* omnivores and meat *is* an intrinsic part of our diet. Indigenous cultures always express gratitude to the animals providing their nourishment. The least we can do is treat our animals with dignity and respect – honor the sacrifice of our animal products: buy local; find a farmer or butcher you trust; purchase animal products from reputable humane farming operations. It is worth the few dollars more and the nutritive quality is superior, too!

The measure of a society can be how well its people treat its animals. ~Mohandas Gandhi

Commercially-Raised Animals (CAFOs)

The Paleo diet emphasizes protein products from animals raised naturally. The quality of the protein depends on what the animal is fed and how it is raised, famously stated by Michael Pollan: *"You are what you eat, eats."*

Factory farms, called CAFOs (Concentrated Animal Feeding Operations), are profit driven so they use the cheapest feed available to fatten up their animals. The health of the animal is an afterthought. Commercial meats, fish, seafood, poultry and eggs from CAFOs are typically contaminated with pesticide residues, antibiotics and hormones. This significantly compromises nutritional quality. Some of this information overlaps with yesterday's discussion on interpreting animal product labels.

Some Problems with CAFO* Products:

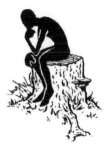

- **Inflammatory Diet:** Feed primarily consists of grains and soy
- **Questionable Feed Fillers:**
    - **Arsenic** is supplemented in pork and poultry
    - **Candy (and other stale human foods)** are fed to cattle and pigs, sometimes *still in the wrappers* (sugar fattens them up plus "fiber" is provided by the plastic wrapper!): hard candy, trail mix, licorice, chocolate bars, french fries, cheese curls, tater tots, peanuts, chocolate chips, cookies, gummy worms, marshmallows, breakfast cereals, orange peels, dried cranberries, etc
        - Ecolonomics Three Surprising Things Cows Are Fed
    - **Sawdust** soaked in nitric acid to help break down the indigestible fiber
    - **Chicken Poop** mixed with feathers, bacteria, antibiotics, even rodent residues
    - **Seafood Byproducts** (guts, scales, heads) most factory-farmed animals do not naturally eat fish
    - **Remnants** from human food production such as orange rinds, almond hulls
- **Synthetic Vitamins:** Less bioavailable and abundant than naturally-occurring vitamins and minerals
- **Agricultural Residues:** Pesticides, herbicides and/or fungicides
- **Unsanitary Living Conditions:** Overcrowding, lack of fresh bedding, poor air quality, questionable practices involving manure disposal and water usage
- **Stressful Conditions:** Cages, crates, tethers, no outdoor access, cannot engage in natural behaviors
- **Antibiotics and, depending on the animal, Hormones or Growth Promoters**

*This information is provided to educate about the broken system of animal husbandry, not to make anyone feel bad about incorporating CAFO products in their diets. Vote with your food dollars by purchasing high-quality animal products when you are able; over time, farms will modify husbandry practices to satisfy demand.

Food is the bedrock of health. Our food choices can either lead to disease or create health and vitality.
~Terry Wahls, MD, author of The Wahls Protocol, Minding My Mitochondria

---

Nutritional Compromise from CAFO Animal Products

✓ High in inflammatory omega-6 fat
✓ Low in anti-inflammatory omega-3 fat (grass-fed beef contains up to 5 times more omega-3 and twice the CLA)
✓ Fat contains residues from antibiotics, steroids, hormones and agricultural chemicals
✓ Low vitamin K2 due to limited access to green foods and sunshine (read about K2 on Days 7 and 16)
✓ Lower vitamin and mineral content due to incomplete and unnatural diets
  o Pasture-raised chicken eggs have more omega-3s and beta carotene than vegetarian-fed
  o Grass-fed beef contains more beta-carotene, vitamin E, iron, potassium, phosphorus and zinc

---

Healthiest Animal Protein Sources:

➢ ***Wild-Caught* Fish/Seafood**: Aquatic animals are able to eat their natural marine diet and live in their natural environment (<u>tip</u>: red or sockeye salmon is always wild caught).

➢ ***Grass-Fed* Beef, Bison, Lamb and Goat**: Anti-inflammatory omega-3s in beef from grass-fed cattle are 7% of the total fat content, compared to just 1% in grain-fed/finished beef (the animal's diet in the last few weeks is extremely important – for full benefit, the animal must be grass-fed *and grass-finished*).

➢ ***Pastured* Poultry/Eggs**: Products from birds that roam freely on a pasture contain more diverse nutrients because they forage for their natural diet including insects, worms, seeds, green plants and grains.

➢ ***Pastured* Pork:** products from pigs raised free to roam in fields and woods, rooting and digging for their natural diet; fat content is higher in anti-inflammatory omega-3's.

➢ **Organ Meats**: liver, heart, tongue, kidney, glands, etc. Evidence suggests organ meats from any animal (even CAFO-raised) are nutrient-dense food sources (more on Organ Meats on Day 23).

➢ **Bone Broth**: Less abundant amino acids such as proline and glycine are found in high concentrations in connective tissues and therefore, bone broth. Drink that broth (or eat that gristle).

Further Reading: ⏺ PaleoLeap Not just the Cows: Pastured Pork and Poultry

No Such Thing as Low-Fat Paleo

Due to decades of anti-fat advertising, many people remain diligent with a low-fat approach when starting Paleo. A "low-fat Paleo" template would restrict both carbohydrates *and* fats, leaving protein as the primary food source. High protein alone does not make a healthy diet and is not sustainable. Fear of fat must be released!

Paleo is Quality Protein, not High Protein

The teeter-totter graphic to the right compares macro-nutrients of three diet options. Note the primary shift is between fat and carb proportions while protein amounts remain virtually identical.

> **Key Point:** Paleo is not a high protein diet. It's a *quality* protein, higher fat and higher veggie diet!

Sometimes eating Paleo may *appear* to be higher in protein simply because buns, pasta or rice are missing. Fill that void with additional vegetables and quality fats, not extra-large protein servings.

> *The quality and digestibility of the protein source are key and ultimately matter more than quantity.*
> ~Nora Gedgaudas, Primal Fat Burner

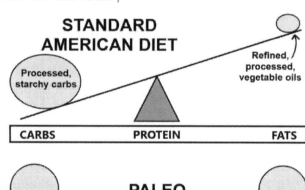

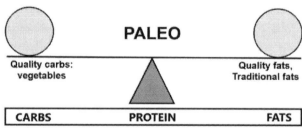

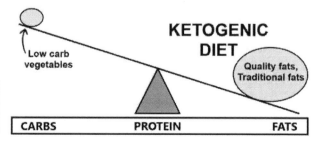

How Much Protein?

A healthy diet clearly includes protein, yet there is major confusion regarding exactly how much is ideal for optimal health. Protein requirements are impacted by age, sex, size, individual genetics, activity levels, physique goals and health status; they will also vary day to day and over time. Unless aiming for peak competitive athletic performance or trying to build *a lot* of muscle, most people do not need to track daily protein intake.

By following our suggestions of incorporating animal protein with vegetables and healthy fats at every meal, protein intake should naturally range between 50-150g/day. Follow an intuitive style of eating and adjust protein intake according to your body's desire and response (review table listing protein deficiency symptoms).

Those Who Benefit from *More* Protein:

- *Athletes/Active Individuals:* More protein can aid muscle building, strength development and major endurance training (marathons and triathlons). Indicators to increase protein include:
  - ✓ Decline of strength or muscle mass (instead of fat) during a weight loss period
  - ✓ Not recovering well from workouts
- *Elderly*: Protein helps maintain strong bones by minimizing mineral loss
- *Dieters*: Higher protein preserves muscle during weight loss and is satisfying (suppresses appetite)
- *Injured*: Rebuilding lost or damaged tissue increases protein requirements

There is no definitive magical number for protein intake; most guidelines include a range plus some qualifiers. Do not obsess over the numbers listed below – they are merely a benchmark to consider.

Benchmark Guidelines for Daily Protein Requirements			
	Sedentary Lifestyle		Active – Highly Athletic Lifestyle
Weight (lbs)	RDA* (*minimum for survival*): 0.36g/lb	Elderly: 0.5-0.6g/lb	Recovering from Injury: 0.7g/lb	Active or Highly Athletic: 0.8-1.4g/lb (Muscle building & intense endurance training are at the higher limits)
125	45g	70g	90g	100 - 175g
150	55g	85g	105g	120 - 210g
175	65g	95g	120g	140 - 245g
200	75g	110g	140g	160 - 280g
225	80g	125g	160g	180 - 315g
250	90g	140g	175g	200 - 350g

*May be lower than *optimal* levels – the RDA only represents basic survival needs

Further Reading:

- ⌐ MarksDailyApple How Much Protein Should You Be Eating?
- ⌐ MarksDailyApple How Much Protein Can You Absorb and Use from One Meal?

Protein Digestion

Strong stomach acids begin the digestion process by 'unwinding' the amino acid chains. Enzymes further break apart protein in both the stomach and the intestine. Several factors influence protein digestion: how well the food is chewed, the acidity of the stomach, the amount and type of protein in the food as well as the quality and quantity of enzymes. If you suffer from digestive distress with protein consumption, trust that this process will improve with gut healing the longer that Paleo is implemented (Digestive Aids are discussed on Day 8).

Critical Components to Protein Digestion:

- ➤ **Extra Water** – If you opt to increase protein intake, be sure to increase fluid intake.
- ➤ **Adequate Dietary Fat** – Protein and fats naturally occur together for a reason in eggs, fish and meats.
- ➤ **Quality Salt** – Adequate amounts of chloride are necessary to produce hydrochloric acid in the stomach and salt (sodium chloride) is the only dietary source. With salt restriction, stomach indigestion occurs from protein stagnation. Seek quality salt with trace minerals: Celtic sea salt, Himalayan salt or Real salt.

Excess Protein Can Convert to Glucose

The body uses available amino acids from any given meal to build protein chains, then incorporates those proteins into necessary structures. Remember, excess protein is not stored. When more protein is consumed than can be used, the liver can convert it to glucose. This is useful to replenish glycogen stores, but there is a risk that this protein-generated glucose can cause an insulin response. However, just because this *can* happen doesn't mean it *will*. For most non-diabetic individuals, the insulin-generating effect of excess protein is not a major concern since glucose is generated 'lower (quantity) and slower' than from carbohydrates.

At the extreme, excess protein consumption can be a very real concern for those with hormonal imbalances or other health complications. Generally, most individuals can process 25-35 grams of protein in one sitting. Recording blood glucose levels is the only way to know if your individual body tends to manufacture glucose after eating large amounts of protein. If you have concerns, keep protein around 25g or less per sitting.

> **Caution**: Excess protein can convert to glucose. Those with diabetes, pre-diabetes, syndrome-X or other compromised hormonal conditions should be particularly mindful not to over-consume protein at one sitting.

A Few Words Regarding Protein Powders

Protein powders technically are not Paleo because they are highly processed. Additionally, most protein powders are whey-based and whey is a component of dairy, which is also not Paleo. However, in special cases (certain athletes, individuals without the ability to chew, individuals needing to consume extra calories), protein powders can be an acceptable and beneficial supplement. As always, source matters.

Problems with Commercial Powders:

1. Protein exists in isolation (without fat to help metabolize it)
2. Heavily processed (in the form of protein concentrate or isolate); likely damaged
3. Loaded with chemicals, artificial sweeteners and flavorings, powdered creamer (trans fat) and MSG

Best Paleo-Friendly Protein Powders:

- ➤ **Gelatin/Collagen** – Preferred from pastured animals, but even lower quality brands are acceptable
- ➤ **Cricket** – Includes the entire insect; high in minerals and fiber
- ➤ **Egg** – Generally made from whites only
- ➤ **Hemp** or **Pumpkin** – Only ingredient should be hemp seeds or pumpkin seeds
- ➤ **Bone Broth** – powdered (or homemade), an easily-digested and quickly-absorbed protein option
- ➤ Though not Paleo, whey from grass-fed or pastured cows is ok if tolerated (preferable to defer the addition of whey until food reintroductions at the end of the program – for now, try collagen instead)

Gelatin/Collagen in the Diet

Collagen is the most abundant protein found in the body – gelatin is simply the cooked form of collagen. Both are great sources of amino acids, offer superb healing for the gut (as in bone broth), support healthy skin, nails, hair and cell structure, and are a great way to replace protein powders.

There are many high-quality brands including Great Lakes, Vital Proteins and products marketed on Paleo websites. Select the unflavored products and consider a hydrolyzed product which dissolves in hot *or* cold liquid. Here are a few ideas for incorporating gelatin into your diet, including unsweetened gummy snacks (after the program you can research gummy snacks sweetened with fruit juice or honey):

- ᐟᕒ OhLardy Easily Add Gelatin to your Coffee or Tea
- ᐟᕒ PrimallyInspired Gelatin! Health Benefits and 6 Ways to Use Gelatin
- ᐟᕒ PrimallyInspired Protein Workout Recovery Shake Using Gelatin
- ᐟᕒ PrimalPalate Gut Healing Gummy Snacks

> **Gelatin on a Budget:** Grass-fed and antibiotic-free is preferred over conventional, but even CAFO-derived gelatin is very healing for the body – the primary problem with CAFO animals is fat compromise, but gelatin is protein, so it's not as much of a concern. Do not let budget restrictions prevent from adding gelatin.

Meat Myth 1: Red Meat Is Unhealthy

Evidence indicates that red meat is one of the healthiest, most nutritious food choices with highly bioavailable vitamins and minerals. So how did red meat get such a bad name? The primary targets of the attack on red meat are its saturated fat and cholesterol content (those topics are detailed on Days 2 and 17).

> *Red meat is not bad for you. Now blue-green meat, that's bad for you!* ~Tommy Smothers

How Anti-Meat Studies Define "Red Meat"

Genuine red meat includes cuts of beef, buffalo, deer, antelope, goat, lamb, bison, etc. However, the studies that attack red meat define it very differently and can include the following:

- Hamburgers (on buns made of refined white flour) with sides of soda, chips/fries made with inflammatory omega-6 vegetable oils
- Pizza with carbohydrate-laden crust plus processed dairy and meat toppings
- Processed or cured CAFO meats such as ham, bacon, sausage, hot dogs, cold cuts, pickle loaf
- Prepared food (with unknown additives and preservatives) such as fast food or frozen entrees

It is highly probable that reported increases in health problems from that kind of "red meat" are caused by the additional carbs and chemicals surrounding it...and not by the meat itself!

Nutritional Advantages of 100% Grass-Fed *and Finished* Beef	
Vitamin B12	A rich source of vitamin B12 which is not found in plants; B12 is vital to total body functioning, prevents anemia and is essential for protein digestion.
Vitamin D	The form in meat is uniquely absorbable and bioavailable.
Other Vitamins	Especially beta carotene (precursor to vitamin A), vitamin E, B-complex and K2
Iron	The form in red meat is absorbed and utilized more efficiently than that found in plant foods. Those with iron deficiency anemia benefit from red meat consumption. However, *those with iron overload conditions like hereditary hemochromatosis should limit all meat consumption*.
Minerals, including Trace Minerals	Zinc (more bioavailable), magnesium, copper, cobalt, phosphorus, chromium, nickel, selenium (antioxidant), potassium (blood pressure regulation), calcium
Fat Content	Naturally leaner than commercial beef; the fat present is high quality
EPA and DHA	High percentage of *anti*-inflammatory omega-3's
CLA	This naturally-occurring fat reduces cancer risk, obesity, diabetes and immune disorders and is found in the fat of wild game and fully pastured animals.

Meat Myth 2: Processed Meats Cause Cancer

The October 2015 'WHO Report' claimed processed meats are as cancer-causing as cigarettes! However, it is apparent that the fine print was overlooked:

1. These findings were based on observational studies where participants reported what they ate based on their memory.
2. There were no control groups.
3. We do not know if the participants had other cancer-causing habits: excessive alcohol consumption, smoking status, lack of exercise, uncontrolled stress response, etc.
4. The studies lumped low-quality CAFO full-of-fillers-meat-in-a-can with quality homemade grass-fed beef sausage or pastured-pork bacon.
5. The document specified only colorectal cancers, not all cancers. The reported 18% increased risk of colon cancer translates to a relative risk of 50/100,000 chance, still rather unlikely.

Paleo Diet: Cancer Protective
- Emphasis on abundant multi-colored vegetables for vitamins, minerals, antioxidants, chlorophyll, fiber and other components to offset carcinogens from *any* source
- Toxic residues are avoided by consuming high-quality animal products or only lean CAFO products
- Awareness/avoidance of fillers and added chemicals in food
- Emphasis on a wide variety of proteins including fish, seafood, beef, shellfish, pork, poultry, wild game, eggs and organ meats

Beware: Despite the noted discrepancies, actual links between red meat, processed meat and cancer do exist *in meats that are charred* or *cooked at extreme temperatures*. Avoid burned or overdone proteins and be sure to eat your veggies!

Further Reading: ThePaleoMom The Link Between Meat and Cancer

Meat Myth 3: Meat Rots in the Colon

Remember that protein is a 3D structure made from a long chain of connected amino acids. Our bodies are designed to efficiently disentangle these chains (by stomach acids) and break them into their smaller components (by enzymes)...long before any meat makes it to the colon!

How and Where Protein Is Digested:

1. **Stomach**: Acids unravel/denature the long protein chains. Nothing *rots* in a vat of highly acidic hydrochloric acid and pepsin!

   > **Concerns about Antacids:** Digestive problems such as GERD and heartburn often occur when there is *not enough acid.* Without an acidic environment, proteins cannot sufficiently break down or pass into the intestine so they putrify in the stomach. The popular medical treatment of reducing stomach acid (antacids) further perpetuates that problem (see Day 8 for info on Healthy Bowels and Digestive Aids).

2. **Small Intestine:** Enzymes efficiently break down protein chains into smaller amino acid pieces that can easily be metabolized. These amino acids are absorbed in the small intestine prior to entering the colon. Bile salts and enzymes break down any accompanying fats.

3. **Large Intestine / Colon:** In healthy individuals, no protein enters the colon because it has all been absorbed in the small intestine. Gut bacteria digest some of the remaining fat. Fats like cholesterol are reabsorbed and excess fat is eliminated in stool.

   > **Think about it:** Our bodies rely on obtaining protein from food sources (it's classified as *essential*). Protein will not be left intact all the way to the large intestine where it can be counter-productive.

Meat Myth 4: Protein Injures Kidneys

'Excess' protein is the amount left over *after* the body incorporates it into body structures and *after* glycogen stores have been replenished. Increasing consumption of higher-quality protein with Paleo is not the same as excess. Even if eating Paleo slightly increases your protein intake, the body adapts*:

1. **Kidney Function Adjusts:** The kidneys become more active which is a normal adaptive response to additional protein in the diet. This is not a pathological condition but is similar to the increased adaptive kidney activity during pregnancy or after someone has donated a kidney.

2. **Kidneys are Not Damaged:** Protein does not damage kidneys in healthy individuals. If that were true, kidney donors would be advised to reduce protein. Though please note, high-protein diets *can* be harmful for those with existing chronic kidney disease (CKD)*.

   > *Unhealthy kidneys lose the ability to remove protein waste and it builds up in the blood. Protein intake for patients with CKD is medically determined by the stage of kidney disease, nutrition status and body size.

Meat Myth 5: Eating Meat Makes You Fat (The Truth: Eating Protein *Supports* Weight Loss!)

This claim stems from two other myths: 'eating fat makes you fat' and 'saturated fat and cholesterol are unhealthy,' neither of which apply to quality protein sources. In fact, sufficient protein *improves* weight loss:

1. **Highest Satiety** - Protein has a much greater satiety value than either fat or carbohydrate and suppresses appetite.

2. **Metabolism Boost** – Protein has 2-3 times the thermic effect of either fat or carbohydrate, meaning that it stimulates metabolism and speeds weight loss. When daily protein comprises 25-30% of total calories, metabolism can be boosted up to 100 calories per day when compared to low protein intake.

3. **Fulfills Protein Requirements** – Because protein is essential, humans have a natural strong appetite for it. If protein is insufficient, people eat more food until protein intake is achieved, then appetite subsides.

4. **Long-Term Success** – Numerous clinical trials have shown high-protein / low-carb diets are more effective than low-fat / high-carb diets for *losing weight* and *keeping it off*.

Meat Myth 6: Eating Meat Triggers Gout

Gout is a painful arthritic condition often called a 'rich man's disease' because they can afford more expensive meats, sugars and alcohol. For most gout sufferers, the primary conditions that lead to gout are inflammation and fructose consumption (more on Fructose on Day 22). Eating a Paleo Diet greatly reduces both these factors.

Paleo Diet Reduces Chance of Gout	
Factors that Lead to Gout	**Paleo Advantage**
Inflammation from Too Many Omega-6 Oils	Better omega-6 and omega-3 ratios: ✓ No crop oils (high in omega-6) ✓ Emphasis on grass-fed and wild-caught meats (higher in omega-3 than farmed versions) ✓ More likely to eat small fatty fish or take an EPA/DHA supplement like fish oil
Inflammation from Too Much Sugar	Significantly lower sugar intake: Avoids glucose from grains, legumes, high-sugar fruits and added sugars
High Fructose Consumption	✓ Reserves fruit as a treat, prefers low-fructose varieties such as berries or citrus ✓ Avoids high fructose corn syrup and agave nectar
Genetic Predisposition	Better body awareness to determine personal triggers

Limit Bouts of Gout:

Predisposed individuals should focus on reducing fructose consumption, maintaining hydration levels, rebalancing the omega-6: omega-3 ratio and limiting/avoiding personal gout triggers (which range from shellfish to red meat to raw spinach to gluten). Unfortunately, there is no pattern to specific triggers – they need to be identified at an individual level. This Paleo Elimination Diet is an excellent method to do so.

Section III: Budgeting and Locating Quality Protein Sources

We've discussed the importance of selecting quality grass-fed and wild-caught animal products, but they are generally higher priced and for some, it's not financially feasible. For those choosing to purchase commercially-raised animal products, they *can* still be healthy! If budget is a concern, carefully-selected factory-farmed products can fulfill your dietary needs...and they are still way more nutritious than grains!

There are two main approaches to maximize nutrition from meats while adhering to your budget:

1. **Purchase Pastured Products at Better Prices**
    a. Buy in bulk (1/4 steer) or on sale (near expiration date) to stock your freezer
    b. Purchase whole chickens/fish versus prepared cuts like breasts, thighs or filets
    c. Opt for roasts versus hand cut steaks
    d. Try less desirable cuts such as heart, tongue or liver
    e. Select ground products with higher fat content (they are cheaper and this fat is healthy)
    f. Use the website ⌐🖑 EatWild to find a farmer near you or one that ships products to your home
2. **Seek CAFO Products with the Highest Nutritional Benefit and Least Inflammatory Risk**
    a. Choose nutrient-dense cuts – organ meats are nutritional powerhouses regardless of source*
    b. Choose lean cuts – fat from factory-farmed animals is highly inflammatory
    c. Select cuts with the highest omega-3 and lowest omega-6 fat
        i. Fish and ruminants (beef, lamb, bison or goat) are best
        ii. Pork is a distant second choice
        iii. Poultry (chicken, turkey) is very high in omega-6 fat; if poultry is a staple in your diet, supplement with omega-3 fish oil (EPA & DHA) or increase wild-caught fish consumption

Further Reading: The Paleo community abounds with suggestions for budgeting meat purchases:
- 🖑 ThePaleoMom If I Can't Always Afford Grass-Fed
- 🖑 ThePaleoMom A Paleo Budget: Priorities and Strategies
- 📖 *The Frugal Paleo Cookbook,* by Ciarra Hannah

> ***Loving Liver:** The liver is essential for purifying the blood and metabolizing toxins. It houses all the nutrients necessary to support these processes, making liver extremely nutritious. Fortunately, the toxins do not remain in the liver – they are shunted to fat cells for storage...part of the reason why fat from CAFOs is inflammatory.

Section IV: Substitutes for Non-Paleo Foods

The following Paleo-friendly substitutions extinguish inflammation created from poor food choices. Many will need to be made at home – abundant recipes online. Do not be surprised if some substitutions fail to satisfy like their commercial counterparts (which are often engineered with sugar or additives to induce cravings). Certain Paleo substitutions have a more palatable taste (such as coconut milk in a cream soup) while others don't, but are just a healthier choice (like kale chips versus potato chips).

Paleo Substitutions for Westernized Ingredients/Foods*	
Butter	✓ Grass-fed butter ✓ Clarified, purified or drawn butter; ghee ✓ Coconut oil – excellent for cooking, frying and baking
Canola and Other Industrial Oils	✓ Grass-fed butter, clarified butter/ghee ✓ Coconut, avocado or olive oils (avocado oil has neutral flavor) ✓ Pastured animal fats
Cream **Milk**	✓ Full fat canned coconut milk is very creamy and a great addition to casseroles (like green bean), curry dishes, omelets or cream of [*insert vegetable*] soup ✓ Other nut milks such as almond, cashew or hazelnut – these are thinner than canned coconut and are excellent milk substitutes for cooking and in smoothies
Cheese	✓ Homemade cashew, macadamia nut, almond milk or zucchini cheeses ✓ Nutritional yeast flakes have a "cheesy" type flavor ✓ Vegan parmesan-style seasoning: Gopal's Rawmesan® or Parma!® ✓ Paleo-friendly cheeses and sauces are found online or in health food stores. Carefully read ingredients to avoid PUFA oils, soy, grains, etc. The following brands have at least one option (though not their entire line of products): • Kite Hill® Soft Fresh Original, Beyond Better® Original Cashew Sauce, Julian Bakery®, Treeline®, Follow Your Heart® select blocks and slices
Tortillas **Bread** **Sandwiches** **Toast**	✓ Wraps from lettuce leaves, lunchmeat or purchased coconut wraps ✓ Red pepper halves, cucumber boat, roasted portabella caps, jicama slices, wedge of iceberg or cabbage, etc ✓ Paleo vegetable latkes (Cooking Assignment #3 on Day 7) ✓ Turn your sandwich into a salad by putting the filling over salad greens ✓ Homemade almond meal bread ✓ Try these satisfying flatbread recipes: ⌁ PurelyTwins The Best Grain-free Paleo Bread Recipe • For an egg-free AIP version: omit eggs and replace with 1/2 Tbsp coconut flour, 3/8 tsp baking soda, 1/8 tsp cream of tartar, 1 Tbsp melted coconut oil, 5 Tbsp full fat coconut milk and pinch of salt ⌁ SlimPalate Cauliflower Tortillas
Pancakes	⌁ BalancedBites Paleo Pumpkin Pancakes from Practical Paleo ✓ Fried plantains: ⌁ StupidEasyPaleo Fried Plantains with Cinnamon
Cereals	✓ Nut/seed granola with coconut or nut milk ✓ Almond meal porridge ✓ Paleo pumpkin pudding ✓ Faux-meal ✓ Other items like fruit and nut butter smoothies, eggs, salad, soup or leftovers

Western Food	Paleo Substitute
Chips **Crackers** **Popcorn**	✓ Cucumber, jicama or carrot slices ✓ Dehydrated sweet potato slices ✓ Baked carrot, parsnip or plantain chips ✓ Kale chips ✓ Go Raw® Flax Snax (check ingredients on flavored varieties) ✓ Homemade plantain or almond-meal crackers
Rice	✓ Cauliflower rice (cooked) ✓ Jicama rice (cold shredded)
Pizza	✓ Meatza – a sausage crust, prebaked then topped like a pizza (omit cheese)
Crust	✓ Make crust-less quiche or shepherd's pie ✓ Line a casserole dish with approved ground sausage/bacon ✓ Line a pie pan with sweet potato slices ✓ Locate an almond-meal-based crust or find recipes online or in Paleo cookbooks ✓ Grab-&-go idea: bake omelet mix in a muffin pan for mini crust-less quiches
Pasta	✓ Julienned and sautéed vegetables (bell peppers, zucchini, daikon radish) ✓ Carrots peeled into "ribbons" ✓ Baked spaghetti squash ✓ Kelp or Shirataki noodles (buy soy-free, legume-free varieties and rinse first) Tip: Check Amazon or a kitchen supply store for spiral cutters or julienning blades – these can cut hard vegetables such as sweet potato or winter squash into 'noodles'
Mayonnaise	✓ Guacamole ✓ Coconut milk for making creamy sauces ✓ Primal Kitchen® Mayo or Chosen Foods® Avocado Mayonnaise ✓ Cooking Assignment #2: Homemade Paleo Mayo on Day 4
Salad Dressing	✓ Olive oil and vinegar or lemon juice ✓ Salsa ✓ Puréed berries ✓ Some commercially-available 100% olive oil dressings: Tessamae's®, Whole Foods 365® Herbes de Provence; Bolthouse® has a few varieties
Soy sauce	✓ Coconut aminos is the best option ✓ Fish sauce works in a pinch (start with a small amount – very salty) ✓ Worcestershire sauce adds salty flavor, but not necessarily the soy sauce flavor

Baking Powder	Usually contains cornstarch and aluminum; aluminum-free is available
	Options to make your own: for 1 tsp baking powder equivalent:
	    a. ¼ tsp baking soda + ½ tsp cream of tarter
	    b. ¼ tsp baking soda + 1 ½ tsp lemon juice (or vinegar of choice)

Breadcrumbs	Make your own by adding seasonings to: ✓ Freshly ground flax, sunflower or pumpkin seeds ✓ Crumbled pork rinds, dried shiitake mushrooms or approved bread/crackers ✓ Almond meal, ground nuts ✓ Paleo starches/flours like tapioca, arrowroot, coconut or potato ✓ Finely ground dried coconut flakes
Cornstarch or Thickeners	✓ Arrowroot flour, powder or starch ✓ Tapioca flour or starch ✓ Potato flour or starch ✓ Gelatin (grass-fed or pasture-raised is preferred) ✓ Coconut flour may work, but is not the best choice as it tends to get lumpy ✓ AFTER program: rice flour

Western Food	Paleo Substitute
Peanut Butter and Jelly	✓ Nut or seed butters on a green apple slice ✓ Try almond, hazelnut, sunflower seed, cashew or macadamia butters
Sweeteners	✓ Cinnamon ✓ Green apple, grated ✓ Occasional unsweetened applesauce ✓ CRUTCH: 100% stevia, hardwood xylitol (not xylitol from corn) ✓ AFTER program: dates, date paste, honey, 100% maple syrup, molasses, stevia, organic sugar or crystalized cane sugar, xylitol from hardwoods, coconut sugar (more about Paleo Sweeteners in Day 28)
Desserts	We are trying to break away from the sugar habit – proceed cautiously: ✓ Fat bombs and other ideas on Day 3 under Food Hacks ✓ Low sugar fruits with coconut crème ✓ Freeze dried berries ✓ 21-Day Sugar Detox treats – search online for "21DSD treat recipes" ✓ 85-100% dark chocolate (add to a fruit if it is too bitter on its own) ✓ CRUTCH: 100% stevia or hardwood xylitol

*Find recipes, Paleo eating ideas and more at 🖰 Pinterest Paleovation

To Do List:

☐ Paleo Mayo needs to be made or purchased by tomorrow

☐ Comfort Food ideas were mentioned on Day 5 – this is an optional cooking assignment. Research an appealing recipe to prepare by Day 10.

☐ Do you need to restock fresh cut vegetables?

☐ Tomorrow is Cooking Assignment #3. Do you have your ingredients?

Cooking Assignment #3: Substituting Veggies for Grain (choose one):

    a. **Rice**: cauliflower, jicama

    b. **Noodles**: consider buying a spiralizer to produce a more authentic noodle appearance/texture

        i. Sautéed: zucchini, sweet potato, yellow squash, carrots, bell peppers

        ii. Roasted: spaghetti squash

    c. **Sandwich Bun**:

        i. Latkes: sweet potato, zucchini, carrots, turnips, etc (you'll also need eggs for these)

        ii. Grilling: eggplant slices or portabella mushroom caps

        iii. Raw: lettuce leaves, cabbage leaves, bell pepper or cucumber

☐ Did you watch a movie or video? Or care to watch another?

Recommended Food Documentaries			
Movies			**Not-so-Boring Taped Lecture Options**
🖰 Food, Inc 🖰 Fed Up 🖰 Fat Head 🖰 Origins*	🖰 Ingredients 🖰 Carb Loaded 🖰 King Corn 🖰 Food Fight	🖰 Killer at Large 🖰 Hungry for Change 🖰 Cereal Killers 🖰 That Sugar Film	🖰 Great Cholesterol Myth (Jonny Bowden) 🖰 Sugar the Bitter Truth (Robert Lustig) 🖰 The Oiling of America (Sally Fallon) 🖰 Minding your Mitochondria (Terry Wahls)

*Directed by Mark van Wijk

Coming Up Soon:

- Tomorrow we talk about dairy and calcium, and cover tips on refrigerator management

Day 7

When you want to quit, remember why you started. ~Anonymous

Today's Topics:

1. Paleo-Wise: Dairy
2. Planning Better for Hunger and Food Efficiency
3. Cooking Assignment #3: Use a Veggie Instead of a Grain

Fast Fare – Use Paleo Mayo
♥ Baby shrimp and mayo salad
♥ Salad mix with olive oil & lemon juice
♥ Broccoli steamed in microwave

What are you eating today?

My Paleo Meals: Day 7			
Meal	**Veggies**	**Protein**	**Healthy Fats**
Breakfast	Green Yellow/Orange Red Blue/Purple/Black White/Tan		
Lunch	Green Yellow/Orange Red Blue/Purple/Black White/Tan		
Dinner	Green Yellow/Orange Red Blue/Purple/Black White/Tan		
Snack	Green Yellow/Orange Red Blue/Purple/Black White/Tan		

I learned that all my allergies and ailments could effectively be 'cured' through the adoption of the Paleo Diet. This way of enjoying food is about getting your digestive system on track, and is not at all restrictive – as some people tend to assume. ~ Mary Shenouda, PaleoChef.com

We've detailed numerous strategies for staying on track:

- Batch-Cooking, Foundation Recipes and 28 Days of Paleo Meals (all in Prep B)
- Restaurant Strategies (Prep D)
- Quick Meals and Alternative Preparation Methods (Prep E)
- Breakfast Suggestions (Prep F)

- 20-Minute Recipes (Day 1)
- Snacks (Day 2)
- Curbing Hunger (Day 3)
- Meal-Building and Fast Ideas (Day 4)
- Substitutes for Non-Compliant Foods (Day 6)

Keep these in mind as you answer the following questions.

What strategies are working well for your lifestyle? Go back and look – what has helped you the most?

1. _____

2. _____

3. _____

What hasn't worked so well and what can you do to change it?

_____

_____

You are 1 week into the program. How is your commitment level?

☐ Strong   ☐ Fair   ☐ Depends on the day   ☐ Weak   ☐ Gone

Remember why you started: Go back to Prep E to revisit your thoughts before beginning this dietary change, as well as Prep C to recall the "Good Health Results" you desire most. Which of your observations and thoughts still hold true to help you complete this program?

1. _____

2. _____

3. _____

Name two positive changes you have successfully implemented so far:

1. _____

2. _____

It's important to recognize and build upon these successes! Each step is a step in the right direction. Even if you are still feeling the effects of low-carb flu, remember that the body needs this time to reset hormones and begin metabolizing fat for energy instead of glucose. Stay positive, stay strong. Change is in progress.

Section I – Paleo-Wise: Dairy

> *My answer to the question of whether dairy is healthy or harmful is, in short: it depends.*
> ~Chris Kresser, author of The Paleo Cure, Unconventional Medicine

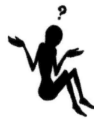

The Dairy Debate

Dairy clearly falls into the *gray area* of the Paleo spectrum. The debate on whether dairy is healthful or harmful will easily go on for decades with no absolute answer. Certain people thrive on pastured, raw dairy such as the Masai herders of Kenya and Tanzania. Much of their nutrition traditionally comes from cattle, including the milk and blood in addition to the meat. For others, lactose intolerance limits their choice of dairy to specific products. And of course, some individuals cannot tolerate even the smallest amount of any dairy.

Dairy for Growth

Animal milk is a mixture of proteins, sugar, fat, vitamins, minerals, antibodies, hormones and growth factors. This distinct mixture of components is a complete nourishment system for baby animals.

As with any sugar, the milk sugar *lactose* elicits an insulin response. However, dairy is unique because it also includes the only protein that triggers insulin: *whey*. Milk is specifically designed to boost insulin levels so it can quickly shuttle glucose, amino acids, fat and vitamins into cells for the baby animal's growth.

This makes dairy a *dual growth stimulant*: the milk itself contains growth promoters *plus* additional growth is generated by the insulin response from lactose and whey. Although this is essential for baby animals, there is concern that the embedded growth, hormonal and immunologic messages are harmful for human adults.

Modern Dairy Concerns

Conventional dairy introduces a new set of concerns. Husbandry practices add chemical residues and modern processing destroys nutritive value. Differences between milk in stores and traditional raw milk are enormous:

1. **CAFO Dairy** – Utilizes supplemental hormones (such as rBGH) which make cows produce more milk.
2. **Homogenization** – Squeezes milk through tiny holes under intense pressure, destroying the architecture of the fat droplets and creating fats that are foreign to most human digestive systems.
3. **Pasteurization** – Heat exposure denatures milk proteins, destroying many beneficial components of milk, including the enzymes that aid in digestion.

Symptoms of Dairy Intolerance

There is significant variation between individuals regarding how well dairy is metabolized, which components cause reactions and what symptoms manifest. The only way to determine personal tolerance is to eliminate all dairy, assess how the body feels without it, then gradually reintroduce one dairy component at a time. If not digested properly, dairy causes inflammation and immune reactions. Symptoms include:

- Itchy skin
- Eczema
- Sinus congestion and phlegm
- Wheezing
- Stomach pain
- Diarrhea or constipation
- Bloating and gas
- Nausea
- Excess ear wax

Dairy Components – Casein, Whey, Lactose and Butterfat

Some components of dairy are problematic to *some* people. Knowing what part of dairy creates negative symptoms helps shape a personalized diet that maximizes health.

A. Casein

Casein is a slow-digesting dairy protein comprising about 80% of total protein in animal milk. This insoluble portion of milk is the main component of cheese and curds. Casein is also used in many food products as a binding agent, even in foods labeled "lactose-free."

> **Cheesy Addiction:** Cheese is mostly casein blended with enzymes. Enzymes partially break down the casein into *morphine-like compounds*!! No wonder cheese is hard to give up.

Casein	
Characteristics	**Problems**
Similar Shape to Gluten	✓ More than 50% of gluten-sensitive people are also sensitive to casein
Binds to Opioid Receptors in the Gut and Brain	✓ Potentially addictive
Slows Digestion	✓ For newborns, this improves absorption, but it's harmful for adults
Casein Structure Varies by Animal Breed	✓ Primary dairy cattle (Holstein) produce A1 beta-casein which tends to cause most of the casein-related digestive problems ✓ Less common dairy cattle (Guernsey, Jersey) produce A2 beta-casein, a structure which humans tend to tolerate better

B. Whey

Fast-digesting whey is a blend of the 20% remaining milk proteins, plus hormones (including growth factors and estrogen) and immunological factors. The hormones that naturally appear in milk are similar in structure to human hormones. In people with leaky gut syndrome or other digestive compromise, those hormones can enter the bloodstream and disrupt hormonal balance.

> **Athletes and Body-Builders:** Many athletes purposely use whey protein post-workout because the insulin effect speeds amino acid delivery and stimulates muscle growth. However, the body is naturally more sensitive for about an hour after a strenuous workout and will absorb any protein at higher percentages for muscle repair and growth. Until your tolerance to dairy is determined, skip the whey protein for post-workout nutrition this month and opt for food-based protein (chicken, fish, eggs, meat) with starchy vegetables (sweet potatoes, beets). If a protein powder is a must, collagen protein is a good choice (more information on Whey in Prep B, Day 6 and the Reintroduction Guidelines on Day 26).

C. Lactose

Lactose is the sugar in milk made from *glucose* + galactose. To break it down, our bodies need the digestive enzyme, lactase, which many people stop producing after childhood. Roughly 65% of all humans are lactose-intolerant. Left undigested, lactose interferes with the balance of gut bacteria and produces digestive consequences such as cramping, diarrhea, bloating, gas, etc.

Lactose Intolerant?	
Post-Program Dairy Options	**Why They Are Less Irritating...**
Raw Dairy	Naturally-occurring digestive enzymes in the milk remain usable if the product is not heat-pasteurized.
Choose Goat, Sheep, Buffalo, Camel or Yak Dairy	Each animal milk has slightly different lactose structure and these forms can be better tolerated in sensitive individuals.
Be Selective with Dairy Products	<ul><li>Restrict milk and yogurt, which are highest in lactose</li><li>Try incorporating butter, heavy cream or cheese which are lowest in lactose</li></ul>

Further Reading: 🖰 ChrisKresser How to Cure Lactose Intolerance

D. Butter / Butterfat / Milkfat / Purified Butter

High-quality, grass-fed butter is perhaps the most amazing component of dairy.

Grass-Fed Butterfat	
Benefit	**Details**
Nourishment	<ul><li>Vitamins, including A, B12, D, E, choline and K2</li><li>Trace minerals such as selenium, zinc, iodine, chromium</li></ul>
Easily-Digested	<ul><li>Butyrate – short-chain fat that is directly absorbed in intestines with no need for gall bladder (read more on Day 2)</li><li>Highly-absorbable forms of fats, vitamins and minerals</li></ul>
Metabolism	<ul><li>Short-chain and medium-chain fats as well as CLA encourage the body to burn fat for energy (more on Days 2 and 4)</li></ul>
Medicinal Properties (highly prized in Eastern Africa and the Indian subcontinent)	<ul><li>Anti-inflammatory, antibacterial, antifungal, antioxidant</li><li>Soothes digestive tract, protects against intestinal infection</li><li>Protects against osteoporosis, obesity, heart disease, cataracts, thyroid disorders, cancer, arthritis, sexual dysfunction, infertility</li></ul>

Further Reading: 🖰 PaleoLeap The Many Virtues of Butter

Compared to other dairy products, butter is very low in irritating proteins and contains no lactose. Butter can be consumed by the average individual without concern of negative health consequences. However, clarifying butter removes the few remaining proteins and is well-tolerated by even highly sensitive people (more on Saturated Fats and directions to make clarified butter and ghee on Day 2).

Eat butter first and eat butter last, and live till a hundred years be past. ~Dutch Proverb

Dairy-Free for a Month

Even if dairy is tolerated relatively well, enough valid reasoning exists to remove all dairy for a month to let digestion rest. Other than grass-fed butter or ghee, dairy products tend to aggravate chronic health conditions and are best avoided until these ailments stabilize. Adhering to the Strict Paleo Protocol will accelerate healing.

Conditions that Benefit from Elimination of Dairy (except butter)	
✓ Chronic Inflammation	✓ Insulin resistance
✓ Leaky gut	✓ Autoimmune conditions*
✓ Gut flora imbalance	✓ Gluten intolerance / sensitivity*

* Use clarified butter (ghee) or an alternative fat if highly sensitive to dairy protein

Isn't Dairy Necessary for Calcium?

Not on a Paleo Diet! Calcium is present in many non-dairy sources in highly bioavailable forms, all abundant in the Paleo Diet. Eating a wide variety of vegetables and protein sources will provide ample calcium. Humans are genetically designed to attain all appropriate nutrients from a hunter-gatherer diet. Consider this: Where does a grass-fed cow get the calcium to produce her milk? From her natural diet – grass!

Non-Dairy Calcium Sources	
Sources	**Specifics**
Dark Green Vegetables	Collard greens, kale, turnip greens, bok choy, broccoli, seaweed
Seafood (esp with bones)	Sardines, salmon, mackerel, shrimp, oysters, mussels, anchovies
Nuts / Seeds	Almonds, hazelnuts, sesame seeds
Sweets	Oranges, dried figs, blackstrap molasses

No Bones to Pick: Canned salmon bones are softened by heat processing and are a great source of calcium. Crush these soft bones directly into a salmon cake recipe – you won't even notice they're there!

Eating Paleo Improves Calcium Nutrition:

There are a variety of reasons why the Paleo Diet easily meets calcium needs:
1. Improves efficiency of calcium absorption so *less calcium is necessary* to satisfy nutritional requirements
2. Contains abundant, calcium-rich foods from non-dairy sources
3. Contains vitamin K2-rich foods which improve calcium metabolism, helping to direct calcium into the bones rather than accumulate in soft tissues.

Factors that Interfere with Calcium Absorption	
Source of Interference	**How Paleo Improves Calcium Absorption**
Phytates	Removes high-phytate sources: grains and legumes
Stress	Significantly less dietary/nutritional stress + improved sleep
Aging	Less oxidation (from eliminating sugars and increasing healthy fats)
Phosphoric Acid (colas)	Eliminates soda
Protein Restriction	Healthy protein levels
Chronic Inflammation	Removes sugars and omega-6 fats, adds anti-inflammatory omega-3 fats
Taxed Immune System	Avoids common trigger foods to heal leaky gut and digestive distress
Weak Stomach Acid	Less reflux, less need for antacid drugs
Deficient Vitamins A, D, E, K	More healthy fats, organ meats, cholesterol-rich foods and sunshine
Mineral Deficiency	Generous vegetables, real salts and careful supplementation

As the gut heals on a Paleo Diet, mineral absorption improves. Don't rely on RDA numbers for calcium needs – they may be higher than necessary because they're based on the western diet which contributes to poor calcium absorption.

Lower Calcium Concerns on Paleo

Lower net calcium is not a major concern within a Paleo Diet for the following reasons:
- Calcium interference is significantly reduced without grains and legumes
- Sufficient alternative-calcium sources are abundantly consumed
- High intake of other critical bone nutrients (more about Bone Health on Day 16)

Good to Know: Individuals who deliberately follow a high-protein diet* excrete more calcium in their urine, raising concerns about calcium deficiency (*Paleo is not high-protein when followed correctly). Even if urine calcium concentration increases while eating Paleo, calcium deficiency is still not a concern because Paleo eaters also *absorb and retain more* calcium due to minimal digestive interference.

Vitamin K2 to the Rescue – Calcium Director

Vitamin K2 is rarely discussed as a critical bone nutrient, but in essence, it acts as a mineral director. Without proper hormonal signaling, not all available calcium readily deposits in the bones – it can float in the blood and accumulate in soft tissues, like joint cartilage (joint achiness and stiffness), arterial walls (hardening of arteries or high blood pressure) and organs (kidney stones). Vitamin K2 reverses this tendency, directing calcium into bone.

Key Point: Vitamin K2 draws calcium out of the soft tissue and places it into the teeth and bones!

Vitamin K1 is found in green leafy vegetables and algae. Sunshine and specialized gut bacteria are required to convert it into vitamin K2. Grazing animals are very efficient with this process and store K2 in their fat. Unfortunately, the human gut biome cannot produce significant amounts of vitamin K2. Therefore, the best way to ensure adequate intake of K2 is by consuming fat products from pastured animals.

Vitamin K2-Rich Foods	
✓ Grass-fed butter and cheese	✓ Pastured bacon
✓ Pastured organ meats	✓ Bone marrow
✓ Pastured egg yolks	✓ Natto (fermented soybean)
✓ Pastured goose liver pate	✓ Homemade fermented
✓ Sardines	vegetables

Most people are deficient in vitamin K2. With the introduction of high-volume, commercial animal husbandry (CAFOs), manufacturers cut costs by using synthetic nutrients. Some nutrients get supplemented while others are ignored. The prerequisite foods for vitamin K2 production (green leaves and sunshine) are not available to confined animals, effectively breeding K2 out of the modern food supply.

How Vitamin K2 Was Eliminated by CAFO Animal Husbandry	
Artificial CAFO Nutrition	**Negative Impact on K2**
Synthetic Vitamin A	▪ Confined animals no longer need to eat the green foods to supply beta-carotene (precursor to Vitamin A), but this eliminated *green grass and leaves that supply K1*
Synthetic Vitamin D	▪ CAFO animals no longer need sunshine for vitamin D, but *sunshine is necessary for conversion of K1 to K2*

Further Reading: 📖 *Vitamin K2 and the Calcium Paradox: How a Little-Known Vitamin Could Save Your Life,* by Kate Rheaume-Blanc

Dairy Substitutes

Many of us simply crave the creamy texture and flavor that dairy products supply in foods like melted cheese, cream sauces, ice cream, butter, etc. Use the following Paleo-friendly dairy substitutes to enhance flavors and texture without adding dairy:

Paleo Dairy Swaps	
Component	**Substitute**
Creamy Texture	Avocado, coconut milk, Paleo mayo, grass-fed butter, some smooth nut butters like cashew or macadamia
Cheesy Flavor	Nutritional yeast, some mushrooms
Buttery Flavor	Butter, clarified butter or ghee (grass-fed always preferred)
Ice Cream	Frozen berries blended with coconut milk

➢ **Coconut Milk** – The number one Paleo dairy substitute. Great for cooking, drinking and adding to coffee or tea, plus it's a good source of healthy fats; the canned variety has the creamiest consistency.

➢ **Nut Milk** – Beverages made from almonds, cashews, macadamia, hazelnuts, etc. Choose unsweetened and organic when possible.

Kitchen Tip – Make Your Own Nut Milk: Soak 1 cup of raw nuts for at least 4 hours or overnight. Discard the water. Place the soaked nuts in a blender with 3 cups of filtered water. Blend for several minutes until smooth. Strain through a cheesecloth or nut milk bag. Refrigerate the milk and use within 3 days. The leftover pulp can be used for baking Paleo muffins, thickening a sauce or rounding out a meatloaf.

Primal Diet – Dairy Inclusions

Based on individual sensitivity levels, certain people can include *select* dairy products in their diet. *Quality* dairy plus Paleo is referred to as the Primal Diet.

Primal Diet = Paleo Diet + Select High-Quality Dairy

After eliminating dairy for a month, the food reintroduction phase allows personal assessment of dairy components to pinpoint how much dairy is tolerated. Here are guidelines to identify quality dairy products:

Selecting High-Quality Dairy	
Issues with Dairy	**Better Choice Solution**
Cattle fed non-native diet of grains and soy creates inflammatory compounds	Grass-fed or pastured dairy products
Pasteurization kills digestive enzymes which help humans digest dairy	Raw dairy (see excerpt below)
Dairy products have insulin-stimulating lactose and whey	Select high-fat products such as heavy cream or butter
Cheese fermentation creates morphine-like compounds which are potentially addictive	Save cheese for a treat
Conventional dairy cows are treated with hormones and antibiotics	Select rBGH-free, antibiotic-free or organic (which is both)
Dairy naturally contains estrogens and growth hormones	Goat milk has much less hormonal impact due to the smaller size of the animal

Fermented/Cultured Dairy

Fermentation increases the shelf life of dairy products, imparting rich flavors and making them easier to digest. The fermentation process rejuvenates damaged proteins, makes minerals more bioavailable and breaks down lactose, so those who are lactose-intolerant can include them in their diet (read more about Ferments on Day 21). Fermented or cultured dairy products include yogurt, kefir, buttermilk, sour cream and, potentially addictive, cheese. Some specialty stores even carry cultured butter.

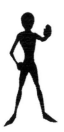

Raw Dairy – Safety First!

Raw dairy is neither homogenized nor pasteurized, so all nutrients are preserved. However, raw milk *must* come from a source committed to cleanliness, protocol and animal welfare. Because tainted milk can contain pathogenic bacteria, local laws often restrict raw milk distribution. To locate nearby trusted raw dairy farms, inquire at local butcher shops, farmers markets or online forums like ⌁ RealMilk.

Further Reading:
⌁ MarksDailyApple The Definitive Guide to Dairy
⌁ ThePaleoMom The Great Dairy Debate

The problem is that we think we have to process dairy to be "healthier" to consume, and we muck it all up!
~Diane Sanfilippo, BS, NC, author of Practical Paleo, 21-Day Sugar Detox

Section II: Better Planning for Hunger and Food Efficiency

Hunger

Still hungry between meals? Snacking is totally acceptable (ideas on Day 2). However, if you are interested in reducing the need for snacks, review Day 3 for ideas to increase satiety with more fat and protein in each meal.

What are your thoughts regarding your hunger levels and snack habits?

_____

Fridge Efficiency Chart:

Perhaps you find that produce in the fridge drawer is neglected or you're looking for a system to identify which foods you (or your housemates) need to save for a recipe. The following template helps you remember which foods need to be used, saved or restocked. A full size Fridge Efficiency Chart is in the Resource Section or printable from ⏼ Paleovation. Place it in a plastic sheet protector; stick it on the fridge and make notes with dry or wet erase markers.

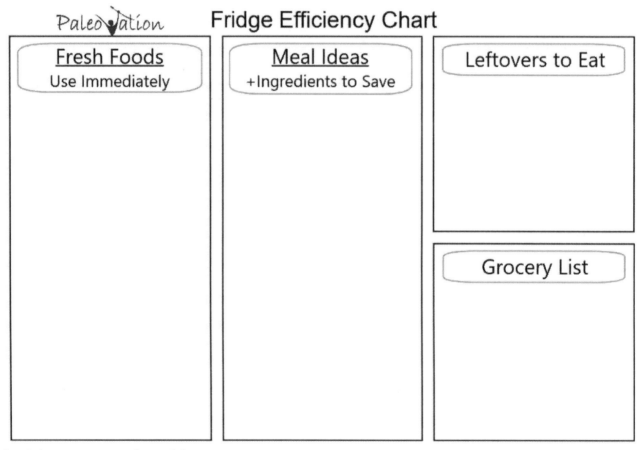

The Crisper Drawer of Death?

Many times, the crisper drawers are loaded with fresh produce...and then forgotten until they're slimy. Rearrange your fridge to open space for vegetables on the main shelves where they are prominently displayed and easy to grab. Reserve crisper drawers for items with a longer shelf-life or those you won't forget to use:

Long-Lived Items to Place in the Crisper Drawer		
✓ Carrots, celery	✓ Nuts and seeds	✓ Liverwurst
✓ Lemons, limes	✓ Nut butter, almond meal	✓ Smoked fish
✓ Garlic, ginger	✓ Cans of sparkling water	✓ Eggs
✓ Curry paste	✓ Kombucha	✓ Bacon
✓ Fruit	✓ Lard, tallow, duck fat	✓ Extra butter

What other strategies will improve your refrigerator efficiency and/or management?
- ☐ Defrost dish – always have something thawing in the fridge
- ☐ Door shelves – keep grab-n-go pouches where you see them
- ☐ Wash fruit and vegetables before placing in the fridge
- ☐ Store fresh herbs upright in an jar of water
- ☐ Use bins to separate and store produce
- ☐ Other: _____

Section III: Cooking Assignment #3 – Using a Veggie Instead of a Grain

An easy way to eat more nutrient-dense vegetables is to substitute them in place of a typical grain serving whenever possible. These alternatives get more vegetables on the plate *plus*, psychologically, make a grain-free meal much more satisfying. Browse these suggestions (you may already have tried some) and prepare a new idea by Day 12.

> *Go vegetable-heavy. Reverse the psychology of your plate by making meat the side dish and vegetables the main course.* ~Bobby Flay, chef

RICE
1. **Cauliflower Rice**
   a. Grate cauliflower first, then cook
      - Grate the cauliflower by hand (box grater) or with a grating disc in a processor
      - Choose how you want to cook it:
         o Sauté in oil over medium heat, then cover to retain steam, ~10 min
         o Microwave in glass bowl for 5 min, stir and microwave 5 min more
         o Toss with oil and spread on a baking sheet; bake at 350° for 15 min
   b. Cook cauliflower first, then chop
      - Partially steam cauliflower florets (don't overcook – won't work if they get soggy)
      - Put florets in food processor with a chopping blade and pulse-cut a few times
   c. Buy frozen cauliflower rice and prepare according to package directions (watch for additives)
2. **Jicama Rice**
   a. Grate the jicama; use raw

BUNS
1. **Veggie Latkes** (make a triple batch because these freeze well – reheat in oven on a baking sheet)
   a. Choose your veggie (sweet potato, turnip, carrot, zucchini, etc)
   b. Grate, then squeeze out as much liquid as possible using a nut milk bag or dish towel
   c. Mix with beaten egg(s) and seasonings of choice
   d. Heat oil in a skillet and drop in veggie batter, press down slightly to flatten
   e. Fry each side until golden
   f. Recipe: MarksDailyApple Vegetable Latkes
2. **Raw Vegetables**
   a. Choose your veggie (bell peppers, cucumber, jicama, cabbage or iceberg lettuce wedge)
   b. Halve and seed, or slice to make bun-sized portions
3. **Cooked Vegetables**
   a. Roasted sweet potato or eggplant slices
   b. Grilled portabella mushroom caps

NOODLES
1. **Spaghetti Squash**
   a. Halve, seed, coat with oil and season. Roast in oven 350° for 45-60min. When the squash is soft, scrape it out with a fork to create the 'noodles' and top with sauce. If the 'noodles' don't scape out easily, cook longer.
   b. Crock pot version: wash the squash (two small squash may fit in your cooker) and pierce 4-5 times with a knife. Put in slow cooker and add about 2 cups of water. Cook on low for 6 hours.

2. **Sautéed Vegetable Strips**
    a. Choose your veggie (sweet potato, zucchini, carrot, sweet peppers, daikon radish, etc)
    b. Choose your cutting style:
        - Vegetable peeler makes fettuccini ribbons
        - Spiralizers typically have various blades for spaghetti or angel hair thickness
        - Grater/grating disc can make smaller 'noodle' pieces
        - Paring knife or slicing blade on processor can make thin julienne strips
        - Purchase pre-sliced bell pepper strips either from a salad bar or frozen section
    c. Sauté grated veggie in skillet with oil and seasoning of choice *or* if you choose zucchini or yellow squash, a hot marinara poured over the top can sufficiently soften the 'noodle'

Paleo Mayonnaise

Your mayo should be complete. How did you use it first? _____

Did you like the taste?   Yes   No   (If not, add additional seasoning or try again with another recipe or oil)

More ideas to use mayo are listed on Day 4. How else will you use your mayo?

_____

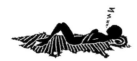

Take Care of You

If you still need some rest, please make time for it. Give yourself permission to slow down. Consider trying a low-carb flu relief strategy. This transition may not be easy, but your body genuinely needs time to heal. Stay strong!

If nothing ever changed, there'd be no butterflies. ~Author Unknown

To Do List:

- ❑ Paleo Comfort Food recipe is still an option
- ❑ The Veggie Grain-Substitute Recipe you want to try: _____
    - ➤ Select ingredients for your Cooking Assignment #3: Veggie as a Grain. For efficiency, you may already have the vegetable in your fridge. Plan to try it by Day 12.
    - ➤ You potentially can overlap this assignment with a comfort food recipe. Examples:
        - Meatza crust made of sweet potatoes
        - Spaghetti noodles made of zucchini spirals
        - Hamburger with latke bun

Coming Up Soon:

- Tomorrow's Topics: Legumes and...perfect poop? Yes, for real!

Day 8

When everything goes against you until it seems as though you could not hang on a minute longer, never give up then...for that is just the place and time that the tide will turn. ~Harriet Beecher Stowe

Today's Topics:
1. Paleo-Wise: Legumes
2. Healthy Bowel Characteristics
3. The Quest for Consistent Poop (and Bowel Health)

Fast Fare – Use Paleo Mayo
♥ Avocado filled with egg salad
♥ Smoked salmon on cucumber slices

Use the following questions to highlight foods from the past week. If you prefer to continue recording meals in the Veggie + Protein + Fat table, download the PDF at ⏚ Paleovation or copy a blank table (Resource Section).

- Name a meal you want to make again: _____

- Name a Paleo food you didn't care for: _____

- What foods and beverages are very satisfying for you right now?
  _____

- How will you continue to plan for vegetables at every meal?
  _____

- Is there anything bothering you about the foods you are currently eating?   No   Yes   If yes, elaborate:
  _____

- Are there any westernized foods you are missing?   No   Yes   If yes, expand on what aspects you're missing (texture, taste, habit) and list some appropriate Paleo replacements or substitutions (check Day 6):
  _____
  _____

- What have been your go-to items for a fast meal?
  _____

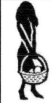 **Fastest Egg Salad Ever:** Who said egg salad had to be made from hard-boiled eggs? If you don't have time to boil and peel the eggs, scramble them instead! Chop the scrambled egg into small pieces and add your homemade mayo, minced onion, celery and seasonings. Serve in a pepper half, on top of salad greens, or use as a dip for veggies or bacon chips.

Section I – Paleo-Wise: Legumes

Legumes are seeds produced within a pod, generally referred to as beans, and include soybeans, lentils, peas, garbanzos, peanuts and more. Although they're touted as excellent plant-based protein sources, the proteins are incomplete – missing some essential amino acids. Legumes are not necessary in a healthy diet – other Paleo foods provide those nutrients found in legumes more efficiently and are less likely to cause digestive distress.

Chemistry Corner: Legumes have the unique ability to capture, or fix, nitrogen from the atmosphere. Because nitrogen is an essential component of amino acids (the building blocks of protein), legumes contain the highest protein content in the *plant* world (yet animal product proteins are more concentrated and higher quality). After harvest, the remaining unused legume plant is tilled back into the soil so its nitrogen can fertilize the next crop. For this reason, many traditional and organic farming practices include legumes in crop rotations.

To Bean or Not to Bean? That is the Paleo Question

Primitive humans had limited access to legumes and the prerequisite methods for proper preparation. Legumes have the potential to significantly contribute to gut irritation and increased permeability of the digestive lining (leaky gut syndrome). This doesn't make legumes entirely bad, but definitely places them in the *non-optimal* food category for humans.

"Intestinal permeability" has been discussed in the medical literature for over 100 years! ~Josh Axe, DC

There are valid arguments for and against legumes because some people tolerate occasional amounts *when they're properly prepared* (next page) while others are completely intolerant. To preserve the integrity of the Strict Paleo Protocol, this program eliminates legumes and their byproducts for 1 month for a variety of reasons:

1. Not a staple in ancestral diets – our genetics have not fully adapted for their ideal assimilation
2. High carbohydrate load
3. Contain antinutrients and FODMAPs (fermentable carbohydrates), causing gas and digestive distress
4. Specific concerns regarding soy and peanut products and their industrial production practices
5. The process of elimination is the only way to determine individual sensitivities

> **Paleo Legume Exception – Green/Yellow Beans, Sugar Snap Peas and Snow Peas:** In general, the legume *seed* contains the majority of the problematic elements, not the pod. When in the pod, the seed contribution is a small fraction with less detrimental impact on health. Therefore, legumes eaten *in the pod* are an acceptable Paleo food – they contain fewer antinutrients and are typically not consumed in high quantities as other beans.

The Legume Debate	
Pros	**Cons**
• **Plant Protein** – one of the best plant-based protein sources available • **Inexpensive** – affordable dietary staple for impoverished areas • **Healthy Soluble Fiber and Resistant Starch** – a good source of both (more in Section III as well as on Day 15) • **High Satiety** – legumes are filling • **Certain Nutrients** – some legumes, like lentils, contain large amounts of folate and reasonable amounts of other vitamins and minerals	• **Incomplete Protein** – legume protein pales in quantity and quality when compared to animal proteins • **Antinutrients** – contribute to leaky gut and mineral deficiencies • **Displace Healthier Foods** – if used as a staple, legumes displace nutrient-dense foods such as vegetables, seafood and healthy fats • **Contain Fermentable Carbohydrates** (FODMAPs, more in Section III) which can cause acid reflux, gas, bloating and other digestive upset, especially for those with bowel disorders or small-intestinal-bacterial-overgrowth (SIBO, see Day 15) • **Significant Carbohydrate Load** – legumes have a high carb-load for the amount of protein, a concern for those wanting to lose weight • **Proper Preparation** – required to reduce antinutrients

Anti-Nutrients

Like grains, legumes also contain antinutrients that interfere with digestion, potentially contributing to leaky gut syndrome and other digestive woes. For people with sensitivities, these toxins cause more harm than good (read more about Lectin and Phytate antinutrients in Prep E).

A. **Lectins** – Short, difficult-to-break-down proteins that all plant seeds contain in varying amounts. These can damage the digestive tract (for example, gluten is a lectin found in grains).
   - Legumes have particularly high concentrations of lectins (especially soybeans and peanuts), up to 10% of the total protein content.
   - Lectins are incredibly resistant to heat – common cooking doesn't decrease their potency; however, soaking, fermenting, sprouting or an *extended* high-heat boil can inactivate a high percentage.
   - Few people take the time for proper legume preparation to reduce lectin content (note that legumes served in a restaurant may not be properly prepared).
   - Physical damage from lectins can accumulate insidiously over time.

> **Legume Gloom:** Red kidney beans (commonly used in chili) contain a lectin called *phytohemagglutinin* that blocks production of stomach acid, contributing to acid reflux and disrupting digestion of proteins. This lectin is toxic and cases of food poisoning have been linked to raw or undercooked kidney beans.

B. **Phytates** – The storage form of phosphorus concentrated in the bran or hull of seeds as part of its protective shell. Phytates bind other minerals and hoard them for seed growth. When they are eaten, they prevent mineral absorption in the gut which contributes to deficiencies.
   - Prolonged soaking of legumes can neutralize most of the phytates, but in unsoaked beans, phytates remain intact through cooking.
   - If meat intake is low, phytates can interfere with iron, zinc and calcium absorption.

> **Paleo Advantage:** After the program, adding a small amount of animal protein to a legume-containing meal can increase mineral absorption despite the phytate content.

C. **Saponins** – These are naturally-occurring phytochemicals found in legumes, quinoa, nightshade vegetables and some herbs like stevia and ginseng. These compounds act as deterrents for parasites and pests.
   ➢ The name stems from the term 'sapo' which is Latin for soap. Saponins have detergent-like properties (ability to make oil and water mix) and can create foam in water.
   ➢ This detergent-like structure allows saponins to easily interact and disrupt body structures comprised of fat and water, particularly cell membranes:
      - **The good:** Saponins have antimicrobial properties – they can dissolve cell membranes of pathogenic fungi and bacteria. Some saponins may also aid nutrient absorption – certain fruit and vegetable saponins selectively increase cell permeability to allow nutrients into the cell.
      - **The bad:** Cell membranes lining the human intestinal tract can be destroyed by saponins, contributing to digestive problems and increased gut permeability.
   ➢ Saponins are generally concentrated in the seed, so large seeds like legumes and pseudo-grains (quinoa) contain *very* high quantities (note: agave also contains large amounts).
   ➢ Soaking, sprouting or cooking legumes *does not reduce* saponin content.

> **Bottom Line:** There is no consensus on whether saponins are beneficial or detrimental to health, but some people appear to be very sensitive to them.
>
> **Our Recommendation** - Eliminate the majority of saponins for a month by following the Strict Paleo Protocol. Then experiment with adding them back to establish individual tolerance levels.

Legume Preparation Recommendations
Soaking, sprouting, fermenting and heating can inactivate and neutralize *most* lectins found in *most* legumes. Only properly prepared beans should be eaten: always soak first, then fully cook or sprout.
1. Soak at room temperature for 18-24 hours or at 140° F for 3 hours. After draining, boil or sprout:
   a. **Boiling** – a minimum of 15-minute boil is needed to break down lectins; do not use a slow cooker.
   b. **Ferment After Cooking** – you may add bacteria to cooked legumes (such as yogurt starter) and ferment a few days to produce enzymes and probiotics to support both digestion and gut flora. (note: fermenting prior to cooking can reduce anti-nutrients but the heat of cooking will destroy beneficial bacteria produced during fermentation).
   c. **Sprouting** – after soaking, simply keep the beans moist with access to air until they start to grow. A common method uses a large, open canning jar lined with a damp paper towel.

> **Hummus Bummer:** Hummus is made of ground chickpeas (garbanzo beans, a legume) and tahini (sesame seed paste). Since legumes are not Paleo-approved, try a creamy substitute made of soaked macadamia nuts, roasted soaked cashews, cauliflower, hearts of palm or artichoke hearts (recipes online). Blend your choice with olive oil, lemon juice, garlic and tahini. You may find these creamy substitutes are better than hummus!

Uniquely Problematic Legumes: Peanuts and Soy

Aside from the concerns with legumes in general, *peanut* and *soybean* products have additional hazards.

A. Peanut Problems

Because of the name, many people classify peanuts as nuts and don't realize that they are actually legumes.

- Unlike lectins in other legumes, peanut lectins are difficult to destroy by any cooking technique.
- Traditional preparation involves an 8+ hour salt-water boil, an unusual practice in western society.
- In agriculture practices, peanuts are frequently rotated with cotton, a textile crop which can be doused with chemical concentrations much higher than food crops. Chemical residues may remain in the soil and can be absorbed by peanuts (that grow underground) the following year.
- Peanuts often contain strains of mold which produce a toxin called *aflatoxin*.
  - ✓ Aflatoxin is one of the most carcinogenic toxins known and increases risk of liver cancer
  - ✓ FDA calls aflatoxin an "unavoidable contaminant" and allows concentrations of 20 parts per billion
  - ✓ Especially a concern for people with mold sensitivities
  - ✓ Aflatoxin increases if peanut crops are stored in warm, humid places where mold thrives
  - ✓ Grind-your-own peanut butter machines generally have high aflatoxin residues, unless they are thoroughly cleaned every day

> **Organic Peanut Products:** These do not have the same issues with chemical pesticide and herbicide residues as conventional peanut products. However, even in organic products, concerns remain about the lectin content from lack of traditional preparation methods as well as the presence of aflatoxin.

B. Soy Suspicions

There continue to be discrepancies in quality, safety and digestibility between traditionally-prepared, organic soy versus modern, industrially-processed soy (especially applicable to chemically-isolated products such as soy protein powders). If soy is added after the program, these concerns can be minimized by proper sourcing.

1. **Soy Phytoestrogens (Estrogen Disruptors)**
   - These plant-based compounds mimic the shape of human estrogen but cannot perform the functions of real estrogen. The body mistakenly believes it has enough estrogen for hormonal balance when it truly does not, leading to hormonal disruption.
   - These are associated with uterine tumors, infertility, male hypogonadism and erectile dysfunction.

2. **Anti-Nutrients in Soy**
   - Soy contains the highest levels of phytates of any grain or legume (more about Phytates in Prep E)
   - Soy anti-nutrients are very resistant to degradation and neutralization.
     - o Phytic acid in soy is *not* neutralized by soaking, sprouting or extended cooking.
   - Soy lectin agglutinates (clumps) red blood cells. Once the red blood cells clump together, they're permanently "stuck" and unable to distribute oxygen.

3. **Other Concerns with Soy**
   - The FDA has never given soy protein the GRAS status ("Generally Regarded As Safe").
   - Industrially-processed soy contains goitrogens which interfere with thyroid function.
   - 95% of the US soybean crop is genetically modified, creating unique digestive concerns (Day 24).
   - A common method to separate the protein and oil involves soaking soybeans in hexane (a solvent extracted from crude oil). The FDA does not require hexane residue testing.
   - Free glutamic acid (MSG) is formed during industrial soy processing (more about MSG on Day 20).
   - Modern processed soy foods contain high amounts of aluminum, a brain toxin.
   - Soy lecithin, an emulsifier, is a byproduct of soybean oil processing; although commonly used in even Paleo-friendly foods like dark chocolate, it's still a problematic form of soy.
   - Vitamin B12 analogs from soy are not absorbed, contributing to B12 deficiency.
   - Soybeans constitute a large portion of animal feed in the meat, eggs and dairy industry, subjecting humans to second-hand soy exposure from commercially-raised animal products.

4. Trans Fat in Soybean Oil

Soybean oil is *the number one source* of fat calories in America today. This fat comprises 10% of total calories in the U.S., despite only being available for the last century!

- Soybean oil is a highly inflammatory omega-6 fat (more about PUFAs on Day 3).
- Soybean oil inherently contains trans fat created during processing and heating (Day 4).
- Soy and its derivatives are present in nearly all processed food: salad dressings, mayonnaise, restaurant foods, baked goods, 'vegetable broth', dark chocolate, etc. Read labels!

Bottom Line: It's best to avoid all soy products including soybean oil, soy lecithin, soy sauce, soy protein, etc.

Is There a 'Safe' Soy?

Organic, fermented products including miso, natto, tempeh and soy sauce, are the best soy choices: organic practices ban GMOs and hexane extraction; fermentation neutralizes enzyme inhibitors and phytic acid; yet, thyroid inhibitors can remain intact. Find a soy company committed to using traditional preparation methods and non-aluminum processing equipment; Eden® Foods is one option. Use soy as a condiment, not a staple.

An Asian Anomaly: Soy is frequently used in Asian cuisine and some of the healthiest and longest-lived humans are of Asian descent. How can soy be so harmful?

- Traditional Asian soy foods are fermented, improving digestibility. Common western soy foods like soymilk, tofu, soy burgers, protein powders, have additives and are rarely fermented.
- The traditional Asian diet is based on bone broth and nose-to-tail eating patterns. Soy consumption is quite small when compared to these other highly nutritious Asian staples.
- Soybean oil, soy protein powder and other highly-processed soy products were never staple foods in the traditional Asian diet.

Bottom Line: The limited amount of fermented soy in traditional Asian diets is offset by the nutritional powerhouses of other Asian food staples. There is no reasonable way to compare this to modern use of soybean products – soy additives are in nearly every processed food!

Section II: Healthy Bowels

Some people find that their bowel function and characteristics change as the program progresses. Uncomfortable gas, constipation or diarrhea can indicate the digestive system hasn't yet adjusted to the influx of healthy Paleo foods. For most, bowel disruption is temporary and subsides as the body adjusts to the increase of abundant, bio-available nutrients and healthy fats.

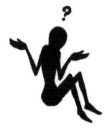

Is There Really a Perfect Poop?

Society has made 'poop' an uncomfortable four-letter word. Yet use of laxatives and stool softeners has become so common that constipation and troubled bowels are now accepted as normal. Though these are common, they're definitely not normal.

So what, exactly, is normal poop, the 'Goldilocks' of excrement? Not too soft, hard, lumpy, watery, skinny, thick, frequent, seldom, smelly, dense, loose, firm, dark, light, urgent, strenuous...but just right.

Your poop is about 75 percent water. The rest is a combination of fiber, bacteria, miscellaneous cells and mucus. The characteristics of your poop will tell you a great deal about how healthy your digestive tract is, everything from the color, odor, shape, size...even the sound it makes when it hits the water and whether it's a "sinker" or a "floater," is all relevant information. ~Sara Eye, Paleo Foundation

Perfect poop has a sausage or cigar shape with smooth sides. Healthy bowels should be emptied daily with minimal exertion and without extreme urgency. The color varies but should be *without* any visible food particles (which can indicate insufficient chewing or improperly digested vegetables).

Poop Chart		
Constipated	**Perfect**	**Diarrhea**
Hard, small clumps	Smooth and cylindrical	Watery, bits of undigested food
Difficult to pass	Little effort to pass	Difficult to hold in
Large diameter	½-1 inch diameter	Loose feathery pieces
Very dense – sinks like a rock	Medium density – sinks or floats	Irregular density – scattered in water

Stool Color Variations

Normal stool varies in color. Bile turns brown as it moves through the colon, so medium brown stool is common. However green stools can also be normal, especially in response to increased green vegetable intake.

- ***Persistent* greenish or yellowish stool** can indicate that the bile did not have enough time to turn brown and the contents are passing too quickly. See options below for slowing digestion by temporarily reducing fat intake or adding soluble fiber to bulk up the stool.
- **Pale gray or greasy stool** can indicate the absence of bile which inhibits the digestion of fats and fat-soluble vitamins. Stool with mucous (clear goopy or stringy substance) can indicate irritation inside the digestive tract. *If these traits persist*, medical attention is needed to rule out problems like clogged bile ducts, low stomach acidity or other digestive disorders.
- **Black stool** can indicate blood in the digestive tract – see a medical professional immediately.
- **Red color** can indicate blood, but this can also be caused by hemorrhoids or large amounts of beets or dark red cherries which will skew the color for a bowel movement or two. See your doctor if it does not dissipate.

Section III: Options to Encourage Healthy Stools

Since the Paleo Diet is drastically different from what most people are accustomed to eating, less than perfect stools are not uncommon during this transition for many reasons: decreased grains, increased fats, not enough vegetables, too much protein, detoxification effect on the system, etc. Eventually the body will regulate on its own, but until then, consider some digestive strategies. Any of the following suggestions can boost digestion, however, due to significant variations in bowel dysfunction, recommendations span the full spectrum of bowel irregularities. Select strategies that are pertinent to your situation and easy for you to incorporate.

1. Slow Down and Chew Longer

This may seem trivial but thorough chewing is the first step in the digestive process. It incorporates saliva and enzymes to start breaking down food and exposes more surface area for stomach acid and intestinal enzymes to target. This subsequently decreases the undigested food particle load on the intestines. Take smaller bites and chew each mouthful to a liquid consistency before swallowing.

2. Boost Digestion *Before* Meals

- **Ginger** – This root stimulates digestive enzymes and bile production which helps with fat digestion. Try freshly-grated root, powdered in capsules, or even a cup of ginger tea.
- **Apple Cider Vinegar (ACV)** – Take a swig of unpasteurized ACV with 'mother' 15-20 minutes before meals to stimulate enzyme production (the *mother* is the home for beneficial bacteria – product labels will designate if the mother is intact). It's fine to dilute ACV in water if it's too harsh to swallow straight.
- **Peppermint** – Available in fresh leaves, oil, tea or capsules (some products have enteric coating to protect the capsule from stomach acid, releasing the contents in the intestines).
- **Horseradish** – Find fresh or grated in the refrigerated grocery section as the shelf-stable products contain additives. Use this to flavor your meals, but know that too much can cause diarrhea.
- **Bitters** – Traditionally, a pre-dinner salad contained bitter greens to stimulate digestion. Either add some bitter greens to the first part of your meal (mustard greens, dandelion, kale, arugula, mizuna) or supplement with traditional liquid bitters. Angostura Bitters are available in liquor stores and you can try 1 tsp before *or* after meals to see which works better.

Living on the edge - that's what I feel like when I don't know what my bowels are going to do next.
~Jane Wilson-Howarth, author of <u>The Art of Staying Clean and Healthy While Traveling</u>

3. Soluble Fiber (more about Fiber on Day 15)

This type of fiber soothes the digestive tract. Though soluble fiber is abundant in fruits and vegetables, the following are acceptable Strict Paleo sources:

  a. **Roots and Hard Vegetables** – sweet potatoes, winter squash, carrots, pumpkin, beets, turnips, rutabagas, parsnips, radish
  b. **Unripe Fruit** – green banana, green plantain, green papaya and green mango
  c. **Some Ripe Fruit** – avocados, unsweetened applesauce (better than just apples)
  d. **Fermented Vegetables** – such as sauerkraut and kimchee (more on ferments on Day 21)
     <u>Note</u>: Even though foods like cabbage can cause gas, fermented versions contain digestive enzymes and beneficial bacteria that partially predigest the vegetable. Ferments are much easier on the digestive system than the raw forms for those who are sensitive to FODMAPs (see below). Regardless, there are some people who don't tolerate any ferments well.
  e. **Soluble Fiber 'Best Practice'** – Although there is not much scientific evidence for this suggestion, many people report feeling better if a soluble fiber is eaten first before other food is introduced into an empty stomach. For example, eat some veggies before indulging in the steak.

The way I see it, if you want the rainbow, you gotta put up with the rain. ~Dolly Parton

4. FODMAP Foods

Some individuals are sensitive to certain foods that can ferment in the digestive tract, collectively called FODMAPs (fermentable sugars and alcohols). Symptoms of sensitivity include excessive gas and other digestive troubles and is often referred to as Irritable Bowel Syndrome (IBS). This following list is not complete, but identifies Paleo-friendly foods that potentially trigger distress for those with IBS.

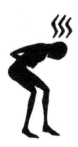

  a. Allium family (onion, garlic, shallot, leek)
  b. Brassica family (cabbage, broccoli, cauliflower, Brussels sprouts)
  c. Some nightshades (peppers, eggplant)
  d. Random other vegetables – asparagus, artichokes, okra, mustard greens, sunchokes (Jerusalem artichokes), beets, dandelion greens, mushrooms
  e. Some fruits – apples, apricot, blackberry, avocado, cherries, figs, mangoes, nectarines, peaches, pears, plums, watermelon
  f. Random spices – fennel, horseradish, wasabi, chicory
  g. Random nuts – pistachios, cashews

> If you suspect FODMAP sensitivity, limit the above foods for 3-8 weeks until the gut lining has a chance to heal. Eventually, try adding single foods back into your diet to determine which are tolerated well. To learn more about determining tolerance, see the Reintroduction Guidelines on Days 25 and 26.

5. Resistant Starch (this works like a fiber; more info on Day 15)

Certain *cooked and cooled* foods develop a compound called resistant starch (RS) which is beneficial for the digestive tract. RS is exactly what it says it is, starch that resists digestion and cannot be broken down into glucose (and therefore has no insulin response). Feel free to eat Paleo sources of RS such as *cooked and cooled* potatoes or plantains (after finishing the Strict Paleo Protocol, cooled rice is another source).

Some people get over-ambitious about RS and choose to supplement with potato starch which can initially cause diarrhea as the system regulates. At this point, let your system first adjust to the Paleo Diet and choose RS from *real food* sources (like potato salad) and hold off on resistant starch supplements.

If one's bowels move, one is happy; and if they don't move, one is unhappy. That is all there is to it.
~Lin Yutang (1895–1976)

6. Digestive Enzymes

Enzymes help break down food during digestion. Although the body produces its own enzymes, sometimes the quantity is insufficient for complete digestion. Additional enzymes can be acquired through foods or supplements.

    a. **Raw foods** – a gold mine of enzymes (<u>note</u>: cooking destroys many of them); incorporate as many low-sugar, raw foods as you can handle:

        i. Raw vegetables, fruits, sprouts

        ii. Raw sashimi, oysters on the half shell, ceviche, lox salmon, pickled herring or rare-cooked meats such as beef steak, tuna steak and liver

        iii. After the program, raw honey and high-sugar raw fruits can be introduced

    b. **Supplements**

        I. Digestive enzymes are found in health food and supplement stores. Follow the bottle directions.

        II. Professional-grade supplements are available online: Two high quality products by the company Pure Encapsulations are detailed in the 'My Picks' tab at PureRXO.com/Paleovation

          • *Digestive Enzymes Ultra*

          • *Digestive Enzymes with HCl* (which includes hydrochloric acid to increase acidity levels during meals; consult a physician before adding HCl if currently taking any prescription or over-the-counter anti-inflammatory medications as there can be contraindications).

7. Change Fat or Protein Proportions

During the Paleo transition, it is common (and healthy) to replace carbohydrate-heavy foods with more fat or more protein. Sometimes, too much added fat (especially coconut oil) will lubricate the system and contribute to diarrhea. At the same time, increased protein tends to cause constipation. Make temporary dietary adjustments to protein or fat intake to ease digestive discomfort, then slowly modify amounts over time. Do not shy away from the healthy fats – just give the body time to adjust.

8. Easily-Digested Foods

Consider increasing consumption of nutrient-rich, easily-digested foods such as cooked vegetables that you tolerate well (purees are gentle), soups/stews, fermented vegetables like raw sauerkraut, organ meats, avocados, gelatin or bone broth. It is okay to skim the fat off the broth if fat appears to be a trigger.

9. Increase Rest and Decrease Stress (Remember "Rest to Digest")

Stress and sleep are discussed at length later in the program, but at this point, just know that proper sleep allows the body time to heal as well as digest. Likewise, increased stress and sleep disruptions can manifest as physical symptoms, including digestive distress.

10. Probiotics

Supporting and populating the good gut bacteria is essential for optimal health. Abundant intestinal flora assists in digestion while producing fuel and nutrition for colon cells. Eliminating dietary sugar starves the bad gut bacteria; at the same time, friendly microbes can be fortified in a variety of ways (more about Gut Health and Probiotics on Day 21):

    a. Incorporate fermented foods such as kombucha, kimchee, raw sauerkraut and water kefir; after the program try dairy kefir or grass-fed yogurt.

    b. Supplement with a high quality probiotic containing 10-50 billion organisms per dose and in a capsule with enteric coating. This coating protects the contents from stomach acid and releases the digestive bacteria properly in the intestine. Refrigerated probiotic products tend to have better potency.

    c. Another type of probiotic supplement contains soil-based organisms (SBOs) from a healthy soil biome. Modern ultra-hygienic culture has reduced exposure to dirt and its associated healthy bacteria. These types of microbes naturally encapsulate in spores which offer stability at room temperatures. Search online for brands such as Prescript Assist® or MegaSpore®.

11. Proper Elimination Posture

Ancestrally, elimination occurred in a flat-footed squat position, but modern humans rarely squat for any occasion. When humans sit upright, bowel contents are retained through an involuntary muscular contraction. The squat position gently opens the pelvic area and relaxes the muscle that holds bowel closed (this doesn't efficiently occur in a seated position, it is specific to a squat).

If bowel movements take a lot of time *or* effort, consider purchasing or making a Squatty Potty® to align the body for proper elimination in the comfort of your own bathroom.

Further Reading

There is no one-size-fits-all solution to consistent healthy elimination. The following article contains numerous links that specifically address other potential digestive issues:

🖰 BalancedBites Healthy Digestion

To Do List:

- ❑ Optional Paleo Comfort Food to make by Day 10 – what are you making? _____
- ❑ Buy ingredients for your Cooking Assignment #3 Veggies as a Grain Substitute; try making this by Day 12

Coming Up Soon:

- An inner look at sedentary behavior
- Tips for effective lunch planning

Day 9

I take a vitamin every day. It's called a steak. ~Robert Duvall, from the movie, <u>Kicking and Screaming</u>

Today's Topics:

1. Paleo-Wise: FREE DAY
2. Planning Paleo-Friendly Lunches
3. Bring Awareness to Sedentary Behaviors
4. Observe Changes in the Body

Fast Fare – Finger Foods
♥ Carrot slices and olive tapenade
♥ Salami
♥ Radishes and green onions

Jot down the Paleo foods you're eating today. Use the 'notes' line to record new food ideas, obstacles, etc.

Meals: _____

Snacks: _____

Beverages: _____

Notes: _____

Section I – Paleo-Wise: FREE Day

With this break from Paleo-Wise reading, here are some ideas to fill your extra time:

- Review earlier topics
- Read a recommended article
- Search online for new Paleo foundation meal recipe – ideas in Prep B
- Grocery run – perhaps try a new grocer or specialty store
- Finish Cooking Assignment #3: prepare a veggie-as-a-grain recipe
- Make a new Paleo recipe (or make more of an established favorite)
- Cut or prepare veggies for the next few days
- Watch a food-oriented documentary – ideas on Day 5

Section II: Lunch Planning

Have you ever stared blankly into the open refrigerator not knowing what to eat for lunch? Here are a few simple ways to quickly pack a lunch and get out the door:

1. Pack dinner leftovers into single serve containers *every night*
2. Prepare a quickly made recipe (ideas below and in the Fast Fare table at the beginning of each chapter)
3. Keep grab-and-go items in the pantry and fridge
4. Use the Lunchbox Template below to generate ideas that meet the Veggie + Protein + Fat plan

Quick Lunch (also called the *Back-Up Plan* when there are no leftovers)
Always stock ingredients for favorite quickly-made recipes or easy grab-and-go items:

Quick Lunch Ideas	
☐ Tuna salad in red pepper halves	☐ Salami or deli meat and olives
☐ Individual guacamole cups and fresh cut veggies	☐ Salad greens
☐ Frozen pre-cooked tuna/salmon cakes	☐ Pre-cooked frozen burger
☐ Frozen leftovers	☐ Scrambled eggs
☐ Hard-boiled eggs and avocado mayo	☐ Jerky and freeze-dried berries

Lunchbox Template
The following template can easily be adapted to match personal preferences and modified over time as food tolerances are determined. Select one item from each category (or two or three from veggies!). It also includes an optional Fruits/Extras section which can remain blank if those are not regularly consumed foods. An example is provided, followed by a blank template to copy and write in your favorites. Printable copy available at
Paleovation.

LUNCHBOX TEMPLATE

Veggies	Proteins
Bell pepper strips	Deviled eggs
Cabbage wedges	Lunch meat
Buttered green beans	Tuna in a can
Cherry tomatoes	Pulled pork
Slaw	Ham
Potato salad	Liverwurst
Cauliflower rice	Breakfast sausage links
Carrot sticks	Bratwurst/hot dog
Roasted veggies	Tuna cakes
Mini bell peppers	Fried fish (with nut flour breading)
Sautéed broccoli	Meatloaf
Kale chips	Mini quiches (bacon wrapped muffins)
Seaweed wrapper	Sweet potato topped like a pizza
Seaweed flakes	Egg salad
Sweet potato puree	Tuna salad in romaine leaf wrappers
Paleo 'cream of broccoli' soup	Stir fry with cauli-rice
Sautéed greens	Meatza
Cauliflower hummus	BLT salad
Half a roasted squash	Meatballs
Marinated mushrooms	Hard-boiled eggs
Raw beet salad	Sardines in a can
Sugar snap peas	Lox rolled around cucumber strips and capers
Baba ganoush (eggplant spread)	Stuffed peppers
Salsa	Taco rolls (taco meat and veggies rolled and baked in cabbage leaves)
Gazpacho	

Fats	Fruit/Extras
Olives	Blackberries
Guacamole	Raspberries
Spreads/dips like olive tapenade	Strawberries
Nuts or nut butters	Cherries
Trail mix	Grapefruit
Spiced nuts	Almond meal crackers
Coconut flakes	Plantain crackers/chips
Coconut butter	Sweet potato chips
Cashew hummus	*Paleo 'breakfast cookie'
Add extra olive oil to entrée/veggies	*Paleo-friendly dessert
Seeds or seed butters	*Paleo banana bread
Pat of grass fed butter	*Fruit leather
Paleo mayo	*Applesauce or other high sugar fruits
	*Pureed fruit in a pouch

*For after the program

LUNCHBOX TEMPLATE

List your favorite foods in each category. Build a lunch by selecting a Veggie + Protein + Fat.

Veggies	Proteins

Fats	Fruit/Extras

Section III: Sedentary Behavior Awareness

The westernized environment is built around convenience and comfort like padded ergonomic seats in vehicles, plush recliners, memory foam and sleep number beds. Unfortunately, all these luxuries encourage inactivity and lounging. The following clichés fit: *A body at rest stays at rest. If you don't use it, you lose it.* Muscles, tendons and other connective tissues will atrophy with inactivity to the point that simple, functional movements such as balancing or bending can become a challenge.

You may already be developing neuromuscular compromises from sedentary behavior. Before discussing the topic of movement and exercise, some basics first need to be addressed. Try the following simple test to assess your present coordination level.

The Rising Test

The ability to stand up unassisted from a seated position may seem trivial, but this simple test measures the body's capacity for overall functional motion. *Your ability to rise unassisted correlates with your longevity*!

1. Start in a seated position
2. Raise both arms out in front of you
3. Stand up unassisted (it's okay to use one hand just for balance purposes)

My Rising Ability
Using one hand or less
☐ Tall stool
☐ Hard chair
☐ Soft chair/couch
☐ Floor (advanced)

Adjust the initial sitting depth to your current skill level – start at a higher seated elevation if your physical ability is limited. For very beginners, please be mindful of balance and use support as necessary. Progress to lower seats at your own rate. Feel free to mark your current level in the table to the right (it will be repeated later in this book for retest purposes).

> **Build Strength Faster:** Consciously incorporate unassisted standing every time you rise from sitting. To progress faster, each time you sit down, practice squatting *almost* to the chair and then stand up again. Repeat 3-5 times.

Practicing this skill will improve dexterity and full body coordination. Even if you passed the test at the most advanced level (from the floor), everyone can benefit from contemplating the degree of sedentary behaviors in their current lifestyles.

Why and How to Reduce Sedentary Positions

Prolonged sitting is linked to many health consequences including back and neck pain, poor posture, obesity, circulation complication and lymph compromise to name a few. Sometimes the culprit is habit linked to sitting – snacking on unhealthy food or extended sitting periods without taking a break to stand or stretch.

- 🖑 PaleoLeap Sitting Part 1: Myths and Truths about Sitting, Obesity and Chronic Disease
- 🖑 MarksDailyApple You Might Want to Sit Down for This

Nearly everyone can benefit from reducing sedentary behaviors. To better grasp how much sitting you do, list three sedentary items on tomorrow's agenda (*not including during meals**) and the length of time you typically allow. Examples include: in a vehicle, at a desk, watching TV, reading, at a movie or at a sporting event. Also note if you typically consume a non-Paleo snack during that time...be honest!

Typical Sitting Time				
Sedentary Task	**Time**	**Non-Paleo Snack?**		
1. _____	1. _____	1. Y	N	
2. _____	2. _____	2. Y	N	
3. _____	3. _____	3. Y	N	

* **Meals Aren't Included When Assessing Total Sit Time:** Proper digestion *requires* a calm, seated state. Remember, "rest and digest." During meals, please assume a relaxed upright position, chew thoroughly, enjoy your food and be grateful for the opportunity to nourish yourself.

Modifying Sitting Behaviors

As you consider the total sitting time for those three tasks, also consider how you might engage more muscle by assuming an alternate posture (ideas below). Even a random minute or two adds up over the course of the day. This is not about breaking a sweat, it's about asking your body to fully support itself on a more frequent basis. The two main goals are to *reduce total sitting time* and *break up prolonged periods* in a single position.

1. Start small. Begin with 1-5 minute increments. Even parking 30 seconds farther from a building adds a full minute of walking.
2. Alternatives to sedentary positions can include anything within your ability level: stand, balance, sway, forward fold, walk, hang, take the stairs, swing a leg, stretch, practice your golf swing, dance in place, hold a plank pose, roll a tennis ball under one foot, tip toe, squat against the wall, etc.
3. Plunging into movements unfamiliar to your body invites opportunity for injury. Modify sitting behaviors at your own pace and add more engaged actions over time.

NON-Sedentary Choices		
Sedentary Moments	**Gentle Alternative**	**More Engaged Action**
Read/listen to a book	Stand	Walk on a slow treadmill 1 ½ -2 mph
Talk on the phone	Pace around the room	Go outside for a brisk walk
Sit at a desk	Wiggle on a Disc-o-Sit® seat mold or use a standing desk	Flat-foot squat on the desk chair or invest in a treadmill desk
Watch TV	Balance on one foot	Standing stretches
Waiting rooms, meetings	Stand in the back	Invite colleagues on a walking meeting
Tie shoes	Sit down on the floor	Forward fold (bent knees is fine)
Brush teeth, wash hands	Stand on one foot	Balance on tip toes
Run errands	Park farther away	Park the car once, walk to several buildings
Fold clothes, chop vegetables	Work standing at a counter	Tip toe walk between tasks
Sit at the playground	Play catch	Hang from the monkey bars
Relieve yourself	Use a Squatty Potty® to elevate feet to a squat	Use a Squatty Potty® and actually hover above toilet seat (check weight limit, first)
Waiting for the microwave	Stretch	Do some countertop pushups

This topic sheds light on how easy it is to let sedentary behaviors dominate our daily lives, yet also demonstrates it is a conscious choice to include more physical activity. It is up to you to 'omit your sit' and preserve your body's functional movements. If you desire to devise a plan to reduce sedentary behaviors, please do that here:

1. How many sedentary minutes do you wish to replace each day? _____

2. List some tasks you plan to replace sitting/sedentary behavior (use the above chart for ideas).

   _____

3. How do you plan to incorporate more muscle engagement? (Can break it into intervals through the day):

   _____

Up for a Challenge? Try a Flat-Foot Squat
This ergonomic resting pose is used every day by toddlers and most of the developing world. Practicing this stance will improve mobility, balance and elimination. Though the intention is to stand with feet flat on the surface and bear the weight in the heels, many bodies have lost this physical capability over time. Modify the squat by adding a lift under the heels, widening the stance, using a wall for support, etc.

More Ideas on the Resting Squat (direct links from ⏯ Paleovation):
⏯ TheShawnStevensonModel The Resting Squat – How Squatting Makes You More Human
⏯ YouTube: How to Restore your Squat uploaded by Original Strength (3 min)

Section IV: Noticing Changes in your Body

Have you noted any significant changes in your body since Day 1? It may still be a little early to notice, depending on your individual health and dietary background. However, scan the following list and check items that seem to be improving:

- ☐ Sounder sleep
- ☐ Less achy
- ☐ Less pain with an old injury
- ☐ Smoother joint movement
- ☐ Fewer headaches
- ☐ Steady energy levels

- ☐ Clearer skin
- ☐ Thinking clearly
- ☐ Lower blood pressure
- ☐ Better stools
- ☐ Easier digestion
- ☐ Less acid reflux

- ☐ Desire to be active
- ☐ Better performance
- ☐ Quicker exercise recovery times
- ☐ Improved range of motion
- ☐ Feel stronger
- ☐ Clothing fits better

Observations:

During the detox process, it is common to temporarily experience increased headaches, zits/blemishes, brain fog or fatigue (similar to symptoms of low-carb flu). These symptoms typically dissipate with a little more time on the Strict Paleo Protocol. If uncomfortable symptoms persist beyond the next few weeks, options to alter your dietary plan will be provided at the end of the month. For now, trust the process and just observe.

What are you happy to see improving?

_____

What seems to be stagnating at this point?

_____

Is there anything that seems to be worse now than when you started the program?

_____

What other improvements do you hope to see?

_____

Bowel Health

Are you taking action to encourage healthy digestion and bowel habits? Select the strategies you already incorporate (review yesterday's text for the specifics):

- ☐ Thorough chewing
- ☐ Digestive aids
- ☐ More soluble fiber

- ☐ Resistant starch foods
- ☐ Digestive enzymes
- ☐ Probiotics

- ☐ More bone broth
- ☐ Squatty Potty®

Is there anything else you plan on trying in the next few days?

1. _____

2. _____

To-Do List:

- ☐ Finish your optional Paleo Comfort Food by tomorrow
- ☐ Practice the Rising Test
- ☐ Try a new Veggie as a Grain recipe by Day 12

Coming Up Soon:

- Learn more about effective movement and exercise
- Discover how to entertain Paleo-style
- Did you accidentally go too low-carb?

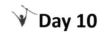 Day 10

Today's Topics:

1. Establishing a Paleo Groove
2. Paleo-Wise: Effective Movement, Exercise and Hydration
3. Have You Accidentally Gone Too Low-Carb?
4. How to Entertain a Crowd, Paleo-Style

Fast Fare – Grab and Go
♥ Jicama slices with salsa
♥ Hard-boiled eggs
♥ Snow peas

Section I: Establishing a Paleo Groove

It takes time to settle into a Paleo routine. In the beginning, each food item must actively be questioned and inspected to verify that it's grain and dairy-free. This skill gradually becomes second nature, plus the motivation to stay compliant improves as you discover what feeling good feels like. This lifestyle development is an ongoing process, so please take a few moments to recognize your accomplishments thus far.

Step 1: Favorite Paleo Foods – Keep foods you enjoy on hand.

What foods/recipes are becoming go-to Paleo favorites?

Breakfasts: _____

Lunches: _____

Dinners: _____

Snacks/Beverages: _____

Step 2: Identify Paleo Strategies – Continually examine which Paleo approaches work for you.

Paleo substitutes that are satisfying (Day 5):

1. _____
2. _____

Restaurant strategies that fit into your lifestyle (Prep D):

1. _____
2. _____

Ways you like to incorporate bone broth (Day 5):

1. _____
2. _____

Quick meals handy in a pinch (Days 1 and 4):

1. _____
2. _____

Snacks you like to keep on hand (Day 2):

1. _____
2. _____

Step 3: Acknowledge your Accomplishments – You have already come a long way!

What have been your biggest changes in eating habits since Day 1?

1. _____
2. _____

Section II – Paleo-Wise: Effective Movement and Exercise

Those who do not find time for exercise will have to find time for illness. ~Edward Smith-Stanley

Time to Move
Following Paleo principles and *eating the way we are built to eat* naturally generates significant health benefits. Unsurprisingly, *moving the way we are built to move* offers similar rewards.

We are designed to move. Movement is crucial for life, evidenced by the muscle atrophy that occurs with inactivity. Proper exercise improves quality of life, reduces risk of chronic disease and cultivates a lean, toned figure. Exercise and movement improve every aspect of health:

Benefits of Movement	
Structural, Functional and Hormonal	
Muscle – increases muscle mass, strength and endurance **Muscle control** – improves coordination, balance, reflexes and reduces risk of injury **Bones** – encourages bone remodeling for stronger, denser bones (especially with strength training) **Joints and Connective Tissue** – increases flexibility, stimulates maintenance/repair of joint cartilage **Weight Control** – more muscle mass increases metabolism, normalizes hormones that regulate hunger **Appearance** – decreased body fat, leaner physique **Posture** – strong core strength improves posture and minimizes ergonomic stresses **Cardiovascular / Circulation** – widens arteries, improves blood flow, strengthens heart muscle, lowers blood pressure and improves full body oxygenation **Anti-Inflammatory** – reduces *chronic* inflammation (despite short-term inflammation such as muscle soreness after a workout)	**Anti-Aging** – slows oxidative damage, strengthens skin and connective tissue (anti-wrinkle!), increases longevity **Digestion** – relieves constipation, reduces heartburn and bloating **Blood sugar levels** – increases insulin sensitivity, improves blood sugar regulation **Cholesterol** – raises HDL, lowers LDL and triglycerides **Healing** – faster and more efficient healing **Sleep** – establishes better circadian rhythms and cortisol cycles for proper sleep support **Mood** – pumps 'feel-good' endorphins into the body; increases levels of neurotransmitters (dopamine and serotonin); improves self-esteem; decreases stress, anxiety and depression (shown to have an outcome equal, if not superior, to the effect of SSRI medication) **Learning / Memory** – increases neurotransmitter receptors associated with learning

Further Reading: ⮐ PaleoFx 9 Hidden Health Benefits of Exercise

The Best Exercise
The best exercise is the one you'll do – which may change over time! Consistency is the key – plan to do *something* several times per week. Start by finding a combination of activities that are fun and enjoyable. There's no wrong way to incorporate exercise.

Sitting is the "New Smoking": While that's not exactly true, research does show that repeatedly spending prolonged hours sitting is detrimental to overall health. Sedentary job positions lead to muscle deconditioning, circulatory compromise, weight gain and loss of function. Changing postures through the day is highly recommended – get up and walk every 30-60 min (set a timer if you must). Even just standing to stretch is a vast improvement over maintaining a single idle position. Standing desks have become increasingly popular and are a viable option to reduce sitting time.

Lack of activity destroys the good condition of every human being, while movement and methodical physical exercise save it and preserve it. ~Plato

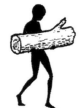

Natural Activities Create Natural Movements

Consider how we are designed to move. Our ancestors were naturally fit because their daily activities created an adequate balance of low, moderate and occasional high intensity movements. Some motions challenged the heart rate, others stimulated muscle development. This is true even with modern indigenous cultures.

Our recent ancestors would be shocked at how little activity our daily lives require with modern conveniences. Grocery stores, running water and automobiles have eliminated a wide range of daily physical activity such as farming, caring for livestock and storing provisions. Even the seemingly 'easy' activity of riding in a buggy required good posture, balance and core muscle engagement.

Laundry Was a Workout: It wasn't too many generations ago that manually washing laundry utilized every major muscle group: hauling water, washing, rinsing, cranking a wringer and hanging clothes outdoors.

How Would a Caveman Workout?

Analyzing early human activities displays a wide variety of full-body movements, some necessary every day and others only occasionally. We can use these concepts to construct a balanced modern workout.

Ancestral Movement Examples	
Motion	**Task**
Walking	Forage, find water, relocate, track prey
Hacking	Chop firewood, prepare food, build shelter, section a carcass, make tools/weapons
Climbing	Trees, rocks, dunes, mountains
Carrying	Water, children, logs, rocks, canoes
Sprinting	Escape, chase, play, race, hunt
Other	Paddle, balance, throw, dance, dig, grab, reach, drag, pound, pull, jump, spar, swim

Building a Better Workout

The goal is not to literally mimic ancestral behavior to become fit...that's impossible. The point is to develop a weekly routine that incorporates a wide variety of natural motions to varying degrees of intensity. Include some movements that *stimulate muscle growth* such as resistance/strength training and others that *target the heart rate* such as cardiovascular exercise.

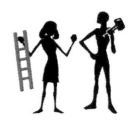

Implementing the combination of cardiovascular plus resistance training techniques provides phenomenal health advantages and quickly increases strength, coordination, balance, endurance, power and speed (plus everything else listed in the Benefits of Movement chart on the previous page). To stimulate ideas for your own personal plan, the chart on the next page offers a variety of movement examples with varying degrees of intensity. Many activities overlap categories. Also, notice the prominence of fun time outdoors...

The message: *Get outside and have a good time – exercise will naturally be part of many activities!*

The key to an effective exercise plan is finding the right balance of how much, how often and how intense to guarantee that you'll *stick with it*. Try whichever movements appeal to you, continually mix it up, sporadically challenge yourself, *rest and recover between sessions* and be amazed by what your body can do!

This approach results in workouts that are fun, engaging and full of variety to prevent boredom or burn out. Don't sweat the details; exercise doesn't have to be about graphs, schedules or beeping gadgets. Use the KISS principle...Keep It Simple Sweetheart!

It's also important to reject any feelings of compulsion, guilt or negativity about sub-par or missed workouts. ~Mark Sisson, author of Primal Endurance

Further Reading: ⌐ MarksDailyApple How to Personalize Primal Blueprint Fitness

Recipe for Full-Body Movement		
Movement Type	**Examples**	**Pointers**
1. Low Intensity Casual activities, gentle movements	Take a stroll, leisurely bike, golf, stand vs sit, stairs vs elevator, wade, fish, stretch, Tai Chi, garden, play catch	• As much as possible each day • Minimum of 2 hours per *week* (only 20-30 min/day, doesn't have to be all at once) • Much more is *much better*
2. More Intensity Activities that break a sweat; occasionally do these even faster or with more resistance	Brisk walk, hike, swim, housework, power yoga, play a sport, Pilates, yard work, dance, slack line, ski, martial arts, paddle, barre class, water aerobics, cardio machines like stair-climber or elliptical, rebounding, ride a horse, skate, bike hills, jog, active profession	• Rotate activities you enjoy • Make time for 2-3 sessions per week of moderate intensity exercise where heart rate is elevated, yet comfortable • As long as you let your body rest and recover *and* it doesn't contribute to injury, do as much moderate activity as you like • Add extra speed/weight about once a week
3. High Intensity Interval Training, also called HIIT (more below)	Jogging stairs, burpees, jump rope, mountain climbers, jump squats or any type of sprinting (run, bike, swim, jump, cardio machine)	• Speed does not matter, go *your* max effort for 20-30 seconds • Recover between sets, ~ 60-90 seconds • Try 5-10 minutes each week - that's all!
4. Strength Training Use body weight, free weights or machines (details next page)	Plank, squat, pushup, pullup, row, deadlift, bench press, curl, crunch	• Okay to start with body weight or supported versions (knees down pushups) • Add free weights or machines as you improve (weighted vest, kettlebells)
<u>Muscle-Building Tip</u>: Complete the movement in a 'slow & controlled' manner on *both* the contraction *and* release.		• Make time for 1-3 sessions per week • Consider consulting a personal trainer

 ### HIIT It – Interval Training

High-Intensity Interval Training (HIIT) is the fastest way to get into shape, stay in shape and burn body fat. HIIT alternates short bursts of very intense movement with short rest periods – heart rate quickly rises then drops with only a short recovery time before repeating. This creates a cortisol/adrenaline rush-and-release cycle which stimulates hormones that promote muscle growth, bone integrity and arterial strength. Short HIIT workouts are completed in just 5-12 minutes and only need to be done once per week. Weight-loss bonus: the full-out effort creates an extended calorie-burn for up to 72 hours after the workout!!!

HIIT is a natural way to move – just watch children playing outside: they'll often cover a mile or two running but rarely more than 30-40 yards at a time. Interval training can be incorporated into many activities – even most cardio machines have built-in interval settings.

Search HIIT Videos and Workouts Online:
- PaleoHacks 10 Effective HIIT Workouts
- YouTube HIIT by BodyRock (many videos, the *Daily HIIT Show* is a series)
- YouTube Tabata videos (20 seconds exercise, 10 seconds rest – for 8 minutes; paced by music)

> *That which is used - develops. That which is not used wastes away.* ~Hippocrates

Increase Muscle, Decrease Size
Muscle is desirable – it uses more energy, even at rest, which encourages weight loss and creates a tighter, defined and more athletic physique. If the goal is to be a smaller size, building muscle should be the primary focus, not just dropping pounds.

> **Muscle Mass Paradox**: A person can *reduce* body size by *increasing* their muscle mass, even though they may weigh the same (or more!) than when they began. DeuceGym Deb's Story

Everyone has heard the cliché, "Muscle weighs more than fat." To many women, that simply creates a fear of building muscle – after all, few modern women want to weigh more. Muscle is indeed, denser than fat, but the key point is *muscle takes up less than half the space of fat!* Developed muscle equates to smaller circumference. For those women who still fear "bulking up," that's impossible because women lack the testosterone necessary for "bulking" – the female result is tight, defined muscle.

> **Paleo Advantage:** By reducing starches and other inflammatory foods in the diet, the body is naturally directed toward burning fat to feed muscle. This is magnified further with even a small amount of strength training!

Strength Training / Resistance Exercise

Strength training is the "fountain of youth" in exercise terms – it affects expression of at least 30 genes that slow the aging process! Muscle is built via strength or resistance exercise. In the past, these exercises were primarily used by athletes to enhance performance and muscle size. However, strength training is now recognized as critical to *everyone's* health and fitness regardless of gender, age or ability.

Strength training involves developing muscle by using weight to generate resistance. Anything that provides an opposing force can do the job – elastic bands, dumbbells, kettlebells, gym machines, a heavy backpack, plastic jugs filled with sand/water or even your own body weight.

Strength Training Exercise Examples	
Chest	Push-ups, bench presses, chest flies
Back	Rows, pull-downs, pull-ups, back extension
Shoulders / Arms	Overhead presses, curls, lateral raises, front raises, upright rows, shoulder rotation (for rotator cuff)
Lower Body	Squats, lunges, leg extensions, hamstring curls, step ups
Abdominals	Crunches, knee tucks, woodchops, planks
Full Body	Planks, squats

A Few Basic Strength Training Guidelines:

1. Pay attention to posture – stand/sit up straight; maintain good form during the exercise. Engage your abs (tighten your core) through the entire movement to protect your spine and improve balance (more about Posture on Day 17).
2. Lift *and lower* weights 'slow and controlled' through the full range of motion, maintaining good form.
3. Breathe! Do not hold your breath.
4. Muscles adapt to resistance over time by getting stronger! Regularly increase intensity by adjusting the amount of weight lifted and/or the number of repetitions (a natural sustainable "maximum" develops with consistency)
5. The last repetition should be uncomfortable but without compromising form (rep recommendations vary between 8-20 repetitions).
6. Rest days are just as important as workout days. Muscles need time to recover and develop. Avoid working the same muscle group two days in a row.
7. Prepare for soreness. Muscles get stressed with resistance training and will be sore while they rebuild stronger. Residual effects of strength training can last up to 72 hours (including the fat-burning effects)!

How to Get Started with Strength Training

Join a fitness center, consult a personal trainer, buy home workout videos, get a fitness app, research YouTube videos, visit the library or find a CrossFit gym – the CrossFit community is closely tied to Paleo principles.

    🖑 BuiltLean 7 Primal Movement Patterns for Full Body Strength
    🖑 PaleoFx Lift Heavy Things: How and Why to Start Strength Training

Tips to Increase Muscle and Decrease Fat (Body Composition)

Body composition compares the proportion of body fat to lean mass (muscle, bone, etc). To create a leaner composition, fat-burning metabolism must be stimulated. These workout strategies assist with that goal:

1. Workout in the morning before breakfast. The body is already in a fat-burning mode because glucose and glycogen supplies are depleted from the overnight fast.
2. To fuel an intense workout and stay in fat-burning mode, use MCT oil pre-workout and skip the carbs.
3. Incorporate strength training with cardio exercise goals – building strength also builds endurance.
4. If you use exercise machines, use the interval program to avoid chronic cardio drawbacks (more below).
5. The body is extra sensitive to food for about an hour after a workout and will naturally shuttle more nutrients into muscle for repair and growth (versus into fat for storage). After exercising, refuel your body with protein and starchy vegetables, such as chicken and sweet potatoes.
6. Allow proper recovery time between workouts to repair and build muscle. Continual stressful workouts can stimulate cortisol which will undo your hard work: excess cortisol signals the body to break down muscle for fuel and retain body fat (more on Cortisol consequences on Day 11).

   🖑 <u>Whole9life</u> Are You Recovering, or Are You Just Resting?

Conventional Cardio Alone Doesn't Work

Cardio exercise certainly offers health benefits such as strengthening the heart muscle. However, most people think that to achieve fitness goals, they must suffer through extended, grueling cardio workouts. Unfortunately, what most fail to realize is that there's a point when too much cardio exercise will not only fail to produce better results, but will actually *worsen* physical conditioning.

Myth: If walking is good, jogging is better; and if 5K is beneficial, then a half or full marathon must be great!

The problem is that long-term cardio exercise (too much, too often) does not allow time for the body to rest, recover or rebuild. This is neither healthy nor sustainable. At some point, cardio *benefits* transform into *stressors*. This point of diminishing returns is termed *chronic cardio* and that, too, varies between individuals.

> **Key Point:** Just because some exercise is good for us, doesn't mean more is better!

Chronic cardio can include any activity done on a regular basis that maintains a steady, elevated heart rate for an extended period of time (jogging, biking, stair climbers, treadmills, elliptical machines). Generally, a cardio session should last between 30-90 minutes, depending on one's stamina and fitness level. Periodically including longer cardio workouts is beneficial, but health risks arise when frequency and length of those long cardio workouts fail to decline.

How Much is Too Much Cardio?

What might be too much for one person is perfectly fine for another. What might be excessive for a beginner could be perfect a year later. The tipping point when a healthy amount of cardio exercise becomes too much depends on multiple individual factors:

- Exercise intensity and frequency
- Fitness level
- Age
- Health status
- Daily activity level
- Quantity and quality of diet
- Quantity and quality of sleep
- Fitness goals

The vast majority of people who exercise sensibly and recreationally will not fall into problems of "too much" exercise. Competitive exercisers, especially those who train for endurance events (like Ironman triathlons, ultra-marathons, century bike rides or multiple marathons in a year) are at a greater risk of developing complications such as chronic tendonitis, damaged joints and muscle wasting from too much exercise.

How Over-Exercising Causes Bodily Harm

Building heart rate endurance is great – it cues the body to strengthen muscles, including the heart. However once *sustain-mode* is reached, the body adapts to that condition and no longer cues additional muscle development. Instead, the body interprets the sustained, elevated heart rate as a stressful event that must be endured (Why is this bear still chasing me?)! Unwanted stress hormones like cortisol are triggered and transform any advantages of the exercise into major body stressors (more about Cortisol on Days 11 and 12).

> *If you don't have answers to your problems after a 4-hour run, you ain't getting them.* ~Christopher McDougal

Chronic cardio forces the body to maintain fight-or-flight mode due to elevated cortisol. This causes free radical damage, systemic inflammation and muscle *breakdown*! On top of the increased stress from the exercise itself, a high-carb diet (often implemented to sustain chronic cardio) further harms the body by raising insulin levels.

Symptoms of Chronic Cardio		
✓ Increased joint pain	✓ Stress-inducing rather than stress-relieving	✓ Systemic body inflammation
✓ Chronic injuries		✓ Excess cortisol triggers insulin and fat storage
✓ Fatigue	✓ Workouts become less effective over time	
✓ Muscle wasting		✓ Lack of motivation
✓ Insomnia	✓ Accelerated aging	✓ Thyroid and adrenal burnout

Further Reading: ⌁ BenGreenfieldFitness Top 10 Reasons Exercise is Bad for You
⌁ PaleoForWomen Do You Exercise Too Much?
⌁ ChrisKresser Why You May Need to Exercise Less

A Warning About Chronic Anything! Many health-conscious people develop addictions to working out – training hours upon hours, yet ignoring recovery time. This leads to chronic cardio, chronic weight-lifting or even chronic yoga. If you love training and are not ready to slow down, consider this advice: ⌁ Whole30 It's Nothing Personal

---

What You Eat Creates Your Physique

To fuel a workout, the body first uses glucose from diet, then stored glycogen. However, after a short time those supplies are depleted, leaving only two possibilities for fuel – *entirely dependent on the individual's diet*:

1. **Burn Body Fat for Fuel:** The fat-adapted metabolism is achieved via a Paleo or low-carb diet. The body regularly switches to burning fat for energy when glucose is not present.
2. **Break Down Muscle Protein to Produce Glucose:** Sugar-burner metabolism results from a high carb (low-fat) diet. The body only burns glucose so muscle is sacrificed while fat is preserved.

Key Point: Exercising does *not* teach the body to burn fat – *only diet does that* (by eliminating sugar/starches)!

Due to the effects of insulin, eating a high-carb (low-fat) diet increases the risk that muscle will be *lost, not built*. When long endurance workouts are added, weight loss may happen but not just fat is lost – muscle is lost too! The result: a transformation from big-and-jiggly into small-and-jiggly (often referred to as "skinny fat").

Furthermore, extended cardio workouts reinforce the sugar burner's craving for more carbohydrates (glucose to refuel). No matter how hard a person tries to outrun a bad diet, they continually have to run farther *and* faster to stay ahead of it. Futility eventually sets in. The urge to refuel with carbohydrates creates a difficult willpower battle and any weight lost is often regained (read more about Fat-Burner versus Sugar-Burner in Prep G).

Exercise Results: Chronic cardio workouts do not deliver as promised in the long run. Fitness is not about exercising longer and harder…it's about exercising *and eating* smarter!

📖 *The Art and Science of Low Carbohydrate Performance* by Stephen Phinney and Jeff Volek
- Mark Sisson, former world-class marathoner, has visited this topic more than once:
    - ⌁ MarksDailyApple The Evidence Continues to Mount Against Chronic Cardio
    - 📖 *Primal Endurance*, details specific strategies for low-carb athletes

Stay Hydrated

The universal hydration rule is to drink 8 glasses of water per day regardless of the body's thirst signals. Though we absolutely need adequate water, conventional wisdom has over-simplified water need. For some people, 8 glasses of water is revitalizing but others may feel like that amount must be forced down. The amount of water necessary for each individual varies with age, body size, level of physical activity, altitude, tendency to sweat, humidity levels, current medications and even the amount of caffeine or alcohol in the diet.

> **Bottom Line**: If you feel low on water, drink more but do not force yourself to consume an arbitrary amount. As a benchmark, the urine of a well-hydrated body is light yellow, while a deep yellow color is normally a sign of insufficient hydration.
>
> ⌐ ClevelandClinic What the Color of Your Urine Says About You

> **Paleo Advantage:** Paleo eaters naturally consume a significant amount of water simply through dietary staples including abundant vegetables and bone broth.

Electrolytes

Electrolytes are mineral salts that dissolve in body fluids and carry an electrical charge. They are used to transfer impulses involved in many bodily functions; but in the context of exercise, the primary roles of electrolytes are body temperature regulation and muscle contraction/relaxation. Sodium, potassium and magnesium are discussed here but calcium and several other minerals are also involved.

Role of Sodium (keep in mind that table salt is *sodium chloride*)

1. **Digestion**
   a. Sodium activates the first enzyme in the mouth, salivary amylase, to break starch into sugar.
   b. Hydrochloric acid (HCl) is produced in the stomach with the chloride part of salt (sodium *chloride*), crucial for all digestion. With insufficient dietary salt (like the low-salt diet advice), production of hydrochloric acid suffers and low stomach acid can result, contributing to symptoms like bloating, belching or even heartburn (enzyme and HCl supplements discussed on Day 8).
   c. Sodium aids in the release of digestive secretions from the gallbladder and pancreas including digestive enzymes and bile.
   d. Sodium neutralizes acidity of foodstuffs in the intestine – the sodium part of *sodium* chloride is used to produce alkaline *sodium* bicarbonate to balance the acidic contents released from the stomach.
2. **Water Regulation** – Water follows sodium: excess dietary sodium causes water retention and loss of sodium (through urine or sweat) results in water loss, risking dehydration.

Salt Needs Change in a Low-Carb Diet

Even the term 'carbo-hydrate' clearly shows that water (hydrate) is linked to carbs. The mainstream advice to restrict sodium is based on a *high*-carb (low-fat) diet which includes associated water retention. However, when sugar and starchy carbohydrates are restricted in the diet as they are with Paleo, there's a diuretic effect as the body changes from retaining both water and salt to discarding them. That's the reason many people lose 4-5 pounds of water weight during the first week of a lower carb diet – and also why it's important to consume enough natural dietary salt while the body is acclimating.

> **Blood Pressure Caution:** With Paleo, the diuretic effect of restricting carbs plus removing heavily-salted processed foods will reduce sodium reservoirs significantly and may affect blood pressure. If you have blood pressure concerns, it's best to monitor it closely (use a cuff) as you change diet and exercise patterns.

Sodium Depletion

Blood is the primary reservoir for sodium. Water follows sodium. If too much salt is lost too fast through urine or sweat, water volume in the blood will drop, compromising circulation and other metabolic functions:

1. **Low Blood Pressure** – Low sodium can contribute to lightheadedness when standing up quickly or fatigue with exertion. If blood volume drops too much, fainting results.

2. **Potassium Deficiency** – Potassium is an electrolyte that works together with sodium to ensure proper fluid balance in the body's cells and blood. When sodium and blood volume drop too low, the kidneys overreact to retain sodium by sacrificing potassium. Because potassium plays a role with building muscle, the resulting potassium depletion can contribute to loss of muscle mass as well as headaches, fatigue and fainting.

   ⤶ PaleoLeap Sodium, Potassium and Paleo

Excessive Sweating

To regulate body temperature in hot conditions, a salty sweat is formed for its cooling effect during evaporation. The primary mineral in sweat is sodium, so both sodium and water are drawn out of the blood when sweat is produced. In cases of excessive sweating, this lowers blood volume (resulting in low blood pressure) and introduces the risk of accelerated mineral losses and deficiencies. Extreme sweating may occur during vigorous exercise, movement in humid conditions and extended exposure to heat as in a sauna or hot tub.

> **Key Point:** If your exercise routine includes significant sweat loss, and/or your version of Paleo is very low carb, be sure to rehydrate with water *and* include sufficient sodium in your diet.

Under normal exercise conditions rehydrating with water is often enough to replenish the blood volume. However, lower-carb diets are a special case – it may also be necessary to replace sodium supplies due to the increased metabolic need for salt. During the transition period, pay attention to hydration levels and salt intake.

When you have sugar cravings, try some sea salt. You may actually be craving minerals! Kim Millman, MD

Muscle Cramps from Magnesium Deficiency

Excessive sweating can lower magnesium stores, although it's a longer-term depletion process than sodium. Magnesium mainly exists in muscles and bones where it assists with muscle *relaxation*. Because magnesium calms muscles, depletion causes muscles to get 'twitchy.' With further stress from exercise, sleep deprivation or poor diet, the twitchiness becomes a cramp.

Magnesium is an effective treatment for muscle cramps and can be applied in the form of topical magnesium oil, Epsom salt soak or oral supplementation (caution: too much magnesium too fast has a laxative effect). It takes time to replenish magnesium reserves and regular dietary inclusion thereafter is necessary to maintain levels.

Electrolyte Replacement

For most people following the Paleo Diet, all that's necessary for electrolyte replenishment is a diverse diet. Simple real-food sources of a few key minerals like sodium, potassium and magnesium ensure sufficient electrolyte reserves. Here are several dietary options:

1. **Quality Salt** – Celtic Sea Salt, Himalayan Sea Salt or Real Salt are a great source of all necessary electrolytes and trace minerals, whereas table salt only provides sodium. When eating Paleo (especially lower carb versions), choose a high-quality salt and use the salt shaker guilt-free.
2. **Vegetables** – Steam veggies rather than boil because minerals are lost in the water – or save the water for other cooking purposes like a vegetable purée or soup base.
   a. **Magnesium** – it's the mineral in chlorophyll – the greener the veggie, the higher the magnesium
   b. **Potassium** – found in dark green vegetables, cruciferous vegetables (broccoli, cauliflower, Brussels sprouts), many orange vegetables (carrots, squash, sweet potatoes) and baked potato with skin.
3. **Nuts and Seeds** – almonds, walnuts, pumpkin seeds, pistachios, cashews, pine nuts, sunflower seeds
4. **Meat and Seafood** – Meat is one of the best sources of both potassium and magnesium; better seafood sources include sockeye salmon and halibut. However, minerals are lost in drippings when cooked. Capture the drippings and add them back as sauce/gravy or save for making bone broth.

> **Bone Broth Electrolytes** – Surprisingly *plain* bone broth is low in mineral content. To enhance the electrolyte content of homemade broth, use a quality salt, include vegetables (keep a bag of stems and peels in the freezer until you're ready to make a batch) and add reserved meat drippings.

Sports Drinks

Effective sports-drink marketing campaigns claim the best way to replenish electrolytes is by drinking their product – which is loaded with sugar, artificial colors and preservatives. Unfortunately, solving one problem by creating another is not a real solution. Special formulas, chemical additives and refined sugars are not necessary to replace electrolytes. And, unless you're a serious endurance athlete, there's no need to add sugar to electrolyte replacement. The chart to the right lists sugar-free options.

Electrolytes *without the Sugar*

Rehydrate with pure, clean water plus one or more:
  ✓ Dissolved pinch of sea salt
  ✓ Bone broth
  ✓ Coconut water
  ✓ Juice from fermented vegetables like homemade sauerkraut
  ✓ Kombucha

  🖐 WellnessMama Natural Sports Drink
  🖐 FoodBabe Secret Behind Gatorade How to Replenish Electrolytes Naturally

Section III: Have You Accidentally Gone Too-Low Carb?

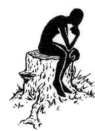

When implementing the Strict Paleo Protocol, some people accidentally go too-low carb by not incorporating enough vegetables. Half of your plate should be vegetables! Though Paleo is certainly lower carb than conventional modern diets, it doesn't need to be 'very low carb.' Carbohydrates from *non-starchy* vegetables do not trigger insulin and can be eaten in unlimited quantities (they are the base of the Paleo pyramid – review Prep B). Carbs from most *starchy* vegetables stimulate only small amounts of insulin at a slow pace (with the exception of white/yellow/red potatoes). Not all carbs are bad – it's the source that matters.

Individuals vary in their carbohydrate needs and the Paleo template provides approximately 50-150 g/day (don't worry, you won't have to count carbs!). If your diet is on the lower end of that range *and* low-carb flu symptoms are not improving by this point, you may feel better by incorporating more carbohydrates from Paleo sources. Are any of these symptoms failing to improve?

☐ Extremely low energy   ☐ Light-headedness
☐ Shakiness   ☐ Muscle fatigue
☐ Dizziness   ☐ Muscle weakness
☐ Difficulty in completing a regular workout   ☐ Nausea

Do you feel like you need more carbohydrates?   Yes   No

Paleo-Approved Carbohydrates

It is completely acceptable to eat more carbohydrates from starchy vegetables. Generally, athletes, larger men and individuals with higher metabolisms can easily metabolize extra vegetable-based starches. For those who want to lose weight, omit white potatoes.

A. Starchy Fruit and Vegetables Examples:

☐ Beets	☐ Taro	☐ Cassava	☐ Butternut squash
☐ Carrots	☐ Jicama	☐ Chestnuts	☐ Acorn squash
☐ Parsnip	☐ Green apple	☐ Eggplant	☐ Spaghetti squash
☐ Rutabaga	☐ Plantain	☐ Onion	☐ Sweet potato/yam
☐ Turnip	☐ Zucchini	☐ Sweet peppers	☐ Low-sugar fruits (still 1 serving daily)
☐ Pumpkin	☐ Kohlrabi	☐ Green banana	☐ Red, yellow, white, gold potatoes

B. Some Higher-Carb Paleo Recipe Ideas:

☐ Butternut squash soup	☐ Plantain chips	☐ Green apples sautéed in coconut oil
☐ Roasted acorn squash	☐ Roasted chestnuts	☐ Caramelized onions and peppers
☐ Pumpkin pancakes	☐ Homemade taro fries	☐ Paleo-friendly smoothie (Day 12)
☐ Paleo carrot muffins	☐ Grated carrot and jicama slaw	☐ Roasted beets and sweet potatoes
☐ Sweet potato puree	☐ Fried plantains with cinnamon	

Bonus: 🖐 FastPaleo Sugar Detox Carrot Cupcake (please don't eat all 12 muffins in one sitting)

Section IV: Paleo Entertaining Ideas

It can be a challenge to preserve Paleo principles when preparing food for a large group, especially if they are not on board with the Paleo Diet. It just takes a little forethought when cooking for a crowd. Do not stress over a menu – guests will love these crowd-pleasing foods! Circle or highlight those that interest you.

Finger Food Picnic or Hors D'oeuvres Party:

- Cured Meats
- Deviled Eggs
- Fresh Cut Veggies
- Olives
- Tapenades
- Cashew Hummus
- Pickles
- Guacamole
- Lox Salmon
- Paleo Chicken Fingers
- Fresh Fruit on Skewers
- Buffalo Wings
- Paleo Dessert
- Roasted, Seasoned Nuts
- Mini-Paleo Muffins
- Almond Meal Crackers
- Pizza-Stuffed Mushroom Caps
- Bacon-Wrapped Figs
- Chips cooked in Coconut Oil
- Almond Butter and Apple Slices
- Trail Mix
- Plantain Crackers
- Meat Satay (marinated and skewered; bake or grill)

Potluck Dishes:

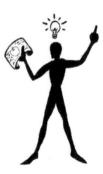

- Beef and Veggie Chili
- Butternut Squash Lasagna
- Meatballs and Zoodles
- Chicken Wings
- Broccoli and Bacon Salad
- Paleo Potato Salad
- Stir-fry with Cauliflower Rice
- Paleo Veggie Chips
- Butternut Squash Soup
- Sweet Potato Puree
- Pulled Pork
- Roasted Root Vegetables
- Meatloaf and Mashed Sweet Potatoes
- Peach and Avocado Salsa

Paleo Grill Out:

Meats

- Wings / Drumskicks
- Pork Chops / Lamb Chops
- Sausages or Hot Dogs
- Lobster Tails
- Scallops or Shrimp Skewers
- Oyster Roast
- Ribs
- Steak
- Fish Filets / Tuna Steak
- Burgers and Assorted Toppings
- Cedar Plank Salmon
- Bacon-Wrapped Meats
- Marinated Chicken Thighs

Veggies and Fruits

- Kebabs (large assortment of bite-sized colorful veggies + cubed steak, pork, shrimp, chicken, etc + maybe a fruit like pineapple or watermelon)
- Vegetables, Garlic and Butter in Foil Packets
- Portabella Mushroom Caps
- Marinated Eggplant Slices
- Grilled Cabbage Wedges or Napa Cabbage Leaves
- Asparagus Spears
- Leeks, Zucchini, Bell Peppers or Sweet Potato Slices (slice length-wise and brush with olive oil)
- Grilled Peaches, Pears or Pineapple Rings
- Ripe Banana Chunks (skewer and toast like a marshmallow...the taste is oddly similar!)

Vegetarian Brunch:

- Veggie Frittata
- Banana / Coconut Faux-meal
- Paleo Muffins
- Pumpkin Waffles
- Cinnamon-Toasted Nuts
- Squash Soufflé
- Roasted Beet Salad
- Paleo Granola and Almond Milk
- Asparagus and Paleo hollandaise Sweet Potato Hashbrowns
- Paleo Pumpkin or Banana Bread
- Fruit Salad
- Dark Chocolate-Dipped Strawberries

Family-Friendly Dinner Ideas

Kids especially love colorful foods *and* building their own meal. If you serve buffet style, simply include non-Paleo foods for the guests (buns, tortilla chips, cheese, sour cream) and omit when building your plate. Easy!

- Taco Bar, Burger Bar, Baked Potato Bar, Nachos Bar, Salad Bar
- Sushi Bar – nori seaweed wrappers with fillings like cauliflower rice, veggies, sushi fish or cooked shrimp
- Sandwich Wrap Bar (place toppings in a butter lettuce, romaine leaf or even a coconut wrap)
- Noodle Bar – Top zucchini noodles, spaghetti squash or sautéed pepper strips with sauces like marinara, Paleo pesto (omit cheese), garlic oil, veggies, bacon bits, sweet potato soup, coconut cream sauce, etc
- Soup Bar – provide the bone broth base and top with meat bits, sautéed veggies, caramelized onion, scallions, fresh herbs, bacon, baby shrimp, coconut milk, fried egg pieces, hot sauce, etc
- Paleo Pizza Bar – crust can be made of meat/bacon, cauliflower, portabella mushrooms, sweet potato, almond meal or coconut flour; precook individual crusts and have guests top theirs how they like
- Rainbow Salad (diced colorful veggies and olives tossed with dressing; the more colors, the prettier it is)
- Eggs fried in a pepper ring (sunny-side up eggs look like flowers)

Jot it Down

Look over the lists above. Circle, star or highlight a few crowd-pleasing ideas that appeal to you, or write down your own favorite entertaining ideas here:

_____

_____

To-Do List:

☐ Cooking Assignment #3: Using a Veggie as a Grain – what will you make by Day 12?

_____

☐ Thinking ahead: Information for Cooking Assignment #4 in tomorrow's text, Jerky *or* Paleo Granola. Choose one (or both). Consider what you'd like to make based on ingredients and supplies you need.
  1. **Jerky in the Oven or Food Dehydrator**
     - Lean ground meat: lamb, beef, pork, turkey, bison – for jerky, the leaner the better
     - Coconut aminos, parchment paper, seasonings; baking sheet or food dehydrator
  2. **Paleo Nut and Seed Granola**
     - Variety of nuts/seeds such as pecans, walnuts, macadamias, hazelnuts, sliced/slivered almonds, cashews, pumpkin seeds, sunflower seeds, etc
     - Oil of choice like coconut, avocado, grass-fed butter; seasonings such as pumpkin pie spice, cinnamon, nutmeg, cloves, salt, hint of cayenne; dried coconut flakes; baking sheets

☐ Anything else (thoughts on hydration, movement, non-sedentary time)?

Coming Up Soon:

- Days 11 and 12 discuss the stress hormone, cortisol, and strategies to lessen its negative effects

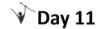

Day 11

Living a healthy lifestyle will only deprive you of poor health, lethargy, and fat. ~ Jill Johnson

Today's Topics:

1. Paleo-Wise: Cortisol Part I, the Stress Hormone
2. Recognizing Personal Stress Symptoms
3. Cooking Assignment #4: Jerky or Granola

Fast Fare – Order Out
♥ Order burrito bowl – double meats, lots of veggies and guacamole (no rice, beans, cheese, sour cream)

What foods are you enjoying the most?

Meals: _____

Grab-n-go: _____

Beverages: _____

Check off the following batch-cooking items you have already incorporated:

- ☐ Meatloaf/meatballs
- ☐ Roasted veggies
- ☐ Bacon
- ☐ Salmon or tuna cakes
- ☐ Fajita steak/chicken & veg
- ☐ Mason® jar salads
- ☐ Roast beef, pot roast

- ☐ Stew, soup, chowder
- ☐ Meatza (Paleo pizza)
- ☐ Paleo pumpkin pancakes
- ☐ Egg salad
- ☐ Paleo unsweetened muffins
- ☐ Pulled pork
- ☐ Taco meat

- ☐ Burgers
- ☐ Whole roasted chicken
- ☐ Shredded beef
- ☐ Tuna salad
- ☐ Chili
- ☐ Nut/seed granola
- ☐ Baked salmon

Has batch-cooking helped you to stay on track?   Yes   No

Have the foundation meals and cooking assignment recipes helped to set up a Paleo meal routine?   Yes   No

It is worthwhile to pinpoint Paleo habits that fit your lifestyle. Please use them to cultivate your Paleo groove. Go back and look over your first 10 days of Paleo eating. Identify two similarities in foods or strategies to easily nourish yourself in a Paleo manner.

1. _____
2. _____

At some point we expect you to branch out from our recipe recommendations and go with your own ideas. Have you made a recipe from an online source? If yes, which site? _____

What do you like about the food you're eating or the way it makes you feel?

1. _____
2. _____

Anything you want to change? And, if that change is non-Paleo, is there a way to make it more Paleo-friendly?

_____

Section I – Paleo-Wise: Cortisol Part I, the Stress Hormone

*Stress is not what happens to us. It's our response to what happens.
And response is something we can choose. ~Maureen Killoran*

Cortisol Affects Diet Which Affects Cortisol

It may seem counterintuitive to elaborate on stress in a book about diet. However, cortisol is a powerful hormone that affects all basic metabolic processes, including cravings and digestion, and is a key player in overall quality of health.

*If you do not manage stress, it will completely undermine all the other positive changes you make.
~Sarah Ballantyne, PhD, author of The Paleo Approach, Paleo Principles*

Energy Management

Cortisol is a steroid hormone secreted by the adrenal glands. It is generally responsible for managing energy levels through the day as well as when an extra energy boost is necessary. To accomplish this, cortisol has the power to control and override core body functions:

1. **Manage Blood Sugar Levels and Insulin Effectiveness** – Cortisol prevents glucose transport into cells by decreasing insulin sensitivity – glucose stays in the blood for immediate energy use.
2. **Regulate Daily Energy Cycle** – Cortisol normally cycles during the day with higher levels in the morning when more energy is required and lower levels at night to allow sleep.
3. **Alter Blood Pressure Levels** – Cortisol regulates salt and water balance – water retention raises blood volume (pressure) which is necessary for quick physical energy burst.
4. **Synchronize Hormones** – Cortisol coordinates interaction of key hormones such as estrogen, testosterone, thyroid and growth hormones.
5. **Monitor Inflammatory and Immune Responses** – Cortisol reduces acute inflammation and pain. This effect is commonly used medically:
   a. **Cortisone Injection** – decreases inflammation at a specific joint or tendon
   b. **Prednisone** – synthetic cortisone used to deliberately suppress inflammatory immune response in autoimmune conditions, allergies, asthma, arthritis, even cancer or transplant recipients
   c. **Topical Cortisone Cream** – anti-inflammatory for skin conditions/rashes: decreases itching and improves healing time

Fight-or-Flight (Short-Term Cortisol Spike)

Cortisol can also be considered a *veto* hormone. It is designed to instantly override normal body functions in preparation for fight-or-flight when faced with an emergency or life-threatening situation (like running from a predator). The human body can produce a ten-fold increase in cortisol when necessary! That critical survival role requires that cortisol be powerful, highly sensitive and immediately responsive to environmental influences. Here's what cortisol does in an emergency:

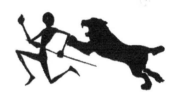

- **Provides a Quick Burst of Energy and Strength**
  - Increases blood glucose by overriding insulin's storage message (creating insulin resistance)
  - Increases blood pressure and heart rate
  - Increases breathing rate
- **Heightens Reflexes and Instincts**
- **Lowers Sensitivity to Pain**

> **After Fight-or-Flight:** When an urgent situation abates, cortisol *should* recede back to normal levels and symptoms *should* dissipate.

Chronic Stress = Health Havoc

Cortisol is clearly crucial for managing *acute* stress – its survival functions are life-saving. Because fight-or-flight requires significant energy, cortisol pulls resources from non-urgent functions such as digestion, healing, growth, reproduction and even cognition (in a crisis, taking time to deliberate over choices is not feasible).

Unfortunately, our bodies classify many details of modern culture as high-stress so the result: cortisol is activated too often, for too long, at wrong times of the day and in the wrong amounts. There's rarely opportunity to return to an ideal, relaxed state to allow symptoms to dissipate. Therefore, the body remains primed-and-pumped, day after day, resulting in a state of chronic stress with chronically-elevated cortisol. The following chart details how survival benefits of cortisol become detrimental when cortisol levels do not recede.

> **Key Point:** What was beneficial for a short-term survival response becomes devastating over time. *Chronic stress will deteriorate health!*

We were never designed to be bombarded with stress or marinated in cortisol. ~Nora Gedgaudas

How Cortisol Affects Body Functions		
Cortisol Action	**Short-Term Benefits (Survival)**	**Chronically-Elevated Consequences**
• Increase blood glucose	Immediate energy source	Sugar cravings, diabetes
• Repress insulin message (maintain high blood glucose)	Keep glucose in the blood for large muscle emergency fuel	Insulin resistance, diabetes, lack of fuel for other cells and bodily functions
• Break down protein to produce more glucose	Additional glucose source from muscles to maintain high energy	Muscle wasting, stunted growth, weak bones and connective tissue, wrinkling
• Elevate heart rate	Pump blood faster	Heart works harder, fatigue
• Increase blood volume	Higher blood pressure for quicker physical action, directed to large muscles	Chronic high blood pressure, fluid retention, salt cravings, vascular headaches
• Accelerate breathing rate	More oxygen for increased blood volume needs	Chronic shallow breaths, light-headedness
• Generate muscle tension	Prepare for extra strength	Muscle cramps, aches, tension headaches
• Reduce blood flow to brain and extremities	Heightened reliance on primal instincts and large muscle reflexes	Slower decision-making and cognition abilities, cold hands/feet, poor circulation
• Digestion slows or stops	Divert blood to muscles	Digestive complications, ulcers, heartburn, irritable bowel syndrome
• Strong anti-inflammatory (short-term)	Pain eliminated – won't interfere with fight-or-flight response	Immune system fatigues causing frequent illness, slow healing
• Reproduction slows or stops	Reproduction isn't critical in an emergency	Infertility, disruption of estrogen and testosterone, loss of menstruation

Cortisol Overrides Insulin – A Hormonal Tug-of-War

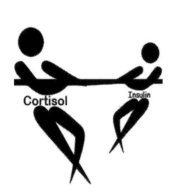

Cortisol   Insulin

Glucose provides the incredible amount of energy required to sustain survival-mode. Blood glucose *must increase* in an emergency. To accomplish this, cortisol overrides insulin in the following ways to keep blood sugar continually elevated:

- Blocks glucose from entering cells (except large muscles needed to run!)
- Increases appetite and cravings for sweet and starchy foods
- Breaks down proteins in cartilage, tendons, ligaments and bone to make glucose

The resulting higher blood glucose level stimulates release of continually more insulin, which the body ignores per 'instructions' by cortisol (that's insulin resistance). This destructive cycle continues until the pancreas stops producing insulin (diabetes).

Key Point: You can eat perfect Paleo, but if stress is not managed, cortisol's effect on glucose and insulin levels will create a blood profile similar to a type 2 diabetic!

The Birth of a Sugar Craving

Cortisol creates sugar cravings! When glucose requirements cannot be met from within the body, cortisol increases the desire to seek glucose from food – in the form of cravings for sugar/starch coupled with an unrelenting appetite. Comfort-food binges during times of high stress are simply satisfying cortisol's demand!

The influx of sugar from a craving boosts insulin...then cortisol must be further increased to override insulin... which then increases cravings for even higher amounts of sugar! With each "sugar fix," blood glucose erratically rises then crashes. In the case of chronic stress, the resulting cortisol-insulin tug-of-war is a daily occurrence. This is as ineffective as driving a car with both the brakes and the accelerator fully engaged at the same time!

> **Belly Fat Fact**: When cortisol is high, it takes even more insulin to drive glucose into the cells. High cortisol *plus* high insulin is insulin resistance and causes waistline weight gain. Belly fat is a symptom of unmanaged stress.

Protein Breakdown = Bone and Tissue Damage

Proteins can be broken down and converted to glucose when necessary. Unfortunately, chronically elevated cortisol accelerates this process. Collagen protein in particular is broken down faster than it can be replenished. Collagen is the key protein in bone, cartilage and connective tissue, so its deterioration contributes to:

- **Weakened Muscles, Tendons and Ligaments** – thus increasing susceptibility to joint injuries
- **Osteoporosis** – collagen loss erodes the bone matrix; excess cortisol also interferes with calcium absorption, further compromising bone integrity (more on Bone Health on Day 16)
- **Wrinkles and Premature Aging** – cortisol-induced collagen loss in the skin is *ten times greater* than in any other tissue

At times of increased stress, it is particularly important to eat collagen-containing foods. Bone broth and collagen supplements are effective options (more about collagen protein and supplements on Days 6 and 16).

> **Strong Bones:** Bone density is improved by reducing chronic stress. Increased dietary calcium when cortisol is elevated won't necessarily be delivered to the bones (Day 16).

Cortisol Preserves Body Fat

To add insult to injury, the hormonal disruption from chronic stress encourages fat accumulation. Body fat is reserved for *future* energy, not immediate needs. In an emergency state, the body prefers glucose for fuel and will protect its precious fat stores, due in part to high insulin which prevents the release of fat for energy. In a state of high cortisol:

- Glucose becomes the body's fuel of choice over fat
- Protein is broken down into glucose – fat stores remain intact

Recipe for Getting Fat Fast:

1. **Eat Sweet or Starchy Food** – glucose triggers insulin which stimulates "fat storage mode"
2. **Eat Fat at the Same Time** – insulin pushes *both sugar and fat* into storage
   (Examples of *glucose + fat*: potato chips, mac & cheese, fries, bread and butter, cheesecake, donuts, ice cream, chips and guacamole, pizza, nachos, crackers with peanut butter, cheesy rice, etc)
3. **Add Unmanaged, Chronic Stress** – cortisol magnifies insulin level which magnifies fat storage

Obesity Formula: (Sugar + Fat) x Stress = Fat Gain

Unmanaged stress creates belly fat! High cortisol directs fat deposits into the belly, liver, back of neck and around internal organs. These areas of fat storage correlate with metabolic syndrome.

Cortisol Interferes with Thyroid Function and Metabolism

When cortisol prioritizes survival functions, the natural consequence is to inhibit non-vital body responsibilities, including even basic metabolic processes. Under normal circumstances, thyroid hormone controls metabolic rate, but in the presence of cortisol, thyroid function will be overridden (creating hypothyroid) as follows:

1. Reduced thyroid hormone production
2. Restricted conversion of inactive thyroid hormone (T4) to the active form (T3)
3. Decreased cell sensitivity to thyroid hormone causing *thyroid resistance* – the body does not recognize or use available thyroid hormone, *even if thyroid blood levels are normal*

Hypothyroid and low metabolism symptoms include fatigue, hair loss, sensitivity to cold, mood disorders, dry skin, difficulty losing weight, memory complications, low libido, irregular menstruation and muscle weakness.

Cortisol Inhibits Immune Function

In the short-term, cortisol functions to *reduce* inflammation in the body – it has the power to suppress the immune system's inflammatory response. This is critical in an emergency because pain interferes with the ability to fight or run.

However, if chronic inflammation persists due to ongoing lifestyle stressors (including a poor diet), cortisol levels gradually escalate as the body futilely attempts to suppress unrelenting inflammation. Ultimately, the entire immune system fatigues at which point, inflammation proceeds unchecked and leads to a myriad of chronic problems (review the Chronic Inflammation topic in Prep A).

> **Pain-Relieving Cortisone Shots:** Although these shots relieve pain in the short-term due to anti-inflammatory effects, *cortisol deteriorates collagen* protein (it is sacrificed for glucose production). Cartilage, tendons, bone and skin in the injection area are prone to degeneration. Repeated medical cortisone shots are strictly limited.

Stress Causes Sleep Deprivation...which Creates Stress...which Causes Sleep Deprivation...

During a survival situation, it is critical to stay awake and alert (falling asleep could get you killed). Although vital in an emergency, this extra awareness is devastating long term when sleep becomes elusive.

On a daily basis, cortisol's *normal* energy management contributes to the circadian rhythm, promoting higher energy in the morning. By evening, cortisol ideally subsides and relinquishes its control to melatonin which assists with falling *and staying* asleep. When chronic stress creates chronic cortisol, the sleep cycle suffers:

- **Impossible to Fall Asleep** - High cortisol levels at night override melatonin.
- **Insomnia Creates Anxiety** - Stressing over lack of sleep further increases cortisol.
- **Cortisol Spikes Again During the Night** - Metabolism revs. Heartrate and breathing rate increase. The brain becomes alert to assess and prepare for danger. Thought patterns race. Glucose needed for fight-or-flight triggers sugar cravings – and the classic 'midnight snack attack'.
- **Cortisol Crashes in the Morning** - After a night of high cortisol, rebound low cortisol in the morning materializes as an energy slump, making it difficult to get out of bed. Coffee and more coffee, anyone?
- **Repeat Daily** - Excessive caffeine interferes with normal tapering of cortisol during the day.

Over time, this destructive pattern is repeated and reinforced. The natural synergistic relationship between cortisol and melatonin is shattered along with any hope for a normal sleep cycle.

> **Break the Cycle:** Many people have more control over sleeping habits than stress load. Prioritizing sleep is one way to reset natural circadian rhythms which will reduce stress and readjust cortisol levels (see Day 13 for Healthy Sleep suggestions).

Chronic Stress Creates Chronic Symptoms

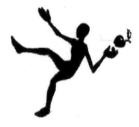

Cortisol response is a normal survival reflex – when the body perceives a potential threat, it quickly and easily initiates fight-or-flight metabolism. Interestingly, the action of cortisol is the same regardless of the *type* of stress: physical, psychological, emotional, short-term, long-term, etc. In a true emergency, the body follows a *release first, evaluate later* approach – there's no time to discern if a threat is real, so the body goes into survival mode even if the threat is merely perceived (the essence of the cliché, "worry yourself sick").

Stress, in and of itself, is not bad. There are times when stress has a positive effect: a work deadline can increase productivity and concentration; athletic performance can improve under pressure. But if stress never dissipates, a cycle of chronic symptoms manifests: elevated cortisol triggers further stress which generates more cortisol.

Additional Reading:

- 🖱 ThePaleoMom How Stress Undermines Health
- 🖱 MarksDailyApple The Definitive Guide to Stress, Cortisol and the Adrenals

Common Manifestations of Excess Cortisol		
Weight Gain	**Weak Muscle and Tissue**	**Skin Irregularities**
✓ Obesity	✓ Fatigue	✓ Stretchmarks
✓ Round 'moon' face	✓ Aches/pains	✓ Thin skin
✓ Belly fat	✓ Thinning limbs	✓ Bruise easily
✓ Neck and upper back fat	✓ Sprains, strains, tendonitis	✓ Wrinkles
Diabetes-Like Symptoms	**Weak Bones**	**Cardiovascular**
✓ High blood sugar	✓ Bone loss, osteoporosis	✓ High blood pressure
✓ High insulin/insulin resistance	✓ Fractures (rib, vertebrae)	✓ Fluid retention
✓ Glucose intolerance	**Reproductive Conditions**	**Mental Health**
Slow healing	✓ Low libido	✓ Cognitive dysfunction
✓ Acne, rashes	✓ Decreased fertility	✓ Moodiness, irritability
✓ Cuts, insect bites, infections	✓ Loss of menstruation	✓ Anxiety, depression

Paleo Advantage: Improving diet is one controllable approach to minimize the effects of cortisol. Here's how eating Paleo significantly reduces stress:

1. **Less Digestive Stress** – Abundant nutrient-rich foods that are easily assimilated
2. **Toxin-Free** – Few antinutrients, antibiotics or other processing chemicals
3. **Stabilized Insulin Response** – Lower sugar/starch intake minimizes insulin resistance
4. **Fat Burning Metabolism** – Lowering belly fat reduces inflammatory compounds produced there
5. **Chronic Inflammation Decreases** – Less demand on immune system, fewer symptoms of chronic illness
6. **Stabilized Mood and Temperament** – Improved production and utilization of neurotransmitters such as 'feel-good' dopamine and serotonin (most produced in the gut!) as digestive lining heals and gut flora normalize (more about Gut Health on Day 21)
7. **Improved Ability to Calmly Respond to Stressors** – Stabilizes normal cortisol levels to prevent escalation
8. **Better sleep** – Less overall stress reverses insomnia

Cortisol Visualization – Chronic Stress Tube (diagram on the next page)

Cortisol is complicated! There is an unending cycle between chronic stress and deteriorating health. The following 3D diagram assists in visualizing and comprehending the enormous impact of chronic cortisol. An extra copy is located in the Resource Section: cut it out, roll the page into a tube and tape in place. Spin it to see how this hormonal imbalance is a self-defeating cycle that perpetuates indefinitely until stressors are reduced.

Chronic Stress Tube Diagram Key:

1. **Chronic Stressors** – the gray ovals are common examples but clearly not a complete list
2. **Black Arrows** – additional side-cycles generated with chronic stress:
   a. Immune system shuts down – frequent illness and inflammation trigger more stress
   b. Energy production increases – triggers insomnia, which itself causes chronic stress (the alternative, relying on sedatives to address insomnia, initiates a stress response as well)
3. **The Two Main Cortisol Messages:**
   a. **Preserve Body Fat** (in an emergency, glucose, not fat is the preferred fuel)
      i. Creates cravings to replenish glucose
      ii. Overrides and inhibits normal metabolism to subdue non-urgent energy needs
   b. **Produce Energy**
      i. Creates cravings for glucose fuel
      ii. Raises blood pressure to move nutrients to large muscles
      iii. Raises blood glucose for quick energy
4. Gray boxes indicate symptoms of chronic cortisol: frequent illness, insomnia, sugar and salt cravings, hypothyroid, fatigue, obesity and eventually diabetes or other chronic disease
5. ***The end result of chronic cortisol is chronic inflammation* which, by itself, is a constant stressor and triggers more cortisol...so the cycle continues.**

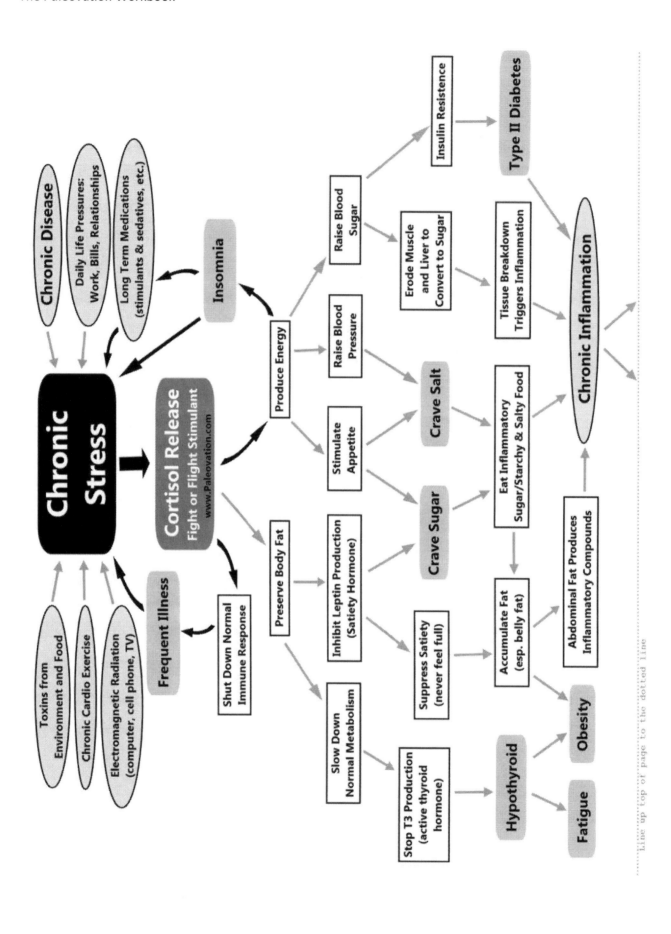

Section II: Recognizing Personal Stress Manifestation

To maintain healthy cortisol levels, stressors must be reduced and stress response must be steadied. Tomorrow we offer strategies to identify hidden stressors as well as calm the stress response. In the meantime, take a moment to evaluate your personal symptoms of stress. The faster you recognize cortisol creeping out of control, the easier it will be to minimize health complications. Checkmark your personal symptoms:

Common Stress Signals – Physical, Emotional, Behavioral			
Physical	**Emotional**	**Behavioral**	**Mental**
☐ Back pain	☐ Short temper	☐ Compulsive eating	☐ Indecisive
☐ Tight shoulders/neck	☐ Worrywart	☐ Alcohol/drug use	☐ Difficulty relaxing
☐ Rapid heartbeat	☐ Forgetful	☐ Social withdrawal	☐ Low libido
☐ Chest pain	☐ Easily agitated	☐ Appetite changes	☐ Little sense of humor
☐ Dizziness	☐ Sweaty palms	☐ Unmotivated	☐ Less creative
☐ Teeth grinding	☐ Nausea/butterflies	☐ Nervous behaviors	☐ Fatigue
☐ Headache	☐ Difficulty breathing	(fidgeting, nail biting)	☐ Insomnia
☐ Heartburn			
☐ Digestive trouble			

Do your stress signals tend to manifest in one category (physical, emotional, behavioral, mental) or across several? List your categories: _____

What do you already do to manage stress?

1. _____

2. _____

Paleo Advantage: Stress and cortisol are an unavoidable part of daily life experiences. However, in the absence of insulin, the detrimental effects of cortisol are *significantly* reduced. Eating Paleo naturally minimizes insulin which subsequently minimizes the negative consequences of cortisol.

Section III: Cooking Assignment #4 – Paleo Jerky *or* Nut-&-Seed Granola

When good food is available, we will eat good food. Both jerky and granola are excellent Paleo staples to have on hand for a quick snack or meal. This is an 'either/or' assignment – you do not need to make both recipes, but no one will stop you if you want to give them both a try!

A. Paleo Jerky

Grass-fed *and* sugar-free jerky is hard to find and expensive. Making your own is simple but there are a few tips to achieve the best outcome. Prepare to make 2-4 lbs in a batch because it shrinks a lot.

Choosing the Meat: beef, lamb, venison, bison, turkey, etc (salmon recipe below)
1. It does not matter which meat you use. Pastured animals are the healthiest option.
2. Generally, the leaner the meat, the better the jerky:
    a. Fat does not 'dry' like the muscle tissue does
    b. With a fatty cut, the fat melts out during the dehydrating process which is messy
    c. Tips below if you happen to have a fattier cut
    d. If you are feeling fancy and fatty, research "Paleo Pemmican" which is a fattier dried meat
3. Ground meat is easier than meat strips:
    a. It is difficult to cut strips of steak to uniform thickness; however, if you have access to a professional slicer (or ask a butcher to slice it) feel free to use evenly-cut strips instead of ground
    b. The final product texture of ground jerky is much easier to chew
    c. Either purchase ground meat or grind your own roast after trimming away fat

General Oven Directions (if using a dehydrator, follow your machine's directions):

1. Choose a large mixing bowl and preheat oven to lowest possible setting (usually 170°F).
2. Mix the ground meat with coconut aminos and choice of seasonings.
3. Lightly grease 1-2 baking sheets with any oil/fat of choice.
4. Evenly spread the mixture on the pan/tray. You want uniform ¼-inch thickness so press down with fingers or roll out with a drinking glass or rolling pin. Alternatively, you also can purchase a jerky gun.
5. Dehydrate in oven until it is solid enough to flip (if it is greasy at this point, pour off grease, put a cooling rack on top of the baking sheet and flip the jerky onto the cooling rack to finish drying).
6. Dehydrate until it is "ready" – a good rule of thumb is that it is still pliable. The jerky continues to dry after it is removed from the oven so take it out before it becomes hard or crispy.

Jerky Recipes:
- ⚙ General recipe: WellnessMama Ground Beef Jerky
- ⚙ Unsweetened salmon jerky: MyGutsy Salmon Jerky

B. Paleo Nut-and-Seed Granola

Consider making a large batch because this tends to quickly disappear. Be careful – granola is easy to overconsume. Limit to one handful-size serving per day. Additional tips:

- Since small seeds, sliced almonds or coconut flakes do not need to toast as long, start roasting the larger nut pieces first, then halfway through the cook time, add smaller/thinner items.
- Serve dry or with coconut milk (adding nut milk would introduce an additional nut serving).

General Directions

1. Choose any variety of nuts or seeds (but no peanuts, they are a legume).
2. Chop the nuts so they are similar in size and will cook evenly (½" pieces are nice). Preheat oven to 350°F.
3. In a bowl, toss the large pieces with melted coconut oil and seasoning (cinnamon, salt, pumpkin pie spice).
4. Spread on a baking sheet and roast for 10 min.
5. While those toast, toss the smaller items with coconut oil and seasoning (coconut flakes, seeds, sliced almonds and, after the program, dried fruit).
6. Remove the pan from the oven. Stir in the smaller ingredients.
7. Finish toasting 5-10 min more. Keep a close eye on it during the last minute or two of cooking (once it is done it burns quickly). Taste-test it to see if it has the right crispness.
8. Remove from oven, granola will toast a little bit more as it cools down.

Granola Recipes:
Select unsweetened recipes or those sweetened with low-sugar fruits to stay compliant with the program.
- ⚙ PassionForPaleo 21 DSD Banola
- ⚙ FastPaleo No Sweet Paleo Granola
- ⚙ AGirlWorthSaving Paleo Pumpkin Granola

To-Do List:
- ☐ Did you practice the Rising Test today? Mark forward progress on the little table on Day 9, Section III.
- ☐ Have you made your veggie recipe that acts like a grain? Enjoy some by tomorrow.
- ☐ Research the recipe you'll use for jerky *or* granola and start gathering ingredients and supplies to make a batch (or two) by day 19. Circle the recipe you want to try: Jerky   Granola   Both
  1. **Jerky in the Oven or Food Dehydrator**
     - Meat of choice, coconut aminos, seasonings, baking sheet or food dehydrator
  2. **Paleo Nut-and-Seed Granola**
     - Variety of nuts/seeds, oil of choice, seasonings, dried coconut flakes, baking sheet
- ☐ Add all necessary ingredients to your shopping list.

Coming Up Soon:
- Tomorrow discusses how to soothe the cortisol response plus some Paleo-friendly smoothie ideas

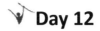

Day 12

I was 32 when I started cooking; up until then, I just ate. ~Julia Child

Today's Topics:
1. Paleo-Wise: Cortisol Part II, Identifying and Managing Stress
2. Calming the Cortisol Response
3. Smoothie Compromise

Fast Fare – Fridge Staples
♥ Hot dogs and kraut
♥ Garlic-stuffed olives
♥ Pepper strips

Are any Paleo foods particularly satisfying today?

_____

Are you getting stuck in a rut anywhere? If so, what can you do to break out of that rut?

_____

Section I – Paleo-Wise: Cortisol Part II, Identifying and Managing Stress

You cannot control the wind, but you can adjust your sails. ~ Yiddish proverb

Modern Stress is Unrelenting

Contemporary lifestyles induce a state of *mild, unrelenting* stress. "Mild stress" may sound innocent but unfortunately, the body doesn't differentiate between degrees of stress – cortisol is released whether the stress is major or minor. It's the duration of the stress (not the degree) that provokes cortisol's detrimental health consequences.

Constant, mild stress never dissipates so cortisol remains chronically elevated and its symptoms never completely subside. This state is so common in modern society that it is often misinterpreted as normal: cortisol can be elevated *even when we think we're relaxed*.

As with the degree of stress, likewise the body cannot discern between *types* of stress. Cortisol is the body's only hormonal stress response and it will be released regardless of the source:

Diverse Stressor Examples	
Physical	Illness, physical trauma, hormonal imbalance, addiction (caffeine, alcohol, drugs)
Social	Relationship/family changes, work pressures, maintaining status quo, sensational news
Psychological	Nagging negative thoughts, holding grudges, PTSD, self-criticism, feeling alone
Environmental	Toxin exposure, air/water/noise pollution, artificial lighting, poor diet, natural disaster

Stress is unavoidable, but conscious awareness of which lifestyle factors could be perceived as threats by your body is empowering – identification of these hidden stressors allows action to minimize them. If these constant, mild "threats" are never addressed, they *will* cumulatively whittle away health.

Reducing Stress

Take a moment to review the Chronic Cortisol Cycle diagram in yesterday's text. In addition to the sheer volume of potential stressors, note that even an increased *reaction to stress* induces more stress! For example, a panic attack is a *reaction* to anxiety that stimulates more anxiety. Health will *always* be compromised by unmanaged stress. This concept is key to understanding the relevance of reducing all stressors within and around the body.

Derailing the stress cycle and reducing cortisol interference is a three-part process:
1. Identify stressors
2. Eliminate or reduce stressors where possible
3. Respond more calmly to remaining stressors

> **Calming the Cortisol Response:** By gradually tempering constant lifestyle stressors, however subtle, the body and mind become much more capable of calmly and rationally addressing the next stress response.

Poor Diet is Chronic Stress

Ironically, poor diet is a prime culprit of chronic stress. Poor food choices set another deteriorating health cycle in motion: low quality foods cause digestive damage, which triggers a stress response, which reinforces poor diet via cravings for inflammatory foods, further interfering with digestion! *This is the reason why eating Paleo is so beneficial to health – it mitigates digestive stress and is a major cortisol reduction strategy.*

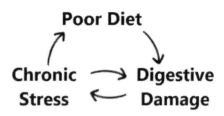

Eating processed and inflammatory foods, even portion-controlled, is highly stressful on the digestive system:
1. **Absorption Interference** – Absorbing available nutrients is challenging
2. **Immune Fatigue** – Combating toxins and non-digestible substances (pathogens, additives, gluten) taxes the immune system
3. **Energy Depletion**
   a. Digesting poor quality foods is energy-intensive
   b. Healing the damage left behind is physically demanding

> **Diet Dagger:** Poor food choices are a major contributor to chronic stress!

Modern Diet Stressors	
Quantity	**Quality**
Excessive Sugar and Starch: pasta, bread, candy, desserts, chips, cereal, bars, shakes	**Difficult-to-Digest Foods**: gluten, artificial trans fats, processed foods, lactose, casein
Excessive Omega-6 Fats: industrialized vegetable oils; processed and restaurant foods	**Anti-Nutrients**: high levels of phytates or lectins especially in grains and legumes
Excessive Volume of Food: "All you can eat," "super-sized," buy-one-get-one-free"	**Toxins**: chemical residues from pesticides, fungicides, hormones, antibiotics, fertilizers and industrial processing methods; alcohol
Insufficient Healthy Fats: a low-fat diet	
Insufficient Nutrients: low vegetable intake; lack of variety of meats, veggies, fats	**Pathogens**: bacteria, viruses, mold and its toxins
	Additives: MSG, colorings, preservatives, etc

> **Paleo Advantage:** Eating Paleo naturally eliminates a large proportion of dietary stressors

Rest and Digest

Digestion is most efficient in a relaxed state. Remember, "rest and digest." However, when digestively-incompatible foods are eaten regularly, they can generate a cortisol stress reaction with every meal, every day. This evokes a triple assault of cortisol's consequences:
1. Cortisol is a stimulant. Its presence fundamentally undermines the *rest-and-digest* state.
2. Cortisol restricts resources for the digestive process because digestion isn't necessary in an emergency.
3. Poor food choices damage the digestive tract, inducing an additional cortisol response.

> **Food Sensitivities = Hormone Disruption:** Consuming food substances to which you are sensitive will automatically generate a stress response that impacts both cortisol and insulin levels.

Excess Body Fat Causes Stress

Excess body fat is strongly associated with joint deterioration, high blood pressure, heart disease, diabetes and sedentary lifestyle – all of which generate stress and increase cortisol. Unfortunately, it's not bad enough that this increases the vulnerability to gain more fat – there's more bad news…

An enzyme present in body fat (especially belly fat) converts *inactive* corti*sone* into *active* corti*sol*. Translated, this means that fat tissue produces its own cortisol which can result in even *more* fat gain! It's another self-defeating cycle: *The fatter you are, the fatter you get!*

Excess cortisone can be concealed inside fat deposits and not be revealed via blood tests. Thus, an individual can suffer high cortisol symptoms yet maintain a completely normal cortisol blood profile.

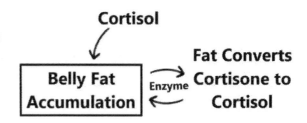

> **Key Point:** Stress reduction is an instrumental part of successful *and sustainable* weight-loss!

Contemporary Environmental Stressors

Modern environments differ vastly from the natural habitat of our hunter-gatherer ancestors. Recent lifestyle changes occurred so quickly that our bodies haven't had time to genetically adapt. Although technological advances in lifestyle comforts and communication are convenient, they generate unintended stress triggers.

While no single stressor in the following list will make or break health, the constant exposure to numerous trivial stressors has a cumulative negative effect on overall stress load. These are just a few examples:

- **Artificial Lighting:** Fluorescent bulbs (some flicker and all contain mercury); lights after sundown delay evening melatonin secretion: back-lit electronics (TV, computer, phone, clock), lamps, street lights
- **Chemicals:** Conventional cleaners, personal care products, fire retardants, air pollution, plastics, heavy metals, residues on foods, anti-bacterial products, molds, medications, air fresheners
- **Noise:** Alert beeps from phones/computers, construction noise, traffic, buzzing electronics, background television news or commercials, loud music, sirens, lawn mower/leaf blowers
- **Electromagnetic Fields:** TV, computers, tablets, cell phones, Wi-Fi, Bluetooth, alarm clocks, hair dryers, microwaves, anything "smart": smart watches, smart meters, performance trackers
- **Other:** Uncomfortable temperatures, non-predictability, crowding, sedentary lifestyle, social isolation, sensory over-stimulation (think casino), severe calorie or nutrient restriction (crash diets), sensational news or politics

Knowledge is power! Recognizing that the body often interprets environmental input as threats gives you the control to minimize those circumstances. Every effort to reduce little stressors eases the intensity of the chronic cortisol cycle.

Lack of Connection

> *When 'I' is replaced with 'we', even illness becomes wellness.* ~Malcolm X

Our ancestors certainly had stress in their lives, but they also had cultural behaviors that connected them to each other, to nature and to themselves. Strong connections relieve stress by satisfying the needs to belong, to live in a safe environment and to establish security and self-esteem. Modern busy lifestyles tend to promote individualization, often neglecting social connection activities unless we consciously make time for them. The following are just a few examples of connections inherent to ancestral or indigenous cultures:

Ancestral Connecting Behaviors	
Connection	**Examples**
Nature	Foraging, hiking, hunting, swimming, paddling, storm watching, star gazing, fishing, barefoot walking, noticing cloud formations, observing animal behaviors, tending pets & work animals, acknowledging moon cycles, seasonal changes and equinoxes
Others	Feasts, bonfires, celebrations, ceremonies, cuddling, co-sleeping, playing games, sharing chores, preparing for battles, caring for community children, respecting elders, storytelling, community activities, sauna, relocating the village
Self	Meditation, quiet time for handicraft, dream interpretation, preparing for rites of passage, women taking solitary time during menstruation, preparing for a hunt, sweat lodge, solitary journey
Spirituality	Ceremonies, healing practices, symbols, sites, narratives, prayers, sacrifices, rituals, fasting, acknowledging gut instincts, expressing gratitude, noticing coincidences

Personal Temperament

Personal perception and outlook drastically change the cortisol response. Pessimism and negative attitudes increase cortisol production while a positive demeanor steadies and normalizes cortisol levels.

Altering Perception Patterns	
Self-Defeating	**Self-Empowering**
Hold grudges, take offense	Release anger, disregard minor annoyances, move forward
Concentrate on what is wrong	Focus on opportunity and gratitude
Impulsively react	Observe, then respond
Complain and blame	Accept and correct

Why questions are self-defeating and perpetuate stress. For example, "Why me?" or "Why does this always happen?" simply invite a "because" answer that is self-deprecating and reinforces a negative situation.

However, a small but *intentional* perspective change can cultivate a more productive outlook simply by replacing *why* questions with *what* or *how*: "What should I do next?" "What do I need to learn?" "How can I improve?" "How will I deal with this situation?" Answers to these questions generate constructive solutions, reverse negative thinking patterns, and begin to resolve a stressful situation.

> *One common thing about great achievers is that they keep asking useful questions every day.*
> *They ask questions like, "what do I want" and "what do I need to do to get it?"* ~ Israelmore Ayivor

Assess Your Personality

In susceptible individuals, chronically-elevated cortisol symptoms such as high blood pressure, taxed immune system, insulin resistance or insomnia contribute to more advanced health complications and even shortened lifespan.

Personality can be viewed as a spectrum of behaviors and traits, with 'type A' on one end and 'type B' on the other. Individuals dominant with type A characteristics *tend* to suffer more stress-related symptoms. Are you at risk? How many of the following traits describe you?

- ☐ Strong need to achieve
- ☐ Finish other's sentences
- ☐ Eat fast, walk fast, talk fast
- ☐ Perfectionist
- ☐ Like to be in charge
- ☐ Feel fulfilled by a high responsibility load
- ☐ Refuse to delegate personal work to others
- ☐ Workaholic, rarely have time for hobbies
- ☐ Dislike the time it takes to listen to others
- ☐ Difficult to sit alone quietly or to meditate
- ☐ Find it hard to say *no*
- ☐ Feel guilty taking time to relax, unwind
- ☐ Always multi-tasking

- ☐ Delays are extremely upsetting
- ☐ Competitive, hate to lose
- ☐ Often impatient with self or others
- ☐ Rarely discuss personal issues or feelings
- ☐ Lose temper if frustrated
- ☐ Obsessively seek approval for a job well done
- ☐ Do not ask for help
- ☐ Struggle to find activities to do during free time
- ☐ Work best (and thrive) under pressing deadlines
- ☐ Don't have time to stop and smell the flowers
- ☐ Repetitive motions (leg bouncing, finger tapping)
- ☐ Usually rushed or pressed for time
- ☐ Believe that stress-relieving tactics are for wimps

If you identify with 13 or more of these characteristics, please prioritize active stress management.

Guru Guidance: A guru told his pupils to meditate 10 minutes per day. One student protested, "I don't have time for that." The guru kindly replied, "In that case, you need to meditate an hour each day."

Section II: Calming the Cortisol Response

> *Life is 10% what happens to us and 90% how we react to it.* ~Dennis P. Kimbro

Calming Strategy #1: Simple Actions

All the following actions interrupt a cortisol surge because they send a strong physiological message of safety, relaxation and reassurance that there's no emergency. Use them when you feel stressed to slow heart and breathing rates, reduce muscle tension, lower blood pressure and improve attitude.

Strategies to Counteract Cortisol	
Action	**Why it works**
Happy Face	A peaceful, calm expression generates endorphins and soothes cortisol. Smiling, laughing or even brushing the lips with fingers stimulates this response. This *fake-it-til-you-make-it* strategy eases stress even when agitated or upset.
Deep Breath	Slow, deep and steady abdominal breaths increase oxygen (including to the brain), release carbon dioxide, relax muscles, stimulate lymph to aid with removing bodily toxins, and trigger the release of endorphins which improves feelings of well-being and provides pain-relief (read more on Belly Breathing on Day 18).
Release Invasive Thoughts	Refuse to replay thoughts over and over again including *What if, I'll never,* and *I should*'ve statements. Acknowledge those thoughts, find gratitude for the purpose they serve, then let them go. If necessary, write down your thoughts to remove them from your head (bonus: the first steps to solution often emerge).
Focus on 5 Senses	Use all 5 senses to tune into your current environment, connect to the present and interrupt runaway thoughts. Try this: identify 1 item you currently taste*, 2 aromas you smell, 3 textures you feel, 4 sounds you hear and 5 items you see.
Be Thankful	Express gratitude for anything: Family, friends, knowledge, abilities, meals, nature, clean water, continued learning, life's experiences. Gratitude improves relationships, health, sleep and self-esteem while reducing aggression. Keep a gratitude jar or journal. Try writing down 3 things you are grateful for each day.

*Maybe a residual flavor from a beverage or toothpaste

Calming Strategy #2: Choosing a Positive Outlook

Anger, bitterness and pent up emotions are highly destructive for both physical and mental health. Suppressed negativity creates tension, heightens sensitivity to stress and stifles a calm response to the next stressor.

At some point in life, everyone experiences negative events beyond personal control, but the *reaction* to them is a choice that *can be controlled*. Anger is a choice. Happiness is also a choice. Choosing joy, love, gratitude or forgiveness even when immersed in a bad situation is a *fake-it-til-you-make-it* strategy that will slow the cortisol surge and minimize health consequences.

> *Holding onto anger is like drinking poison and expecting the other person to die.* ~Buddha

This skill is built over time – start with some practice scenarios. Were you awoken by your partner's snoring or child's nightmare? Choose to become angry or choose to think of how much you love them and are fortunate to have them near. Are you stuck in traffic? Choose to beat yourself up for selecting that route or choose to play some happy music and tap your fingers on the steering wheel. Has someone formerly hurt you? Choose to harbor resentment or choose forgiveness because you deserve to be free.

> **Improve with Practice:** It's not easy to remain cool or level-headed, but that's no excuse for not trying. *Selecting a calm response is an indispensable tool for relieving stress.*

📖 *The Book of Joy: Lasting Happiness in a Changing World,* by His Holiness the Dalai Lama and Archbishop Desmond Tutu, teaches how they personally cultivate a positive demeanor amid hardship or suffering.

Calming Strategy #3: Establish Modern Connections

Many of the previously noted ancestral connections to nature, the self, others and spirituality are still available today. We can complement those with additional modern ideas:

Modern Connecting Behaviors	
Connections	**Examples**
Nature	Get outside: Walk, bike, ski, garden, show-shoe, picnic, interact with a pet/animal, visit an aquarium or animal shelter, decorate with nature (shells, crystals, cut flowers, houseplants), use natural scents indoors, sunbathe, pick up litter, shop at outdoor farmers' markets, camp, look out the window upon waking, learn to identify bird calls, plant a tree, practice earthing*
Others	Smile at strangers, phone/text your loved ones, organize a potluck, join a club or support group, enroll in a class, volunteer, look people in the eye, attend community presentations, give gifts, write a letter/card, give a compliment, set aside some one-on-one time with someone you love, ask for help, offer to help, make time for physical affection, share a meal with a neighbor
Self	Device-free time, listen to music, affirmations, breath work, restorative yoga, qi gong, tai chi, artistic expression (dance, play music, paint, write a poem, adult coloring books), read a pleasure book, hot bath, journal, leave your "comfort zone", self-love, self-forgiveness, meditative crafts like knitting or tying fishing flies, write down goals, rephrase negative thoughts in a positive manner, brainstorm your bucket list
Spirituality	Meditate, pray, keep a journal, sit in silence, listen to calming music, immerse in nature, read a spiritual/inspirational text, join a spiritual or meditation group, pay attention to coincidence, chant, sing, attend spiritual gatherings and ceremonies

*Earthing: The practice of grounding the body either by touching the earth with bare skin or by using an electrically grounded earthing pad, mat or sheet. The theory is that harmful free radicals in the body can easily use the free electrons available on the surface of the earth rather than stealing electrons from bodily tissues

📖 *Earthing: The Most Important Health Discovery Ever,* by Clinten Ober

🎬 *Grounded*, by Dr. Joseph Mercola and Steve Kroschel

Reconnect to Relieve Stress

Using the tables listing both modern and ancestral connections, jot down the ideas that appeal to you most:

Connect to Nature: _____

Connect to Others: _____

Connect to the Self: _____

Connect to Spirituality: _____

Are you currently lacking connections in your environment?   Yes   No

Do you need to prioritize strengthening your personal connections?   Yes   No

Calming Strategy #4: Acknowledge Cortisol Rushes

If you find yourself unable (or unwilling) to pacify a cortisol spike, at the very minimum stop and *consciously acknowledge* the cortisol surge. Pay attention to how it feels to you: jitters, muscle tension, temper rising, fast breathing, mind racing, heartbeat quickening, etc.

Recognizing cortisol in this manner will help identify the symptoms of cortisol manifestation in *your* body as well as how often your stress levels intensify during the day. The more you acknowledge and understand your stress response, the easier it is to recognize minor stress triggers.

Some cortisol calming strategies are categorized in the next table. Look back at your personal stress manifestations noted yesterday, Day 11: physical, emotional, behavioral and mental. The strategies that work best for you may lie within the same category. Check off any strategies that are relevant for you:

Additional Stress Relieving Ideas

Body Management
- ☐ Exercise regularly
- ☐ Allow the body and brain to rest, relax
- ☐ Get adequate sleep or naps
- ☐ Work on breath control
- ☐ Get a massage
- ☐ Enjoy a hot bath (bonus w/Epsom Salts)
- ☐ Try a spa treatment
- ☐ Try alternative therapy like acupuncture or hypnosis

Environment Management
- ☐ Rearrange furniture
- ☐ Beautify with flowers, candles, artwork
- ☐ Buy houseplants
- ☐ Burn incense, diffuse calming essential oils
- ☐ Declutter and organize space
- ☐ Take a vacation, even if just an overnight
- ☐ Take a break from news/TV

Time Management
- ☐ Rank responsibilities and schedule priorities first
- ☐ Put stress-relieving activities on today's To-Do list (chart inserted)
- ☐ Learn time- or stress-management via book, seminar or class (available online or through a library or community center)

Mental Management
- ☐ Pick your battles, based on which ones matter in the long run
- ☐ Focus on the bright side, see the glass half full
- ☐ Laugh at self/situations
- ☐ Avoid simultaneous life changes, when possible
- ☐ Learn bio- or neuro-feedback techniques
- ☐ Consider a course in anger management
- ☐ Practice visualization
- ☐ Try a recorded guided meditation
- ☐ Hire a professional for further coping strategies

Awareness and Action: Recalibrate Your Cortisol

Unmanaged cortisol release is a multifaceted predicament tied to everything from personality to diet to lifestyle routine. Review all the cortisol calming strategies in Section II. Identify which recommendations you already use in your lifestyle (underline or highlight the text if that helps) as well as those you can implement as long-term strategies (perhaps circle, star or highlight in another color). If you need a place to write down your thoughts space is provided in the To-Do List later today.

Further Reading in this Book:
- ↯ Sleep Topic on Day 13
- ↯ Toxin Caution Topic on Day 20
- ↯ Chronic Cardio Exercise on Day 10
- ↯ Cortisol, the Stress Hormone, yesterday Day 11

Bio-hacking Stress Resources:
- 🎧 Bulletproof Rhonda Collier: Hacking Stress with HRV Sense #84
  Excellent podcast discusses how stress changes the timing between heartbeats, also known as Heart Rate Variance (HRV). Includes strategies to measure HRV and restore steady beat patterns.
- 🖱 Bulletproof Best Biohacking Apps: Multiple apps to monitor stress (and sleep) levels.

> **Every Little Bit Counts:** Calming the cortisol response restores energy to proper digestion, growth, learning, fertility, healing, immune function, circulation and eventually, hormonal balance. Your health depends on it!

Section III: Smoothie Compromise

Drinking snacks/meals is not necessarily encouraged because digestion and *brain recognition of eating* starts with the chewing process. However, we realize some people want to include smoothies in their routine, so here are basic guidelines for building a smoothie that is Paleo-friendly.

Chew the Smoothie!

As odd as that sounds, chewing sends a signal to the brain so it acknowledges the body is eating – this improves the hormonal signals that control hunger and proper digestion. Chewing also mixes saliva and enzymes into the food to begin the digestive process.

Smoothie Building

The best approach is to handle smoothie ingredients like a normal meal: *Veggie + Protein + Fat*. The following list offers inspiration for building a healthy smoothie. Remember that smoothies don't have to be sweet – many combinations are savory and delicious.

Some ingredient ideas overlap: for example coconut milk can be the fat *and* the liquid. Also remember that your daily nut and fruit serving could easily be used up in a single beverage. Again, this is a compromise – drinking meals is not exactly Paleo. Regardless, we just want to provide tools to make these dietary choices accessible.

- **Veggies:** Greens, peppers, cucumber, tomatoes, celery (contains sodium for flavor), cooked sweet potato, pumpkin, carrots, butternut squash, beets, etc. Canned, frozen or baby food purees are quick.
- **Protein:** Nut butter, gelatin/collagen, raw or soft-boiled eggs (if queasy about raw eggs, Day 4 has pasteurization info), beef protein powder or…consider cricket flour!
- **Fat:** Coconut milk, coconut oil, avocado, nut butter, coconut butter, MCT oil, bacon drippings
- **Liquids:** Ice, nut milk, coconut milk, coconut water, bone broth, spritz of lemon or lime
- **Sweeteners:** Fresh or frozen berries, coconut water, grated green apple (stevia if you must, as a crutch)
- **Flavors:** Cinnamon, ginger, pumpkin pie spice, sea salt, nutmeg, anise/fennel, clove, cocoa, citrus zest, vanilla bean, cayenne, turmeric, mint, any pure extract (almond, orange, vanilla, etc.), essential oil (citrus, lavender, peppermint, clove)

Further Reading:

- BalancedBites FAQs Is Protein Powder Paleo
- MarksDailyApple 5 Sweet and Savory Primal Shakes (omit whey, sweeteners)

Savory Bacon Smoothie: ½ cup sweet potato purée, ¼ cup coconut milk, 1-2 Tbsp melted bacon drippings, 2-4 slices crispy bacon (depending on thickness), small handful of ice cubes, and dash of cinnamon and nutmeg

---

To-Do List:

- ☐ Put together your ingredients for jerky or granola and make a batch by Day 19
- ☐ Anything else (try a smoothie, mark Rising Test progress in Day 9, try a new Paleo carb source in Day 10)?

_____

- ☐ [Optional] If you want to organize your stress reduction techniques, please use the table below:

Identify Personal Cortisol-Reducing Actions	
Successful strategies I already use	1. _____ 2. _____ 3. _____
New strategies I can immediately try	1. _____ 2. _____ 3. _____
Future strategies I can implement with a little prep work	1. _____ 2. _____ 3. _____

Coming Up Soon:

- The importance of sleep and tips to induce a good night's rest
- How to refresh the recipe routine

Day 13

[On low-fat diets]: *No diet will remove all the fat from your body because the brain is entirely fat. Without a brain you might look good, but all you could do is run for public office.* ~George Bernard Shaw

Today's Topics:
1. Eat More Vegetables
2. Paleo-Wise: Sleep
3. Monitoring Physical and Emotional Changes
4. Fresh Recipe Ideas (avoid the mid-program doldrums)

Fast Fare – Leftover Cauli-Rice
♥ Fried cauliflower rice with diced veggies and egg
♥ Breakfast sausages

Log today's meals if you wish:

Meals: _____

Snacks: _____

Beverages: _____

Section I: Eat More Vegetables
Through the program more vegetables have been included in your daily routine. List the vegetable recipes you've made, including the grain substitute recipe you tried. Circle your favorites (if any):

_____

_____

Do you think these could become permanent menu items? Why or why not?

_____

Select strategies to use so you always have vegetables and veggie grain-substitutes on hand:

Vegetables in General
☐ Prepare double or triple batches of recipes to have planned-overs or stock the freezer
☐ Visit a farmer's market for fresh, local produce
☐ Invest in a CSA (Community Supported Agriculture – you get a vegetable box from the farm each week)
☐ Plan one day per week for meal prep and process enough veggies for seven days
☐ Create a special section on your grocery list for the vegetables you intend to buy
☐ Plant your own garden, container garden or rent a plot in a community garden
☐ Stock up on non-perishable options like frozen, canned or jar veggies
☐ Choose a "breakfast" vegetable to keep on hand like sweet potato hash or sautéed peppers and onion
☐ Collect pre-cut veggies from a salad bar – use in recipes at home to save prep time
☐ Save prep time with prepared salad mixes, peeled & cubed squash, grated carrots, chopped onion, etc.
☐ Purchase containers of fresh-cut veggies and throw away the dip
☐ Add coleslaw mix to a stir fry

Veggie Grain-Substitutes:
☐ Invest in a spiralizer for zucchini noodles
☐ Research a spiralizer cookbook (online, bookstore or library)
☐ Purchase frozen grated cauliflower to use as rice
☐ Contact your local grocer hot/salad bar to request adding cauliflower rice or sautéed pepper strips
☐ Buy pre-sliced carrots to use as crackers
☐ Make wraps out of blanched collard green leaves
☐ Use grilled/roasted portabella mushroom caps as a bun
☐ Keep a spaghetti squash on hand for spaghetti

Section II – Paleo-Wise: Sleep

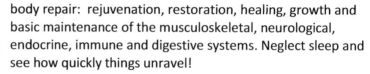

Consequences of Poor Sleep
• Increased Cravings for Salt, Sweets, Carbs
• Brain Fog
• Decreased Insulin Sensitivity
• Weight Gain
• Weakened Skin Elasticity (wrinkles!)
• Impaired Judgment
• Slower Reflexes / Impeded Coordination
• Compromised Athletic Performance

Quality sleep is essential for good health. This is the time for body repair: rejuvenation, restoration, healing, growth and basic maintenance of the musculoskeletal, neurological, endocrine, immune and digestive systems. Neglect sleep and see how quickly things unravel!

Individuals with sleep deprivation are more susceptible to disease, hormonal disruption, depression, obesity, cognition difficulties, compromised immune system and lower overall quality of life.

Sleep Less, Weigh More

Chronic stress and sleep deprivation are mutually reinforcing: stress triggers cortisol, a stimulant, which interrupts sleep and the resulting sleep loss is stressful which triggers more cortisol. This is another vicious cycle that wears down every major bodily system. If the cycle perpetuates uninterrupted, cortisol's impact on cravings for foods high in sugar, starch and salt becomes difficult to control – the impact of poor sleep on insulin resistance can do every bit *as much damage as a diet full of sugar*!

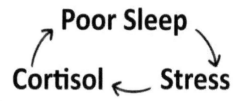

In addition to obesity consequences of increased cravings and insulin resistance, sleep deprivation also causes changes in the brain (via dopamine metabolism) consistent with food addictions and binge-eating disorder.

🖑 <u>ThePaleoMom</u> The Link Between Sleep and Your Weight

Sweet Dreams or Not-so-Sweet Consequences:
Sleep deprivation puts the body in a pre-diabetic state, which can lead to weight gain and compromised health.

Why is Sleep So Elusive?

Sleep is regulated by hormones that cycle through the day, mainly melatonin and cortisol. Both hormones are highly sensitive – they fluctuate with and respond to environmental cues. However, if the wrong cues are sensed and hormone levels become abnormal or erratic, the delicate balance of that natural cycle will collapse.

Melatonin

Melatonin is secreted by the pineal gland in the brain and is the primary hormone responsible for sleep. It is regulated by the body's internal clock and is produced in response to darkness. Melatonin starts increasing after sundown and peaks during the night; then at sunrise it drops, inducing wakefulness.

Circadian Rhythm

Melatonin and cortisol engage in an inverse relationship over the course of each 24-hour period. When cortisol is rising, melatonin declines. As cortisol levels drop off, melatonin increases. That cycle is part of the circadian rhythm and is tied closely to the sleep/wake cycle.

- **Cortisol:** Peaks in the morning, providing energy to start the day, then gradually declines until bedtime
- **Melatonin:** Starts to climb in the evening, sustains higher nighttime levels to support sleep, then drops off early morning

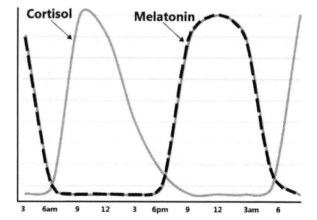

Markers of a Healthy Circadian Cycle

Dietary choices, environmental triggers, hormonal imbalance, unmanaged stress and even personality traits can disrupt the sensitive hormonal equilibrium and compromise sleep. In modern culture, interrupted sleep is so common that its true magnitude and impact is not realized.

Many live with sleep deprivation symptoms and often disregard them as normal or even blame them on other factors. Because sleep disturbance is so common, we have forgotten how to recognize genuine healthy sleep patterns. This table contrasts traits of sufficient sleep versus sleep debt.

Sleep Health	
Markers of Healthy Sleep	**Indicators of Disrupted Sleep**
• Fall asleep easily • Sleep through the night • Fall back asleep easily if woken • Effortlessly wake up refreshed and energized • Feel alert all day long • Concentrate easily during the day • Good memory • Maintain a positive mood/attitude • Improved work performance • Energized, quality workouts • Feel refreshed by a nap, not more tired • Heal efficiently from injuries or overuse • Satisfaction with sleep quality • Healthy libido • Sleep a consistent number of hours • Consistent bedtime and wake time • Do not sleep too much *or* too little	• Unable to calm thoughts when trying to sleep • Stay up too late and get a 'second wind' • Sleep disorder such as sleep apnea, snoring or frequent upper-respiratory infections • Unwillingly wake up too early in the morning • Need daytime stimulants or nighttime sleep aids • Fatigued or achy throughout the day • Memory or concentration difficulties • Often emotional and/or irritable • Work swing shift or night shift • Poor movement or coordination (trip frequently) • Doze off while reading, sitting, TV time, driving • Frequent illness; heal slowly • Chronic expectations of disturbed sleep • Always hungry, especially for sweet and salty foods • Travel across time zones frequently • Seasonal Affective Disorder (SAD) or depression • Stubborn mid-section weight

Supporting the Cortisol-Melatonin Cycle

The modern lifestyle makes it challenging to establish a strong sleep cycle because the key hormones in charge of sleep are also readily influenced by outside factors. The balancing act between cortisol and melatonin is often disturbed and cortisol easily becomes dominant:

1. Uncontrolled stressors prevent the cortisol letdown
2. Insufficient melatonin production tilts the balance in favor of cortisol

Erratic cortisol levels result in a high-and-low energy rollercoaster throughout the day, which many people try to manage artificially with caffeine, sugar and medications. Unfortunately, these interventions further disrupt the hormonal interaction and perpetuate the imbalance. A better approach is to support proper melatonin production by evaluating and modifying modern environments.

Melatonin Disruptors

To properly support the sleep cycle, it is crucial to identify individual sensitivities to melatonin disruptors and employ lifestyle modifications to reduce them. Factors that disrupt melatonin production or function include:

Environmental Influences
- ✓ High cortisol levels or unmanaged stress
- ✓ Electro-magnetic fields (EMFs) from household electronics
- ✓ Jet lag or shift work
- ✓ Exposure to bright light at night
- ✓ Fluoride exposure has also been implicated

Digestive and Dietary Influences
- ✓ Alcohol consumption
- ✓ Caffeine consumption
- ✓ Deficiencies in the amino acid, tryptophan
- ✓ Reduced dopamine levels (related to digestive conditions such as leaky gut, IBS, food intolerances/allergies or dietary stressors)

Melatonin Supplement Warning: These gentle supplements can be used *occasionally* to overcome jet lag or work through a non-typical low-sleep situation. However, if continued long term, the body naturally adjusts to the influx of melatonin by suppressing its own production. Use only on occasion as they create dependency.

Lights Out, Melatonin In

The melatonin cycle is closely tied to natural daylight. Bright sunshine emits the full color spectrum of light and daytime is the *only* time the blue-spectrum is naturally present in high levels. Physiologically, blue light tells the brain it is time to be awake. When the brain senses the blue frequency, it actively suppresses melatonin production to keep the body alert and prevent daytime drowsiness.

In the evening, the sun's spectrum shifts from blue wavelengths to the red/amber frequencies of sunset, cuing the brain to boost melatonin production and prepare for sleep. Light emitted from candles, torches and oil lamps supports the onset of sleep because fire produces the same wavelengths as the setting sun.

However, modern artificial lights emit the full color spectrum, including the daytime blue frequencies (sometimes in atrocious levels). When exposed to artificial lighting after dark, the brain is literally tricked into believing it's still daytime, and therefore blocks melatonin production until all lights are out.

With widespread light pollution, the brain rarely senses a full shift out of the blue light spectrum. Melatonin will be suppressed and cortisol levels will be maintained well into the night. How many of these affect your evening:

- ☐ Indoor lights and lamps
- ☐ Cell phone screens
- ☐ Tablets
- ☐ Televisions
- ☐ Nightlights
- ☐ Clocks

- ☐ E-book readers
- ☐ Security lights
- ☐ Motion detectors
- ☐ Street lights
- ☐ Radio towers
- ☐ Parking lights

- ☐ Stand-by and power buttons on electronics
- ☐ Passing vehicle headlights
- ☐ Indicator lights on outlets or smoke detectors
- ☐ Decorative seasonal lights

Not-so-Bright Idea: Energy-efficient CFLs and LEDs emit more blue light than old-school incandescent bulbs (which are no longer available).

Reduce Night-Time Exposure to Blue-Light

With increased dependence on modern technology, it's impossible to completely give up electricity or devices. The good news is that computer programs and apps can automatically adjust a screen's blue light emittance based on the sun cycle of the current location. Some electronics have built-in settings. Most programs have a 'disable' feature for working on color-sensitive projects or watching a movie in full color.

Free Blue-light Blocking Software:
- ⌐ Website: JustGetFlux
- ⌐ Apps: Twilight or Night Shift

Blue-light Blocking Glasses (inexpensive)
Certain amber-colored glasses block the blue wavelengths. Wear them for 2-3 hours before 'lights out' to stimulate melatonin production. To select a pair, carefully read online reviews to verify blue-light blocking or see link from ⌐ Paleovation, Day 13 (P.S. You do not need to wear them while asleep)

Further Information on Light Pollution
The lack of darkness in our electrified world means very few have witnessed a truly dark night:
- ⊕ YouTube "Light and Health" uploaded by IntDarkSkyAssoc
- ☐ *End of Night,* by Paul Bogard: Both a short promo video and longer taped lecture are available:
  - ⊕ YouTube End of Night uploaded by Paul Bogard

Is there anything more refreshing than a good night's sleep?

Paleo Lifestyle Supports Sleep

The cortisol-melatonin relationship can be disrupted by neurotransmitter deficiency, hormonal imbalance, toxin exposure, dietary deficiencies and a high stress load. Your efforts to incorporate Paleo Lifestyle habits are already working to improve each one of these factors and ultimately improve sleep health.

Paleo Benefit	How it Encourages Sleep
Heals the Gut	A healthy gut supports dopamine and serotonin production and absorption, essential for melatonin production. A leaky gut is healed by removing typical inflammatory foods *plus* incorporating bone broth, fatty fish and gelatin.
Less Dietary Stress	Easily-digestible and nutrient-dense foods provide the body with appropriate building blocks and prevent dietary deficiencies. This reduces stress placed on the digestive system, lowering excess cortisol.
Less Chronic Cardio	Replacing chronic cardio workouts with a variety of low-, moderate- and occasional high-intensity movements supports normal cortisol levels.
Balances Hormones	Removing starches and sugars resets insulin and leptin signaling which, in turn, supports normalization of other hormones including cortisol and melatonin.
Less Toxin Exposure	Reducing processed foods lowers exposure to dietary chemicals/toxins that typically create stress and interfere with hormonal signaling. Numerous followers of the Paleo Lifestyle also take interest in reducing exposure to environmental toxins (see more on Day 20).

Dietary Tips for Better Sleep

Although eating an anti-inflammatory Paleo Diet is a great baseline for improved sleep, here are a few more dietary considerations that may assist with achieving a more restful night.

1. **Organ Meat and Seafood** – Melatonin is made from serotonin which is made from the amino acid tryptophan. While all animal protein sources contain tryptophan, organ meat and seafood have a higher concentration while also having less of other competing amino acids.

2. **Fatty Fish** – The omega-3 fats (DHA and EPA) help support circadian rhythms by improving both brain health and resilience to stressors (with sufficient omega-3s, less cortisol is secreted in response to stress). Fish is also high in vitamin B6 necessary to make melatonin.

3. **Slow Digesting Carbs** – Sleep is extremely sensitive to blood sugar fluctuation. The brain prefers a small, steady, reliable glucose supply overnight. Without it, the brain will spike cortisol to raise the blood sugar level (which also wakes us up). A healthy complex carbohydrate at dinner, such as sweet potatoes, slowly releases glucose to the bloodstream and keeps the brain satisfied all night long. In contrast, a bowl of ice cream before bed causes blood sugar to spike then crash, which initiates a cortisol spike.
   🖑 Balanced Bites FAQs: What Are Good Paleo Carbs to Eat?

4. **Glycine-Containing Foods (especially bone broth)** – Glycine is an amino acid found in gelatin that also acts as a neurotransmitter and increases serotonin levels. Glycine-rich foods help normalize circadian rhythms to improve sleep quality. Connective tissues (gristle), gelatinous meats (shanks, oxtail, ribs, feet, necks) and skin are abundant sources of glycine. You can eat these directly or opt for bone broth, gelatin or collagen powder. Try a mug of bone broth an hour before bed.

5. **Magnesium** – This mineral is a natural muscle relaxer that also supports healthy sleep. Incorporate magnesium-rich foods like dark greens, nuts and seeds, avocado, banana, dark chocolate, artichokes and salmon. After the program you can also try yogurt and kefir, legumes and goat cheese.

6. **Finish Eating 2-3 Hours before Bedtime** – In general, eating suppresses melatonin so late-night snacking correlates with negative effects on sleep quality. Ideally, finish your last meal at least two hours before going to bed.

7. **Caffeine** – On average the half-life of caffeine is five hours. This means that there can be about one fourth of the first caffeine dose in your system *ten hours* after you drank it. Limit consumption, especially after noon.

Recommendations to Induce Restful Sleep:

Sleeping habits are more reasonable to control than our stress load. It's often the best entry point to sway the "cortisol-stress-poor sleep" cycle. Fortunately there are countless lifestyle interventions to improve sleep health.

✓ Checkmark the items you already do to support healthy sleep

X Items you are willing to try

X/✓	**Healthy Sleep Behaviors**	
	Make sleep a priority	Poor sleep = poor bodily function
	Aim for 8 hours *asleep in bed* each night	Do this until your best pattern is established, individual sleep needs generally vary between 7-9 hours per night
	Establish a reasonable bedtime	To avoid the cortisol surge of a 'second wind' (these tend to occur around 11:00pm, so try to be asleep around 10:30)
	Control nighttime artificial light exposure	Use softer lighting and minimize use of electronics after sundown, consider setting an alarm to turn off devices 2-3 hours before bed
	Wear amber-tinted glasses 2-3 hours before bedtime	To filter out blue wavelength in artificial light
	Go to bed at the same time every night	To set the body's internal clock, even on weekends
	Follow the same sleep routine each night	To reinforce patterned signals to prepare the body for rest
	Utilize relaxation techniques	Experiment with controlled deep breathing (inhale, pause, exhale, pause), reciting a mantra, guided imagery or meditation
	Avoid escalatory news, stories or tv shows right before bedtime	Violent, scary and negative news or plot lines can elevate cortisol
	Skip afternoon naps if interfering with onset of nighttime sleep	Nap earlier in the day
	Keep a sleep log	Identify sleep-disrupting patterns/triggers including sleep and wake times, exercise type and amount, diet and drinks for the day, stress levels and any other modifications you are trying
X/✓	**Healthy Sleep Environment**	
	Keep room slightly cool	Encourages the onset of sleep
	Darken your room	Hang blackout shades, cover/unplug things that emit light, wear an eye mask
	Control the noise	Play meditative/sleep music, use a white noise machine or fan, wear ear plugs
	Use calming scents	Such as lavender, chamomile or ylang-ylang
	Replace electric lamps	Use amber and red tinted bulbs or lampshades, or use candlelight after sunset
	Keep extremities warm in cool weather	The more circulation to the hands and feet, the less time it takes to fall asleep; use socks, mittens or hot water bottle at your feet
	Reduce electro-magnetic fields (EMFs), <u>tip</u>: a power strip is a quick solution	Use airplane mode, turn off or unplug sources of electromagnetic radiation: Wi-Fi routers, nightlights, clocks, Wi-Fi ready devices like printers, tablets, computers, smart TVs, cellphones, etc
	Change your alarm clock if you must use one	Try an analog clock or find a digital one with a red/amber display and gentle/gradual alarm tone; consider placing the clock across the room or use a red projection display on ceiling/wall
	Consider sleeping alone	Especially if your partner, child or pet is disrupting your sleep
	Make the bedroom a sanctuary for bedroom-only activities	Use the bedroom for sleeping, relaxing and sex; keep TV, work projects and social media checking out of the sleep environment

X/✓	**Healthy Sleep Nutrition**	
	Follow the Strict Paleo Protocol for a few days	If your sleep becomes compromised due to poor dietary choices or unexpected stressful events
	Avoid stimulants	Caffeine, nicotine, chocolate or tobacco, especially after noon
	Avoid alcohol prior to bedtime	During the night a rebound effect from detoxification can increase restlessness and even cause 2-3 hours of early morning insomnia
	Avoid bedtime snacks	Especially sugar/starch based; blood sugar crashes can trigger cortisol surges, prevent the onset of sleep or interrupt deep sleep
	Always eat starchy veggies at dinner	These slow-digesting carbs provide steady release of glucose to sustain brain activity throughout the night
	Magnesium	Try magnesium-rich foods listed above, supplements (citrate or malate), Epsom salt baths or topically-applied magnesium oil
	Increase percentage of seafood and organ meat in your diet	Increases tryptophan concentration, a precursor to melatonin
	Increase percentage of fatty fish	Helps support circadian rhythms, reduces cortisol intensity
	Increase bone broth or gelatin	Increases serotonin levels to help normalize circadian rhythms
	End dinner 2 hours before bed	Eating suppresses melatonin release
X/✓	**Healthy Morning Routine**	
	Attempt alarm-clock-free	Initially on weekends or vacation days, then graduate to every day
	Expose yourself to bright lights upon waking in the morning	Sunlight or sun lamps are best; just 10-20 minutes of bright morning light can encourage stabilization of the sleep cycle
	Eat breakfast within 1-2 hours of waking	Even a small breakfast can help establish hormonal and circadian cycles
X/✓	**Healthy Daily Activity**	
	Schedule physical activity during the day	Finish any intense exercise 2-3 hours before bedtime
	Manage stress the best you can	Uncontrolled cortisol swings are detrimental for sleep
	Follow stress relief recommendations	Journal, quiet bath, read for pleasure, etc; revisit the text on Day 12 for more suggestions to calm the stress response

Get your Zzzz's ASAP

1. Rate your current sleep quality: poor   1   2   3   4   5   excellent

2. Has your sleep improved since starting the Paleo Diet?   Yes   No

3. In which area(s) are you already making strides toward better quality sleep:

   Sleep Behaviors   Environment   Nutrition   Morning Routine   Daily Activity

4. In which area(s) do you still need improvement: _____

5. Which recommended steps will you take *tonight* to help encourage sound sleep:

   a. _____

   b. _____

   c. _____

6. Which additional actions can you implement over the next few days:

   a. _____

   b. _____

   c. _____

Resources on Improving Sleep (direct links available from ⌐ Paleovation)
- ⌐ MarksDailyApple How to Manufacture Your Best Night of Sleep
- ⌐ Bulletproof How to Hack Your Sleep: The Art and Science of Sleeping
  (note: MCTs are Medium Chain Triglycerides which occur in coconut oil or in concentrated powder/oil)
- ⌐ Bulletproof The Best Biohacking Apps for Stress, Sleep
- ⌐ PaleoLeap Is Polyphasic Sleep for You?
- 📖 *Sleep Smarter*, by Shawn Stevenson

Magnesium Resources
- ⌐ DrAxe Top 10 Magnesium Rich Foods Plus Proven Benefits
- ⌐ WellnessMama How to Make your own Magnesium Oil
- ⌐ SeaSalt Epsom Salt Uses and Benefits

Section III: Monitoring Physical and Emotional Changes

Physical Changes

The low-carb flu should be subsiding by this point and your body may already be demonstrating how well it's adapting to Paleo-style eating. What improvements have you noticed after almost 2 weeks?

- ☐ Sounder sleep
- ☐ Less achy
- ☐ Less pain with an old injury
- ☐ Smoother joint movement
- ☐ Fewer headaches
- ☐ Steady energy levels

- ☐ Clearer skin
- ☐ Thinking clearly
- ☐ Lower blood pressure
- ☐ Better stools
- ☐ Easier digestion
- ☐ Less acid reflux

- ☐ Desire to be active
- ☐ Better performance
- ☐ Quicker exercise recovery times
- ☐ Improved range of motion
- ☐ Feel stronger
- ☐ Clothing fits better

This is the same list from Day 9. Go back to compare how just 4 additional days on the program has added to your success. What differences surprise you?

_____

_____

What do you still hope to improve?

_____

_____

Emotional Changes

Your gut flora is starting to reflect the changes in your diet. More than 90% of serotonin (a feel-good neurotransmitter) is produced and absorbed in the gut. Surprisingly gut flora balance has *everything* to do with your mood. Can you feel the effect emotionally? How have you been feeling lately?

- ☐ Happy/joyful
- ☐ Agreeable
- ☐ Interested/engaged

- ☐ Energetic
- ☐ Content/fulfilled
- ☐ Calm/relaxed

- ☐ Alert
- ☐ Full of wonder
- ☐ Tranquil/peaceful

- ☐ Confident
- ☐ Eager
- ☐ Clear-headed

The opposite would be in this list

- ☐ Discontent/unhappy
- ☐ Tense/edgy
- ☐ Alienated

- ☐ Feisty
- ☐ Hostile/aggressive
- ☐ Hesitant

- ☐ Troubled
- ☐ Grumpy
- ☐ Withdrawn

- ☐ Unstable
- ☐ Apathetic
- ☐ Anxious

Do not be surprised if you are a little bit of both. These things take time to change. Thoughts?

_____

_____

Section IV: Fresh Recipe Ideas

To beat the *mid-program doldrums*, here are a few recipe inspirations – a collection of familiar favorites that have been "Paleo-tized." Check any that interest you and read the recipes online (direct links available from ⍟ Paleovation):

☐ Paleo Gyro Meatballs – Consider making 3-4 lbs at a time to ensure leftovers with minimal additional effort. Feel free to add more seasonings, the lemon flavor is lovely. FYI a cookie scoop (meatball-sized ice cream scooper) makes this job super quick, plus the meatballs are all the same size and cook evenly.
  > ⍟ PaleoCupboard Paleo Gyro Meatballs with Tzatziki Sauce

☐ Paleo Crabcakes – Garnish with pre-made guacamole if you don't have time for the red pepper sauce.
  > ⍟ IBreatheImHungry Low Carb Crabcakes with Roasted Red Pepper Sauce

☐ Paleo Pizza – There are many Paleo crust recipes out there, beware the ones made of straight starch such as tapioca (tapioca starch/flour is okay in small proportions, but limit starches during the program).
  > ⍟ SarahFragoso Everyday Paleo Pizza
  > ⍟ PaleOMG Leftovers: Meatza My Way **(includes variations like fajita, breakfast, etc)**

☐ Paleo Noodles – How about new zucchini noodle ideas?
  > ⍟ PaleoOMG Zoodles and Squoodles Pizza Casserole
  > ⍟ CookEatPaleo Garlic Roasted Shrimp with Zucchini Pasta

☐ Paleo Mini Apple Quiches – Though the recipe title sounds like muffins, these are more like semi-sweet apple quiches. Bake these in silicon muffin cup. Parchment paper muffin cups work amazingly well (and you can reuse the liners 2-5 times). Keep the apple chunky for best results. Freezes well.
  > ⍟ BalancedBites Easy Recipe: Apple Streusel Egg Muffins

☐ Paleo English Muffins – Try these for a snack or add to a meal. Great for mini pizzas! FYI, baking powder contains corn starch. The recipe below uses the baking soda + vinegar option. Another option is: 1tsp baking powder = ½ tsp of baking soda + ¼ tsp of cream of tartar. Adjust up or down for your recipe.
  > ⍟ BeautyAndTheFoodie Quick Paleo English Muffins

☐ Healthiest Ice Cream – Made from caramelized butternut squash...not super sweet, but the salty crunchy coconut/nut topping combination makes this a real treat during the program.
  > ⍟ RealEverything Healthiest Ice Cream Ever

☐ Blueberry Crumble – From 21 Day Sugar Detox, the lemon really makes the other flavors pop.
  > ⍟ BalancedBites Easy Recipe: Fresh Blueberry Crumble

☐ Carrot Cake Pudding – Okay to substitute the carrots with any cooked orange-fleshed veggie (butternut squash, sweet potato, pumpkin, etc). Canned pumpkin is super quick.
  > ⍟ PaleOMG Sugar Detox Carrot Cake Pudding

The idea is to shake up the recipes you are using. Paleo foods do not have to be dull, tasteless or repetitive. Have these suggestions given you other ideas to research (maybe your own favorite)? If so, write them down:

_____

To-Do List:
  ☐ Put together your ingredients for jerky or granola and make a batch by Day 19
  ☐ Look up the recipe for one of the Paleo-tized favorites above. You don't necessarily have to make it, but it may spark ideas on how to stock your pantry and freezer.
  ☐ Anything else (stress relief ideas, sleep support purchase)? _____

Coming up soon:
  • Identifying some common Paleo mistakes (like going overboard on nuts)
  • Ideas for Paleo-friendly crunchy snacks

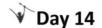

Day 14

> *When it is obvious that the goals cannot be reached, don't adjust the goals,*
> *adjust the action steps.* ~Confucius

Today's Topics:

1. Common Paleo Pitfalls
2. Nuts and Crunchy Paleo Snacks
3. Paleo-Wise: FREE DAY

Fast Fare – Canned Goods
♥ Pumpkin smoothie with coconut milk and collagen/gelatin powder
♥ Canned green beans & lemon pepper

Any special notes about what you are eating today?

_____

_____

Identify your best strategies for nourishing yourself over the last two weeks. Here is what we've provided so far: Batch-Cooking and Foundation Recipes (Prep B), Restaurant Strategies (Prep D), Quick Meals (Prep E), 20-Minute Recipes (Day 1), Meal-Building and Fast Ideas (Day 4) and Substitutes for Non-Compliant Foods (Day 6).

1. _____

2. _____

Is a certain meal or snack giving you trouble (difficult to plan breakfast, finding lunch-on-the-go, etc.)?

_____

If so, how can you adjust for that in the next two weeks? Review strategies here: 28 Days Paleo Meals (Prep B), Breakfasts (Prep F), Veggie Guide (Day 1), Snacks (Day 2), Paleo Fat Bombs (Day 3), Lunchbox Template (Day 9).

_____

_____

Remember those 5 foundation recipes from Prep B? Are some still serving as your foundation?   Yes   No

Of the 5, which foundation recipes will you continue to include in your rotation?

_____

Which of the foundation recipes need to be replaced (didn't like the taste, too much prep time or becoming bored with the same foods)?

_____

Did the recipe selections from yesterday spark any new ideas?   Yes   No

If you need to replace a foundation meal or just want to try something different, list a new recipe here. To avoid overloading yourself with tasks, consider adding only 1 or 2 recipes now. Put the ingredients on your list.

_____

Section I: Common Paleo Pitfalls – Too Little versus Too Much

Although the core Paleo Template is standard, individual differences require tweaking the guidelines to achieve maximum personal benefits. For example, some people digest and burn carbohydrates very well (common in larger men and athletes) while others thrive better with lower carbs but higher amounts of healthy fat (ketosis).

During the transition to Paleo with the focus on introducing new dietary practices, sometimes Paleo behaviors or habits can unintentionally stray out of a healthy range and limit the effectiveness of the Strict Paleo Protocol. To improve personal results, the following two tables detail common deviations from the Paleo Diet and Lifestyle along with suggested adjustments (especially valuable for those who are not responding as expected).

Contemplate your current routine and circle or highlight relevant modifications to improve your approach.

Too LITTLE	
What's Lacking	**How to Modify to Include More**
Healthy Fats	The fear of fat runs deep. When reducing grains and legumes in the typical western diet, there's a substantial calorie deficit which is impossible to replace solely via Paleo vegetables and proteins. Fuel must come from fat to stimulate burning fat. Include traditional fats in every meal and snack (coconut oil, animal fats, olives, avocado, limited nuts). Eat fat liberally – eventually your optimal range will emerge. 📖 *Eat Fat, Get Thin,* by Mark Hyman, MD
Vegetable-Based Carbohydrates	For some people, the carbohydrate reduction during the Paleo transition is too drastic and can negatively impact energy levels. Consider increasing starchy carbs from vegetable sources. Include a wide variety of carrots, squash, sweet potatoes, plantains, beets, parsnips, etc (more on Day 10). Caution: white potatoes are an option but trigger insulin similarly to grains – add sparingly.
Variety	It is common to rely on a handful of favorite meats and veggies, but if the diet lacks variety, it also lacks nutrients. To minimize dietary boredom and maximize nutrients, include a diverse range of foods: • **Vegetable**: select a new color or herb to try; visit the farmer's market; mix into recipes like stir-fry, meatloaf, frittatas, casseroles, etc • **Protein**: beef, chicken, pork, sausage, lamb, bison, goat, turkey, duck, duck eggs, quail eggs, various fish, shellfish, mollusks, canned seafood • **Fat**: olives, avocados, nut butters (1 serving daily), coconut flakes, coconut butter, butter sautés, Paleo mayo and Paleo hollandaise • **Spice**: fresh or dried herbs and seasonings, garlic, turmeric, ginger, etc • **Foods often avoided**: unusual herbs, organ meats, sardines, mollusks Branch away from common favorites with these alternatives: ➢ **Ground beef:** loose sausage, ground poultry, bison, pork, lamb or shrimp ➢ **Tuna:** fresh fish, baby shrimp, sardines, canned salmon, smoked oysters ➢ **Baby carrots:** sticks of celery, broccoli stem, parsnip, kohlrabi or jicama ➢ **Spinach:** watercress, dandelion greens, collards, mustard greens, seaweed
Sodium	Salt is an essential part of a healthy diet and body. Sodium becomes detrimental with too little or too much intake (general recommendations are somewhere between 1 – 2.5 tsp daily!). Most excess salt in the western diet lurks in processed food, but those are eliminated with Paleo. Although it may feel as though you are adding too much salt, it's highly unlikely. Salt your food to taste; use a high-quality salt with trace minerals (Himalayan, Celtic or Real Salt) and consume potassium-rich foods such as sweet potato, avocado, broccoli, spinach or squash (more about Sodium on Day 10) 🖱 ThePaleoMom Is Salt Paleo?
Movement	Humans are not designed to sit all day long, nor are they designed for excessive chronic cardio workouts. Incorporate a variety of sensible movements to improve metabolism, range of motion and circulation.
Sunshine, Playtime, Sleep, Relaxation and Stress Reduction	Stress is one of the biggest offenders to good health...excess cortisol levels literally unravel the benefits of a healthy diet. Unmanaged stress reinforces the hormonal disruption between insulin and leptin, leading to weight gain! Make time for de-stressing in whatever ways work best for you.

Every day may not be good, but there's something good in every day. ~Author Unknown

Too MUCH	
What's Overabundant	**How to Modify to Reduce**
Nuts & Nut Products (nut milk, meal/flour, fruit and nut bars)	Nuts contain the same types of antinutrients as grains and legumes, not to mention a high calorie-load. Because they're a common go-to snack, many people over-consume nuts and nut products. Soaking, then dehydrating nuts neutralizes some of the antinutrients, but nothing will change their dense source of calories. Reduce serving size and limit to one serving per day.
Fruit & Fruit Products (dried fruit, juices)	Historically fruit was only available seasonally, less sweet than modern varieties and not nearly as fast to consume (seedless grapes or watermelon are much quicker to eat than their seeded cousins). Though *some* fruit is a part of a healthy diet, it is easy to over-consume. During the program, fruits are limited. In the long run, select *whole* fruit servings and keep concentrated sugar sources, such as juice and dried fruit, to a minimum.
Flour-Based Foods (tapioca starch, nut meal, arrowroot starch, cassava flour, etc)	To recreate favorite savory foods such as muffins, pancakes or pizza crust, many recipes use Paleo-friendly 'flour.' Although technically Paleo, some concoctions are overly starchy, plus they tend to be hyper-palatable and easy to overeat. Are they better for you than grain-based starches? Yes. Does that make them healthy? No. Consume these only occasionally.
Reliance on Protein	Paleo incorporates high *quality* protein, not high *quantity*. Though it's easy to over-indulge in juicy beef or salmon steaks, burgers, sausages, etc, consciously make vegetables the bulk of the diet (at least half your plate).
Chronic Cardio	Modify workouts with suggestions on Day 10. Slow down, plan rest days, add more leisure activity, shorten workouts, try HIIT or begin resistance training.
Frequent Crutches (sweeteners, alcohol, extra serving of sweets)	We happily suggest 'crutches' to ease the transition to a Paleo Diet. However, if these crutches are utilized too often, they slow down the hormonal regulation between insulin and leptin. The fewer the crutches, the shorter the path to optimal health.
Obsessing over Details (orthorexia – unnatural fixation with healthful eating)	There are fine lines between awareness, discipline and fear. A month of the Strict Paleo Protocol is a time to focus on the details but, for some, it opens a path of food obsession complete with guilt, fear and stress. Human metabolism is adaptable and resilient to minor dietary adversity – there is no need to control every single dietary or environmental factor to ensure good health. In fact, the stress of obsession with perfection causes more health damage than simply allowing minor dietary deviations! Careful reintroduction at the end of the month (explained on Days 25 and 26) will help establish your personal dietary baseline, around which sporadic deviations are reasonable. ☞ Orthorexia The Authorized Bratman Orthorexia Self-Test ☞ BalancedBites Are You Paralyzing Others with Paleo Perfectionism

Does your current routine include any other "too little" or "too much" strays you wish to modify? Explain.

1. _____

2. _____

> Sometimes it's helpful to simply return to the basics:
> ## Meals Built on Veggie + Protein + Fat,
> ## 1 (optional) Nut Serving, 1 (optional) Low-Sugar Fruit Serving
> Within this basic meal-building guideline, variety and portion sizes can be tweaked.

Section II: Nuts for Nuts?

Nuts and seeds are a great go-to Paleo snack, but they are also easy to over-indulge, pack a lot of calories and contain some antinutrients just as grains and legumes do. Continue to limit nut/seed servings to one per day and try some of these options to encourage healthy nut consumption:

1. **Reduce Anti-Nutrients:** Soak or sprout raw nuts and seeds, then roast or dehydrate
   - ⌔ WellnessMama The Importance of Soaking Nuts and Seeds
2. **Slow Down, You're Eating Too Fast:** Buy nuts or seeds in the shell to lengthen your portion satisfaction
3. **Satisfy the Crunch Desire:** If you miss the crunch, replace with other crunchy snacks below
4. **Search Other Nutty Flavors:** Add nut-free but umami-rich foods and flavors (more below)
   - ⌔ MelJoulwan 10 Paleo Flavor Boosters

Crunchy Paleo Snacks

Homemade is best, but a wide variety of Paleo-friendly products are available. Some of these foods are easy to over-consume so stick to a single serving. If you are looking for a fatty animal product (for example, pork skin to make cracklins), pasture-raised is best. Select products made with coconut oil, avocado oil, palm oil, pasture-raised animal fats and a lesser extent, olive oil, as these stand up best to heat.

Nut-Free and Crunchy Paleo Snacks		
✓ Kale chips ✓ Plantain crackers ✓ Raw veggies: carrots, cucumbers, jicama, celery, kohlrabi, cauliflower ✓ Fried salami, prosciutto or pepperoni slices ✓ Pickles ✓ Thin, well-done jerky	✓ Bacon crisps or bits ✓ Toasted coconut chips (large flakes crisped in the oven) ✓ Crispy chicken skin either from roast chicken or deliberately re-crisped in the oven ✓ Veggie chips from taro, yucca, plantain, sweet potato or zucchini	✓ Pork rinds or cracklings, US Wellness Meats and Galactic Hog Skins are high quality brands (FYI, 'scratchings' from the UK usually contain wheat) ✓ Toasted or roasted seaweed ✓ Freeze-dried berries or green apple (limit serving size) ✓ Cauliflower popcorn

Nutty Flavor Substitutes

Some of these ingredients have a nutty flavor. Others have the 'umami' factor (along with the flavors of sweet, sour, salty and bitter, *umami* is a distinct savory flavor the tongue can detect). Adding these to your meals will complement the other flavors.

1. Browned butter or ghee
2. Nutritional yeast
3. Cricket flour (yikes!)
4. Minced, cooked mushrooms
5. Seed-based spices like coriander, cumin, fenugreek, mustard, poppy or sesame
6. Toasted sesame oil
7. Roasted turnips or sunchokes (Jerusalem artichokes)
8. Caramelized onions or roasted garlic
9. Dried (and powdered) shiitake mushrooms
10. Toasted or dried seaweed flakes
11. Coconut aminos

Section III – Paleo-Wise: FREE DAY

Are there any topics that you want to re-review or explore further? Take a moment to thumb through previous days' subjects and consider reading any overlooked links.

To-Do List:
- ☐ Put together your ingredients for jerky or granola and make a batch by Day 19
- ☐ Add ingredients for new foundation recipes to your shopping list
- ☐ Anything else (new lifestyle tweak, stress relief)? _____

Coming Soon:
- Fiber is the topic of Day 15...what is it? Do we need it? Where do we find it? What fiber should we avoid?
- Tomorrow you could expand your culinary knowledge with *spatchcock* – what in the world???

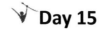
Day 15

Today's Topics:

1. Paleo-Wise: Fiber
2. Half-Way Hooray
3. Cooking Assignment #5: Roast a Whole Chicken

Fast Fare – Canned Pumpkin
♥ Pumpkin soup: broth, coconut milk, pumpkin, spinach and curry powder
♥ Shrimp cocktail

Reflections on today's menu (Was enough food on hand? Are leftovers key to your success? Any improved strategies for including a wider variety of vegetables? Are you remembering to eat the full rainbow?). Notes:

_____

_____

On Days 9 & 10 we discussed options for reducing sedentary postures and adding different styles of movement and exercise. Have you successfully incorporated some of these movement ideas in your routine?   Yes   Not yet

Section I – Paleo-Wise: Benefits of Fiber

Eat vegetables. Lots of them. ~Sarah Ballantyne, PhD, author of <u>The Paleo Approach</u>

What Exactly is Fiber?

Dietary fiber is a non-digestible carbohydrate found in plant foods such as vegetables, fruit, whole grains and legumes. Generally, it forms the cell wall structure which acts as the skeleton for the plant. Human digestive enzymes cannot break down fiber into simpler components, so it passes through digestion mainly intact.

Most fiber sources are a combination of soluble, insoluble, fermentable and non-fermentable fibers. Each has benefits, but it's very difficult to disentangle the overlap. By following the Paleo meal template of Protein + Veggie + Fat, the large rotation of vegetables that make up roughly half of every meal will undoubtedly provide a balance of all fiber varieties.

> **Key Point:** Fiber comes in many varieties and all have benefits. As long as fiber is attained from anti-inflammatory whole-food sources, there is no one variety that is better than another.

Anti-Inflammatory Whole-Food Fiber Sources	
Source	**Examples**
Root Vegetables / Tubers	Carrot, sweet potato, beet, radish, Jerusalem artichoke, jicama, onion
Leafy Greens	Kale, collards, spinach, mustard greens, dandelion greens, mizuna
Foods with Edible Peel/Pod	Zucchini, apple, pear, some winter squash, okra, root vegetables, green beans, snow peas, sugar snap peas
Foods with Edible Seeds	Berries, sunflower seeds, pepitas (pumpkin seeds), nuts, figs, flaxseed
Cruciferous Vegetables	Broccoli, cauliflower, cabbage, kohlrabi, Brussels sprouts
Properly Prepared Legumes*	Soaked and boiled or sprouted beans: lentils, split peas, soup beans

*Non-Paleo source, might be tolerated after the program (more about legume preparation on Day 8)

Feed the Flora

The *number one benefit of fiber* is it feeds probiotic bacteria in the colon. These good bacteria produce enzymes which ferment fiber, yielding beneficial byproducts such as *short-chain fatty acids* and vitamins B and K2 (more about vitamin K2 on Days 7 and 16).

The resultant short chain fats produced by the flora are the primary energy source of cells lining the large intestine, making these fats *vital* for colon health. They are easy to digest and offer the entire body an alternative to glucose as an energy source (more about Medium- and Short-Chain Fats on Day 2).

Other Benefits of Short Chain Fats:
- Appetite suppressant; assists with weight loss
- Potent anti-inflammatory and anti-cancer effects; used as treatment for inflammatory bowel diseases like IBS, ulcerative colitis and Crohn's disease
- Increase absorption of calcium, magnesium and iron
- Maintain gut barrier integrity and decrease gut permeability

What's in a Name? Butyrate is one of the beneficial short-chain fats produced by the gut flora. Interestingly, the richest dietary source of butyrate is hidden in its name: BUTYR-ate...Butter! Choose grass-fed, of course, and enjoy this tasty Paleo-friendly fat without guilt.

Fiber Features

Finally, conventional wisdom got it right! Fiber has many benefits. The main difference between mainstream fiber recommendations and Paleo is sourcing (beware grain or legume sources due to the inflammatory effect).
- Fiber-containing foods slow the release of glucose to the bloodstream, reducing insulin spikes
- Fiber presence helps regulate the pace of peristalsis, the rhythmic colon movement for stool passage
- Soluble fiber tends to be readily used by the good gut bacteria
- Certain fibers bind toxins or surplus hormones in the digestive tract, aiding with removal
- Insoluble fiber protects normal recycling of bile salts and cholesterol which prevents accidental elimination of essential fats and fat-soluble vitamins A, D, E and K (more about Cholesterol on Day 17)
- Some insoluble fibers have anti-inflammatory effects, decrease liver triglycerides, increase fat metabolism, normalize blood sugars and promote normal body weight
- Certain insoluble fibers increase absorption of calcium and magnesium to improve bone health

Can't Handle Fiber? Some individuals with bowel disorders cannot comfortably process fiber. For these individuals, cooked vegetables tend to be the best tolerated source of fiber, especially in the beginning. Over time on the Paleo Diet, beneficial gut flora will gradually be replenished and nourished to assist with raw vegetable digestion and improved colon health. In the meantime, a supplement (fiber or resistant starch, more later) may be beneficial short-term until healthy gut flora are restored (more about Gut Flora on Day 21).

Caution: Processed Industrial Fiber

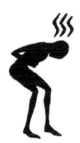

Food manufacturers take advantage of the many benefits of fiber by using slogans like "high fiber" or "added fiber" to make their products appear healthier. However, the fiber used in processed and packaged foods is a different variety – usually inexpensive industrial fillers (think wood pulp or cotton).

These fibers are isolated from the plant and do not produce the same benefits as whole-food sources. Whether advertised or not, these filler fibers are in nearly all processed foods and act as stabilizers or volumizers. They hold water and/or maintain shape to replicate a fattier texture or make the product appear more substantial.

Identify Industrial Fibers: These are labeled under obscure names such as agar-agar, algae, alginate, β-glucan, cellulose gum, carrageen, fructooligosaccharides, guar gum, hemicellulose, kelp, lignin or pectin.

Problems with industrial fiber:
- May *contribute* to obesity. Isolated fiber rapidly absorbs water and expands in the stomach – up to 5 times its original size – which pacifies the appetite for a short while. Unfortunately, it also stretches the stomach chamber. Each subsequent meal requires more and more fiber *or food* to create the same full feeling.
- Fiber fillers tightly hoard water, preventing the body from access to it and contributing to fluid malabsorption conditions.

Laxative Labels

Many laxatives rely on fiber as a primary ingredient. Be careful – not all fiber is created equal. Some fibers *do* relieve constipation but others *cause* it! Additionally, laxatives often contain industrial filler fibers (listed above).

1. **Soluble Fiber** - Dissolves in water and absorbs water to form a gel-like material in the gut, adding bulk to the stool. This acts as an appetite suppressant by *slowing* the movement of food through the digestive system. The end result is that soluble fiber can *cause* constipation, not relieve it! These fibers include psyllium, inulin and vegetable gums such as guar gum. <u>Note</u>: Most industrial filler fibers significantly retain water so they also fall in this category and have a digestive deceleration effect.

2. **Insoluble Fiber** - Does *not* dissolve in water so it passes through the digestive tract quickly. This tends to accelerate the movement of material through digestion which could be a beneficial treatment for constipation. Insoluble fibers include cellulose, pectin and lignin.

> *Our gut flora? Those trillions of "foreign" cells residing along our digestive tract that actually outnumber our native human cells? To those guys, certain types of fiber are food to be fermented or digested.* ~Mark Sisson, author of <u>Primal Blueprint</u>

Resistant Starch – Gut Flora Food

Recall that starch is simply glucose molecules linked together, easily broken apart by human digestive enzymes. However, there exists a unique starch structure that resists digestion and instead, acts like a fermentable fiber. This *resistant starch* passes through the stomach and small intestine unscathed until it reaches the colon where *it feeds the friendly bacteria* (which then generate the beneficial short-chain fat, butyrate). Resistant starch promotes the health of the *entire colon*! Examine the many benefits of resistant starch:

Health Benefits of Resistant Starch (RS)	
Reduces Blood Sugar Levels	**Feeds the Good Gut Flora**
• Lowers blood sugar levels after meals – this effect continues *through the next meal* • Reduces fasting blood sugar • Improves insulin sensitivity • Increases satiety (appetite suppressant) reducing food intake in subsequent meals	• RS is a prebiotic, feeding friendly gut bacteria • Preferred fuel of the gut bacteria (not glucose) • Preferentially feeds the good gut flora over pathogenic bacteria • Increases good bacteria population, normalizing the ratio of friendly to pathogenic bacteria
Improves Gut Function	**Fuels Colon Cells**
• Increases colon cell growth • Increases dietary magnesium absorption • Reduces leaky gut permeability • Improves integrity of the digestive tract • Inhibits circulation of toxins present in gut	• Colon bacteria ferment resistant starch into gases and short-chain fatty acids • Butyrate, a short-chain fatty acid, is the preferred fuel for cells lining the colon • Exceptionally *anti*-inflammatory for the colon

There are multiple varieties of resistant starch, but the primary natural sources come in two forms:

1. **Naturally-Occurring Raw Starch** – This is incompatible with human digestive enzymes – found in raw potatoes, green plantains and unripe bananas (<u>Note</u>: This *only* occurs in the *raw* or *unripe* forms. Cooking or ripening these foods will decrease the amount of resistant starch).

2. **Retrograded Starch** – Sometimes digestible starch undergoes a process called retrogradation: after being cooked, the cooling process crystallizes the starch, making it *resistant* to digestion. This is found in some *cooked-and-cooled* foods including potatoes, plantains, parboiled rice and legumes.

There are two ways to add RS to your diet...from real foods or by supplement (detailed in the following table). Though most colons will benefit from resistant starch, it is always preferable to consume it from real-food sources first and to eat RS along with other fiber-rich foods. Please notice a few real-food sources also have a high carbohydrate load that can negatively affect insulin levels. Please proceed with caution when adding foods such as potato salad (limit to an occasional serving).

Resistant Starch Sources		
Whole Food Sources		**Supplement Sources**
Raw potatoes	Yams	Potato starch (but *not* flour or flakes)
Cooked then cooled potatoes	Cooked then cooled legumes†	Plantain flour
Green bananas	Cooked then cooled rice†	Green banana flour
Plantains	Parboiled rice†	Cassava/tapioca starch
Cashews	Raw oats†	Mung bean starch† (at Asian grocer)
Root vegetables/tubers	Raw mung beans†	High maize starch† Not advised

† Non-Paleo sources determined by individual tolerance. They may be useful for you after the program.

Supplementing with Resistant Starch*

A resistant starch supplement may be temporarily appropriate for some individuals: those with insulin resistance, those who have difficulty digesting fiber-rich foods or those who are simply avoiding extra carbohydrates for weight-loss purposes. Here are a few tips if choosing to add a resistant starch supplement:

- ✓ Consume it raw or slightly warmed. At temperatures above 130°F, resistant starch reverts to digestible glucose (so making muffins out of plantain flour destroys the RS - darn!)
- ✓ It takes 2-4 weeks for the colon to adapt and boost short-chain fat production; be patient for results
- ✓ Expect some increase in bowel gas while the body acclimates
- ✓ Rotate several supplements to vary the starches; this prevents over-feeding one group of gut flora
- ✓ Any time a fiber supplement is added, fluids (caffeine-free) must also be increased
- ✓ Start slowly! 1 *tsp* – 1 *Tbsp* daily; acclimate before you increase, too much too fast can cause painful gas
- ✓ A common final dose range is 15-30g of RS daily (for potato starch, which contains 8g per tablespoon, that would be 2-4 Tbsp per day)
- ✓ Sprinkle RS supplements on meals, mix into drinks or incorporate in sauces, dressing or gravy
- ✓ If painful symptoms develop, discontinue supplementation or read tips below for SIBO

RS Supplement Caveat: A resistant starch supplement is not an excuse to avoid vegetables! Consume it with other fiber-rich foods and only plan to take it temporarily until gut flora are better established.

* Supplementing RS in rodents with current cancerous tumors increased tumor size. No studies have been done on humans but we do not advise supplemental RS in cancer patients. Stick with real-food sources.

RS Strategies for SIBO (Small Intestine Bacterial Overgrowth) or IBS (Irritable Bowel Syndrome)

Normally gut bacteria primarily populate the colon (the last portion of the intestine). However, if bacteria or fungi from the colon migrate, overgrow or invade the small intestine earlier in the digestive tract, they can ferment resistant starch prematurely. This triggers negative digestive reactions like gas, bloating, cramps, diarrhea or constipation. Strategies to help with symptoms:

1. **Incorporate Probiotics** – Taking probiotics with resistant starch may alleviate discomfort
2. **Digestive Enzymes** – Those with bowel disorders may benefit from a temporary enzyme supplement (quality enzyme supplements available at ⚘ PureRXO.com/Paleovation)
3. **Reduce the Dose** – Start with a low RS dose (¼ tsp) and gradually increase as the body acclimates
4. **Eat It in Real-Food Form** – Choose real-food sources of resistant starch to test tolerance but be mindful not to over-consume high amounts of carbohydrates
5. **Consume Alongside Fiber-Rich Foods** – Consuming RS with a vegetable-rich meal helps to spread the RS throughout the colon for more evenly-distributed fermentation and butyrate availability

Further Reading (direct links available from ⚘ Paleovation):

- ⚘ ThePaleoMom The Fiber Manifesto (a 6-part series)
- ⚘ Healthline Resistant Starch 101
- ⚘ ThePaleoMom Modifying Paleo for Small Intestinal Bacterial Overgrowth

In understanding the basics of digestion, you'll discover who's in charge. Here's a hint, it's not you.
~Nancy S. Mure

Section II: Half-way Hooray!

Wow! Look how far you've come! Take a moment to thumb through your responses since Day 1. Notice changes in physical health, attitude, ability to build meals, comfort level with adding more fats, and increased knowledge or understanding about nutrition, lifestyle choices, low-carb flu symptoms, stress response, etc.

What have you loved about your experience so far? Anything is fair game: *not* counting carbs, becoming better informed, finding a new favorite food, using the Veggie + Protein + Fat meal template, physical changes, etc.

_____

_____

What have you disliked about the program? Again, anything is fair game.

_____

_____

Have your taste buds changed at all?   Yes   No
Are there any Paleo foods that are becoming more delicious to you as time goes on?

_____

_____

The Paleo Lifestyle is more than just diet change, it includes strategies to support full body health: incorporating proper body movement, reducing and managing stress levels, emphasizing appropriate sleep, and establishing connections to the environment. Which specific lifestyle recommendations have been most beneficial for you?

_____

_____

What is something that has surprised you about yourself during this transition (ability to heal, curiosity about Paleo-Wise topics, strength of commitment level, attitude toward food, openness to trying new ideas, etc)?

_____

_____

Reward Your Progress!

To have successfully remained on the health-rejuvenating Strict Paleo Protocol for 14 days deserves a reward! Unfortunately, our culture tends to associate celebrations and rewards with sugary food, alcohol or money. Obviously, this is not the time to pop open the champagne or indulge in a frosted cake. And though it's gratifying to treat yourself to an expensive spa treatment or special purchase, rewards do not have to require a financial investment. Find a reward that warms your soul. Here are a few examples to stimulate your thought process – there are many more ideas online. Check any that interest you and/or record your own ideas afterward.

☐ Take a bike ride	☐ Binge-watch a great TV series	☐ Schedule in a hike in a nature area
☐ Make a gratitude list	☐ Research your family tree	☐ Cook a meal for someone in need
☐ Enjoy a long bath	☐ Put fresh sheets on the bed	☐ Find an online guided meditation
☐ Paint a picture	☐ Get some projects done	☐ Set aside quiet time for yourself
☐ Do some puzzles	☐ Watch a classic movie	☐ Go geocaching (use GPS geocaching.com)
☐ Learn a new craft	☐ Attend a free community class	☐ Take and share some digital photos
☐ Dance	☐ Read an entertaining book	☐ Visit a free historical site, zoo or museum
☐ Volunteer	☐ Have a grill-out with friends	☐ Play cards/games with the neighbors
☐ Rest and relax	☐ Browse your photo collection	☐ Visit an animal shelter or play with a pet
☐ Rearrange furniture	☐ Call someone you miss	☐ Explore a new section in your library
☐ Do a home spa day	☐ Check out a community calendar	☐ Learn a foreign language (sites/apps)

Are there any other non-food rewards that would feel great to you right now? If so, list them here:

_____

Your *Body* is Rewarding You!

Now is the perfect point to reflect on the positive changes happening in your body. The longer you stay on the Strict Paleo Protocol, the more your body heals. It also increases the odds that your new habits will evolve into a long-term healthy lifestyle. Here is what's changing deep inside your body:

1. **Fat-Adaptation** – The last two weeks have limited the amount of glucose available to your body so now you are beginning to metabolize fat stores for energy.
2. **Less Hunger** – Since insulin surges are now a thing of the past, the body is better able to respond to both the insulin signal and even more importantly, the leptin signal (which identifies when we're full). The body eventually loses those potent, physical hunger pangs, but even if hunger surfaces during the day, its unfavorable symptoms are reduced: less light-headedness, jitters, nausea or urgency to get to food.
3. **Sounder Sleep** – You should be noticing some subtle sleep changes by this time, either falling asleep faster or getting back to sleep more easily if awoken. This is due to restoring hormonal balance, reduction of cortisol and increased ability to correctly cycle melatonin.
4. **Even and Steady Energy** – Because burning body fat provides steady energy all day long, that afternoon energy slump should be easing.
5. **Less Stress** – Nutrient-dense, anti-inflammatory foods reduce digestive stress and overall stress load.
6. **Healing Leaky Gut** – By removing common disruptors to the gut lining (anti-nutrients, toxins, gluten) the intestinal wall is beginning to repair. Not only will the intestinal lining become more competent at selecting which items pass through to the blood stream, but the immune system will not need to constantly respond as inappropriate particles sneak into the blood. Surprisingly, this also improves the production and absorption of feel good neurotransmitters (serotonin and dopamine) within the gut.
7. **Better Gut Flora Balance** – Limiting glucose starves the pathogenic organisms in the gut. Consuming short-chain fats like grass-fed butter and adding more vegetables (with associated fiber) feeds the beneficial microbes. The overall balance of gut flora will continue to improve.
8. **Less Inflammation** – You may or may not notice that inflammation is steadily decreasing during the program. It won't be long until joints are more fluid, and range of motion improves. That is just one clue that the entire body is less inflamed, including arterial walls, the digestive tract, the brain, the lymph system...everything!

Health Knowledge – With a better understanding of why a Paleo Diet is beneficial to health, you can consciously make better food choices. What are your thoughts about the rewards your body is providing so far?

_____

_____

Section III: Cooking Assignment #5 – Roast a Whole Chicken

The American culture roasts turkey every Thanksgiving, but why limit this type of cooking project to just once per year? Roasting a whole chicken is a pivotal skill within traditional cooking. Meat cooked on the bone is more flavorful *and more nutritious* than the boneless, skinless counterparts.

Roasting a chicken is an easy way to feed a group or whole family, stock leftovers for the fridge/freezer and as a bonus: acquire bones for bone broth. Even non-cooks and beginners are highly successful with this project!

Suggestions for Efficiency:

- Consider roasting two chickens at the same time for oven efficiency and leftovers
- Roast some vegetables on a separate rack while the bird cooks
- Arrange your oven racks *before* preheating so you have enough space to accommodate all the pans
- A meat thermometer is handy
- Though not necessary, some people prefer to use disposable gloves for handling large pieces of meat

General Process:

1. ***Read the weight of the bird*** before you throw away the label – cook time depends on weight
2. Remove the giblets tucked into the cavity of the bird
    a. Rinse them and reserve or freeze to add to bone broth later
    b. Alternatively, fry the liver or heart in a pan with a little oil and seasoning
3. Smell the chicken
    a. Neutral smell = It is fine, no need to rinse
    b. 'Off' smell = Rub it clean under gently running water
    c. Still bad? = Clean it again, especially in crevices and inside the cavity (a weak smell is fine to cook but a persistent, strong smell indicates a rotten bird)
4. Season with salt, pepper, herbs, lemon or other flavors (optional: to flavor the meat directly, loosen the skin at the neck and use your hands to spread the seasoning between the skin and muscle)
5. Optional: Let the bird come to room temperature before cooking (approximately 1 hour)
6. For crispy skin, rub the bird with olive oil, grass-fed butter or coconut oil and roast at 425°F for the first 30 minutes, then drop the temperature to 350°F for the rest of the roasting time
7. For super juicy breasts (but not so crispy skin) roast upside down
8. Roasting time is determined by weight of the bird (20-30 minutes per pound at 375°F) and isn't done until the juices run clear when pricked with a skewer
9. Start checking your bird's temperature about 20 minutes before first suggested "done time"
10. Check every 10 minutes until it reaches **165°F** in the thickest part of the thigh and base of breast
11. Let the bird rest for 15-20 minutes before carving – the meat stays juicier
12. Save all bones, giblets and extra bits for bone broth

Spatchcock a Chicken – *Spatchcocking* or *spattlecocking* is the process of flattening the bird into a single layer for faster, more even roasting or grilling. This can reduce cooking time by 25-50% and all the skin comes out crispy (whereas a roasted bird is only crispy on the top side)! You will need a pair of scissors or kitchen shears.
   ❀ Technique: YouTube Spatchcock Chicken Technique uploaded by Food Wishes
   ᗧ Recipe: ItalianFoodForever Golden Brown Roasted Spatchcock Chicken

---

Recipes:
   ᗧ NomNomPaleo Julia Child's Classic Roast Chicken (excellent play-by-play)
   ᗧ PaleoLeap 20 Creative Recipes for Roasting a Whole Chicken (beware: some have sweeteners or fruits)
   If it's too hot outside to turn on the oven, set up a slow cooker:
      ᗧ PaleoCupboard Slow Cooker Rotisserie Chicken

Carve the Bird:
The easiest way to learn to carve a bird is by video. The first video is more thorough including portioning for serving and the secret location of the 'oysters' on the backbone:
   ❀ YouTube How to Carve a Chicken - Jamie Oliver's Home Cooking Skills (~5min)
   ❀ YouTube America's Test Kitchen How to Carve a Whole Roast Chicken (~2min)

To-Do List:
   ☐ Gather ingredients for jerky or granola and make a batch by Day 19
   ☐ You have a full week to purchase and roast a chicken (or two); finish by Day 23
   ☐ Attain a meat thermometer; digital ones are fantastic!
   ☐ Anything else (movement, reward, etc)? _____

Coming Up Soon:
   • Bone Health – there's a lot more to it than calcium
   • If you're getting bored with unsweetened beverages, we've got options for you

Day 16

Some things you have to do every day. Eating seven apples on Saturday night instead of one a day just isn't going to get the job done. ~ Jim Rohn

Today's Topics:

1. Paleo-Wise: Bone Health
2. Unsweetened beverages

Fast Fare – Just Sauté
♥ Zucchini noodles and marinara
♥ Canned mussels

What are you eating today? Does it follow the Veggie + Protein + Fat template?

_____

Are you beginning to get the hang of this? If not, re-read the Paleo strategies you noted on Days 10 and 14 to support your personal transition. Identify and list any areas to redirect your focus and keep you on target:

_____

Section I – Paleo-Wise: Bone Health

To thrive in life, you need three bones: a wishbone, a backbone and a funny bone. ~Reba McEntire

The hard, compact outer surface of bones gives the illusion that the skeleton is simply a lifeless frame. On the contrary, bones are active and dynamic, complete with blood vessels, nerves and softer inner components that all require a myriad of high-quality nutrients.

Bone Functions

The most obvious role of the skeleton is to provide the body's structural framework. Muscles, tendons and ligaments attach to the structure, allowing for mobility. Other bone functions include:

- **Vital Organ Protection** – Encasing the brain, spinal cord, heart and lungs
- **Blood Cell Production** – Blood cells and platelets are produced from bone marrow cells
- **Mineral Storage** – A large percentage of minerals (including calcium and magnesium) are present in bones which can be accessed (or leached!) when dietary intake is insufficient for bodily functions

Calcium – The Throne of Bone

Effective marketing has elevated calcium to the king nutrient of bone health. Indeed, calcium is the most prominent of the bone minerals, but it is not the *only* mineral for strong, healthy bones.

> **Reality Check:** The rate of osteoporosis in the United States is the highest in the world despite having the highest level of calcium supplementation! Calcium is *not* a one-size-fits-all solution to bone integrity. There's so much more to quality bone health. ᗡ WellnessMama The Problem with Calcium Supplements

Calcium Clarifications

Because calcium is so prominently marketed in modern cultures, it's important to understand some basics about this mineral to put its role in proper perspective.

1. **Calcium Interference**

   Simply consuming more calcium is *not* the key to strong bones. To increase calcium content in bones, the pathway between intestinal absorption and the intended endpoint (deposited in the bone) must be free from interference. Minimizing sources of interference is equally, *if not more*, important than purely focusing on the quantity of calcium intake.
   - Grains and legumes contain calcium-trapping phytates that prohibit mineral absorption
   - Deficiencies of vitamins D3 and K2 disrupt calcium's placement into the bone (more later)
   - Bone tissue is mineralized collagen, the same protein as the surrounding tendons and ligaments. Chronically elevated cortisol with high stress targets collagen breakdown (read more on Day 11).

> **Cola Culprit:** Aside from the fact that soda is high in sugars and displaces water consumption, the phosphoric acid unique to colas (both regular and diet) binds to calcium and magnesium in the digestive tract. Regular consumption of phosphoric acid is associated with lower bone mineral density (BMD).

2. **Calcium Supplements – More is Not Better**
   In the absence of other critical cofactors, calcium is not necessarily directed into the bone and can instead deposit in soft tissues including muscles and joints (contributing to chronic stiffness) and even arteries. In fact, isolated calcium supplements have been shown to *increase the risk of both arterial calcification and heart disease*! Calcium supplementation is not effective when its synergistic nutrients are ignored.

   > **Key Point:** Swallowing is not the same as absorbing. Merely ingesting high amounts of calcium does not guarantee it automatically deposits into the bones.

3. **Dairy is *Not* the *Only* Good Source of Calcium**
   Dairy foods do contain calcium, but it's attained at a potential health cost (review Dairy topic on Day 7). One common criticism of the Paleo Diet is the lack of dairy foods, falsely equating this absence to low calcium intake and a higher risk for bone deterioration. On the contrary, studies show eating Paleo *improves* bone density. How is that possible?

Non-Dairy Calcium Sources
Turnip or collard greens
Broccoli
Kale
Bok choy
Canned fish (with bones)
Almonds
Oranges

   - There are many non-dairy sources of calcium available (see table).
   - Paleo foods naturally include synergistic calcium cofactors and other essential bone nutrients.
   - Proper hormonal regulation throughout the body means mineral deposits are normalized and properly formed (more later).
   - Without interference from phytates in grains and legumes, a higher percent of calcium is absorbed so less total dietary calcium is necessary (more on Grains and Legumes in Prep E and Day 8).
   - Many traditional cultures consume dairy-free diets yet maintain lifelong healthy, strong bones.

Regulating Calcium Deposits

In addition to calcium as a raw material, there are several key regulators necessary to shuttle calcium and other minerals into their appropriate places.

1. **Vitamin D3** – This "sunshine vitamin" is actually a hormone manufactured when the skin is exposed to UV light. It plays a pivotal role in maintaining normal blood levels of calcium by promoting its absorption from the intestine, thus limiting the need to withdraw calcium from bones. Many studies show that without Vitamin D3, supplemental calcium has no effect whatsoever on preventing bone pathologies.
   - ✓ **Not Enough Sunshine?** Consider a quality D3 supplement since dietary sources alone rarely supply sufficient amounts (vitamin D3 is found in fatty fish, liver, egg yolks, raw dairy and cod liver oil). Ask your healthcare provider for a blood test to check vitamin D levels and determine proper dosage.
2. **Vitamin K2** – Properly distributes calcium by relocating it out of soft tissues and depositing it into bone and teeth. Vitamin K1 is the plant form that is converted to K2 by healthy digestive bacteria. This happens to some degree in the human gut but, much more efficiently in the gut of a grass-fed cow (more about K2 on Day 7).
   - ✓ **Source Matters:** Grass-fed butter/ghee is a good source of vitamin K2 but conventional butter has little. Vitamin K2 is also found in pasture-raised egg yolks, liver and sardines.
3. **Parathyroid Hormone (PTH)** – This hormone acts as a director to maintain proper blood calcium levels. It does this by regulating how much calcium is stored in bone, how much gets absorbed during digestion and how much is excreted by the kidneys. When PTH acts to raise calcium levels in the blood, it has access to the stores in the bone and can leach calcium and weaken bone structure when necessary (deficiency of vitamin D3 contributes to this process).

4. **Estrogen** – This female hormone helps the bones retain minerals. Estrogen deficiency stimulates bone breakdown but not rebuilding. Deficiency (common in menopause) also restricts calcium absorption and increases risk of conditions such as osteoporosis.

The Skeleton Crew

Each bone is a living structure comprised of minerals, proteins, fats and vitamins wrapped in a firm frame laced with blood vessels and nerves. If any of these components are undernourished, bone integrity is weakened.

> **Chicken Soup for Bone Health:** What's good *for* bones comes *from* bones. We are genetically adapted to attain a large proportion of bone-building nutrients directly from eating bones and cartilage. The best source of these essential nutrients is bone broth...so Great-Grandma's chicken soup really *was* healing!

1. **Minerals:** Our ancestors thrived on mineral-rich foods grown in mineral-rich soil (or by eating the animals that grazed on such plants). Unfortunately, the modern diet and commercial farming methods no longer satisfy our complete mineral needs. Factors contributing to the high prevalence of mineral deficiencies include:
   - Industrial agricultural practices fail to replenish vital trace minerals into the soil, focusing instead on only three: N, P, K (nitrogen, phosphorus and potassium, as seen on most fertilizer bags).
   - High grain and sugar consumption in the modern diet displaces intake of mineral-rich vegetables and fruits.

   Magnesium Deficiency – This deficiency is widespread because sufficient amounts are *difficult to attain in modern food*. Magnesium is a key mineral that builds the bone matrix structure. Additionally, it contributes to muscle relaxation and is required for more than 300 biochemical reactions within the body. When blood magnesium levels drop, it is leached from the bones.

Bone-Building Essentials	
Minerals	**Vitamins**
Calcium	Vitamin D3
Magnesium	Vitamin K1 and K2
Phosphorus	Vitamin A
Iron	Vitamin C
Boron	**Proteins**
Zinc	Collagen (gelatin)
Potassium	Glucosamine
Sodium	**Fats**
Copper	EPA and DHA
Glandular Function	**Lifestyle**
Parathyroid hormone	Sleep
Estrogen	Resistance exercise

> **Solution:** Buy local organic produce or grow your own. High-quality mineral supplements can fill in the gaps.

2. **Proteins:** With primary focus on minerals, amino acids are often overlooked as critical bone components.
   - **Collagen** – 30% of the dry weight of bone is made of collagen protein. Collagen formation requires a regular supply of amino acids along with adequate vitamin C to incorporate them.
   - **Glucosamine** – High concentrations are found in cartilage and connective tissue.

> **Paleo Advantage:** In cooked form, collagen protein is called *gelatin*. It's naturally present in homemade bone broth along with glucosamine and many other bone-building components.

Build Bones with Exercise

The ideal exercise to improve bone density will stress them with a heavy load. Bones respond to physical stress by strengthening and reinforcing their structure. The best examples are:
   - **Resistance Exercise** – Movements that incorporate pushes and pulls against some kind of resistance. This may be lifting free-weights or dumbbells, using weight machines, pushing and pulling elastic bands or even using body weight as with pushups, planks, lunges or pull-ups.
   - **Weight-Bearing Exercise** – Any exercise done on the feet is weight-bearing, even low-impact varieties, because the bones in the legs support the full body weight. Examples include walking, dancing, climbing stairs, martial arts, etc. Attention to proper alignment and posture during those activities correctly places the stress on the skeletal structure.

- **Yoga** – During yoga practice, the body weight is manipulated across support from the arms, legs or both. Most classes combine compressing, twisting, lengthening and inverting actions which stress and stimulate bones from virtually every possible angle. Other yoga benefits include increased flexibility and improved balance, both of which help prevent falls and bone fractures.
  ⏧ YogaUOnline Yoga for Osteoporosis - An Interview with Loren Fishman, MD, and Ellen Saltonstall

  ➢ **High-Impact Exercise** – The force of the impact stresses bones and triggers the bone rebuilding process, making them stronger. Any physical activities that include impact and vibration fall in this category (jogging, running, jumping, hopping, many sports, etc).

> **A Note about Biking and Swimming:** Some exercises are neither weight-bearing nor high-impact: for example, swimming and cycling do not require the body to support its weight. Bone building will not be stimulated if there is little stress on the skeletal system. If these are your main exercises, either increase the intensity to create full muscular tension on the bones or rotate with other weight-bearing activities to maintain bone integrity.

Bone Building

Bone is constantly *remodeling*, a process of breakdown and rebuilding. When conditions are right, bones can be rebuilt denser and stronger at any point in life! Here's what's needed:

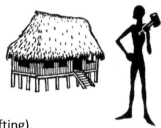

1. Ample availability of bone-building components
2. Reduction of factors that interfere with bone growth
3. Proper hormonal balance to encourage growth (via quality diet, sunshine, stress reduction, etc)
4. Appropriate stress on the bone from physical exercise (especially weight-lifting), full range-of-motion stretches and weight-bearing movements in general

> **Bone Remodeling:** This 4-minute video describes how bones are built and maintained, as well as factors that interfere with the process. The *glucocorticoids* mentioned in the video include the stress hormone, cortisol, and certain steroid drugs such as prednisone (as an aside, this video was produced by a pharmaceutical company):
> ⊛ YouTube: Bone Remodeling and Modeling uploaded by Amgen

Factors that Limit Availability of Bone Components

Maintaining bone integrity is complicated! Multiple body functions are involved with placing the proper nutrients into the bone matrix. Here are a few more factors that interfere with proper bone metabolism:

1. **Gut Damage** – Mineral absorption normally happens in the small intestine and requires a properly functioning gut lining. Compromised digestion in conditions such as leaky gut, irritable bowel syndrome or Crohn's disease prevent absorption of ingested nutrients. Osteoporosis is prevalent with celiac and other autoimmune diseases because nutrient absorption is poor.
2. **Grain-Based Diet** – Grains are both mineral-deficient and phytate-rich (their antinutrients trap dietary minerals). Therefore, high consumption fails to provide essential healthy bone components.
3. **Low-Fat Diet** – Fat-soluble bone vitamins such as D3 and K2 require some dietary fat to be properly metabolized. The popular low-fat diet prevents their uptake, compromising bone health.
4. **D3 Interference** – Cholesterol molecules stored under the skin are converted to vitamin D3 when stimulated by the sun's UV rays. D3 deficiency is common due to societal obsession with lowering cholesterol as well as dowsing the skin with sunscreen to block UV rays. Certain drugs can also interfere with the conversion thereby contributing to softer, more fragile bones.
5. **Insufficient EPA and DHA** – These omega-3 fats are essential and an integral part of bone marrow, yet many people do not consume sufficient quantities through diet alone. The primary dietary source is fatty fish (more about EPA and DHA on Day 4).
6. **Unmanaged Stress** – Excess cortisol stimulates bone breakdown and blocks rebuilding, resulting in osteoporosis (more about Cortisol on Day 11).

Paleo Lifestyle for Strong Bones

The Paleo lifestyle naturally promotes strong healthy bones via many diverse channels:

1. Encourages abundant veggies and fruit – organic sources contain more key bone minerals
2. Emphasizes pasture-raised or wild-caught animal products for higher concentrations of bone-strengthening vitamins and minerals plus appropriate protein intake
3. Incorporates bone broth for a natural source of collagen protein and glucosamine
4. Removes phytate mineral traps present in grains and legumes
5. Heals a leaky gut to increase mineral and nutrient absorption
6. Increases healthy fats for better mineral and vitamin metabolism as well as bone marrow integrity
7. Incorporates movement and exercise to maintain bone strength
8. Promotes outdoor playtime for some sun exposure (vitamin D3) and stress reduction
9. Encourages healthy sleep habits to support overall stress reduction and proper body restoration

Additional Dietary Recommendations for Strong Bones

To maximize micronutrients for bone integrity, consider incorporating more of the following foods:

➢ **Bone-in Fish** – Canned sardines and salmon supply omega-3 fats EPA and DHA, vitamin D and calcium
➢ **Grass-fed Butter** – Grass-fed (but not grain-fed) provides vitamins K2, D3 and some EPA and DHA
➢ **Bone Broth** – Excellent source of gelatin (cooked form of collagen) and glucosamine
➢ **Plentiful Vegetables** – Eating a wide variety of high-quality organic or locally-grown produce boosts:
  • Minerals – like magnesium and potassium
  • Vitamin C – necessary for collagen formation
  • Calcium – most green vegetables like leafy greens are high in calcium
➢ **Scarce Fat-Soluble Vitamins** – Include foods high in vitamins K2 and D3 (sardines, organ meats, grass-fed butter, pasture-raised egg yolks) or select a high-quality supplement
➢ **Additional Mineral- and Vitamin-Dense Foods** – Incorporate organ meats, mollusks, shellfish, leafy greens, seaweed, nuts, seeds, etc

Supplements for Bone Health

Some individuals may be interested in smart supplementation to hedge their bone health. It is important to remember that *you cannot supplement your way out of a poor diet*. To maximize bone integrity, focus must also be placed on improving overall diet, adding weight-bearing exercise and eliminating factors that interfere with bone metabolism.

Bone Health Supplements*	
Nutrient	**Details**
Minerals	Magnesium is the most important mineral to supplement. Select a magnesium supplement with high bioavailability such as citrate or malate.
Proteins	✓ Glucosamine†‡ and/or collagen are available at ⌐ PureRXO.com/Paleovation ✓ Great Lakes Gelatin and Vital Proteins both carry high quality collagen and gelatin products
Healthy fats	EPA‡ and DHA‡
Fat-soluble vitamins	Vitamin D3, Vitamin K2‡
Specifically-Designed Bone Health Products	Some supplement companies specially blend nutrients for bone health. The following examples are available at ⌐ PureRXO.com/Paleovation: 'Calcium K/D'‡ (calcium + vit K+ vit D3), 'PureHeart K2D'‡ (vit K2 + vit D3), 'OsteoBalance' (multi-minerals + vitamins D3 and C)

* Products available at ⌐ www.PureRXO.com/Paleovation for those wanting direct access to a high-quality source; More information on choosing nutritional supplements in the Resource Section
† Precautions for those with shellfish allergy – shellfish-free varieties are available
‡ Speak with a medical provider if you are taking blood thinners

Further Reading (direct links to all recommended reading available from ⌐ Paleovation)**:**

- ⌐ Reread the Dairy topic on Day 7
- ⌐ MarksDailyApple 8 Primal Rules for Building Better Bones
- ⌐ ChrisKresser How to Keep Your Bones Healthy on a Paleo Diet

Section II: Unsweetened Beverage Boredom (UBB)

Are you suffering from a case of UBB? Addiction to sweet and sugary beverages is common, including fancy coffee drinks, sodas, energy drinks, shake mixes, protein powders, fruit juices, smoothies or even herbal tea with honey. Here are a few drink suggestions to add variety while also limiting sugar:

Low-Sugar Drink Options	
Beverage	**What Is It?**
Kombucha	A fermented tea which contains probiotics. Sugar is necessary for the fermenting process (but the bacteria 'eat' most of it). Find a brand that does not add fruit juices or sugar to the *final* product. GT's, Serenity and Master Brew are popular choices. Homemade is another option. ⌐ KombuchaKamp What is Kombucha ⌐ OraWellness How to Drink Kombucha and Not Destroy Your Teeth
Sparkling Water	Carbonated water itself is flavorless (also called soda water or seltzer). Many brands add natural flavors which may appeal to you. Only buy unsweetened varieties with the ingredients carbonated water and natural flavor. La Croix, San Pellegrino, Perrier and Klarbrunn are popular brands.
Spa Water	Place fruit, herbs or vegetables in a pitcher of water so the flavors infuse and the water doesn't taste so plain. Try strawberry-kiwi, cucumber-mint, blueberry-basil, citrus-thyme, cinnamon-ginger-pear, etc.
Herbal / Green Tea	Many herbal and green teas have gut healing, anti-inflammatory and/or detoxification benefits. Try ginger, turmeric, milk thistle, nettle, dandelion, burdock, mint, chai, lemon, detox tea blends or another favorite.
Beet Kvass	For those inclined, make this fermented drink of beets, salt and water. ⌐ HolisticSquid Beet Kvass Myth Busting (and Recipe)
Coconut Water	The liquid inside a coconut contains many electrolytes – it's also naturally sweet. This is the sweetest beverage that is program friendly. Limit to a cup per day. Watch for added sugar or preservatives in commercial products.
Coconut Milk	The coconut milk is released from the flesh. You can make your own with dried coconut flakes, hot water, a blender and cheesecloth. Refrigerated commercial brands likely contain additives. Canned products tend to have fewer preservatives. If canned coconut milk is too thick, just water down. ⌐ AutoimmuneWellness Creamy Coconut Milk
Unsweetened Nut Milks	Almond, cashew, hazelnut, macadamia, etc. Again, watch for additives or make your own. Reminder: this counts toward your nut serving for the day. ⌐ AgainstAllGrain Homemade Almond Milk 2
Black Coffee / Black Tea	These options may be bitter on their own, but they are sugar-free.

Approved Specialty Drinks

- **Paleo Latte:** Heat full-fat canned coconut milk, place in a jar or blender and shake/blend until it's foamy. Add to coffee or tea for a light and creamy beverage.
- **Sun Tea:** In warm weather, use the sunshine to brew tea. Fill a large pitcher or canning jar with water and add a handful of tea bags (about one bag per cup of water). Cover, then set outside in the sun for 2-8 hours. When brewing is done, discard the tea bags and chill in the fridge. Nearly every kind of tea makes a delicious sun tea. Tip: Brew double-strength (2 bags/cup) and add ice later for an iced sun tea.

8 Great Coffee and Tea Ideas

Ideas to spruce up unsweetened coffee or tea:

1. Place cinnamon or pumpkin pie spice in the coffee grounds or tea ball when brewing
2. Brew a weaker cup of coffee/tea to reduce natural bitterness
3. Use a cold brewing technique such as a toddy or sun tea to reduce acidity
4. Enjoy iced coffee and iced tea to decrease bitterness
5. Add coconut milk as a creamer
6. Add coconut cream (this is what rises to the top of the canned coconut milk) as a super creamer
7. Make it Bulletproof® and whip in grass-fed butter and coconut oil or MCT oil
8. Add a splash of vanilla and/or dash of cinnamon which has a natural sweetness

To-Do List:

☐ Gather ingredients for jerky or granola and make a batch by Day 19
☐ Purchase and roast a chicken by Day 23
☐ Anything else (stress relief, new drink, sleep habit)? _____

Coming Up Soon:

- Days 17 and 18 cover the topics Cholesterol and Heart Disease to dispel concerns that a Paleo Diet is not heart-healthy
- Posture tips and belly breathing – these have a digestive and cortisol-reducing benefits

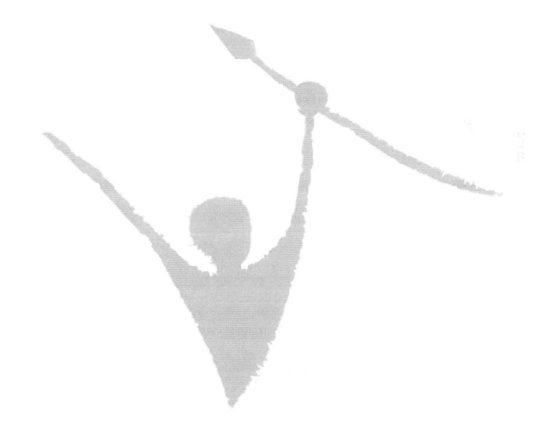

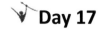

Day 17

Today's Topics:
1. Paleo-Wise: Cholesterol
2. Posture Check

Fast Fare – Bone Broth
♥ Bone broth – egg drop soup
♥ Celery sticks with almond butter

Of all the Paleo foods eaten today, what's most delicious? _____

Browse your food highlights since Day 1 to look for patterns of favorite veggies, snacks, recipes, etc. How is this presence (or absence) of patterns influencing your Paleo experience? _____

Section I – Paleo-Wise: Cholesterol

The 'cholesterol-as-indicator-of-heart-disease' hypothesis has been "the greatest scam ever perpetrated on the American public." - Biochemist George Mann, MD, co-developer of the Framingham Heart Study

Cholesterol Conundrum

It has been confirmed – cholesterol was wrongly targeted as a health-destructive nutrient. Until just a few decades ago, the human diet always contained substantial amounts of cholesterol and fats from animal products, eaten liberally. Unfortunately, rewinding recent decades of negative propaganda and obsession over blood cholesterol values is a daunting task. Maybe this will help:

> **Fact Retract:** The 2015 Dietary Guidelines, published by the USDA and Health & Human Services, removed limits on dietary cholesterol! According to the report, "Cholesterol is not a nutrient of concern for overconsumption."

Note that the cholesterol and heart disease association has always been called a *hypothesis*. As defined by the Webster dictionary, a hypothesis is "a proposed explanation made on the basis of *limited evidence* as a starting point for further investigation." If cholesterol and fat truly caused heart disease, why then have rates of heart disease continued to explode despite five decades of low-cholesterol and low-fat dietary practices?

Interestingly the low-fat dietary dogma restricted cholesterol and fat intake while it simultaneously encouraged the consumption of grains, sugar and industrially manufactured oils. Increases in heart disease parallel amplified consumption of those highly inflammatory non-Paleo foods, not consumption of fats or cholesterol.

Cholesterol – Essential, Not Evil!

Cholesterol is so vital to health that the body does not rely solely on dietary sources for supply...*all cells can produce it*! Cholesterol is a *major* structural building block used throughout the body. Modern practices to restrict cholesterol interrupt the proper function of every one of these critical structures:

Cholesterol Structures in the Body	
Structures	**Cholesterol's Contribution**
Hormones	• Essential base of steroid hormones: testosterone, estrogen, cortisol, adrenaline, etc
Brain	• Aids in memory, learning and neurotransmitter synthesis • The brain houses 25% of the body's cholesterol
Nerves	• Forms *myelin*, the insulating sheath around nerves for efficient neural transmission
Bile	• Breaks apart large fat globules in the small intestine, crucial for digestion • Aids absorption of fat-soluble vitamins A, D, E and K
Vitamin D	• Cholesterol in the skin converts to Vitamin D when exposed to UV sunlight
Cell Membranes	• Creates structural integrity and fluidity of cell membranes • Adds strength and stability to cells; locks in water and nutrients (anti-wrinkle!) • Helps the skin provide a protective barrier against microbes

Point to Ponder: Vitamin D3 is manufactured when the sun's rays stimulate cholesterol in the skin. If cholesterol is reduced via low-fat diet or medication, wouldn't vitamin D levels also suffer? Vitamin D deficiency is widespread and linked to heart disease, osteoporosis, depression, cancer, difficulty losing weight and poor physical performance.

Healing Properties

Cholesterol also has an anti-inflammatory healing role and supports immune function by attaching to bacterial toxins until immune cells can clear them. There's more: cholesterol works as an antioxidant protecting brain and blood cells from free radical damage. Cholesterol is *beyond vital*.

Recycled Cholesterol

A perpetual supply of cholesterol is necessary for optimal health and the body takes this need quite seriously. Neither dietary sources *nor* internal production of cholesterol can sustain the body's requirement, so humans have evolved mechanisms to reabsorb and recycle cholesterol.

> **Did You Know:** The small intestine reabsorbs up to *90%* of existing cholesterol, returning it to the liver via HDL for reuse (more on HDL and LDL later).

So...if the body carefully preserves this vital nutrient, what led to the belief that naturally-occurring cholesterol is detrimental to heart health? It's a case of mistaken identity: cholesterol is found at the scene of the crime.

Cholesterol – Duct Tape for the Arteries!

When a blood vessel is harmed, cholesterol is sent to the scene; it covers the area to protect it from further damage. Cholesterol then assists in patching and healing the lesion. In a healthy body, the injury heals, inflammation ceases and cholesterol is cleared from the location.

Analogy: Blaming cholesterol for causing arterial damage is like blaming the fire truck for causing a fire!

However, in an unhealthy body, healing may be stunted and inflammation can persist. In this situation, additional cholesterol accumulates on the arterial wall as a protective Band Aid. Not only does this narrow the artery, but it also increases the risk that some cholesterol will become oxidized. This harmful, *oxidized* cholesterol triggers plaque formation and hardening of the arteries.

Arterial Plaque - A Result of *Oxidized* Fat

Just because cholesterol is present at the site of a plaque (for repair purposes) doesn't mean it *caused* the plaque. Cholesterol's role in healing is natural...up to the point when it becomes oxidized. To be clear, cholesterol oxidation only occurs in already health-compromised, inflamed arteries. The *oxidized* version further damages the artery, fuels even more inflammation, instigates yet another cycle of destruction (more cholesterol is sent for repair purposes, only to become oxidized) and contributes to pathological plaque formation.

Oxidized offenders are not limited to just cholesterol – any oxidized fat can damage arteries (these were discussed in detail with PUFAs on Day 3). Destructive oxidized cholesterol and fats are found in certain processed foods:

Causes of Arterial Plaque	
Substance	**Dietary Sources**
Oxidized Cholesterol	• Highly processed cholesterol-rich foods like powdered eggs and powdered dairy products (like powdered milk and cheese) • Read labels – these are commonly used as ingredients and flavorings
Oxidized Fats	• Unstable industrial PUFA oils exposed to light/heat during processing and storage including canola, soybean, corn, safflower, cottonseed, vegetable oils • Foods cooked in industrial oils (they oxidize further when heated) • Deep-fried foods in reheated restaurant oils (fried chicken fish & chips, fries, etc)

Manufactured Foods Contain Oxidized Cholesterol

We've mentioned heat as a cause of fat and cholesterol oxidation. Fortunately, the temperatures commonly employed during home cooking do not significantly contribute to this process. Additionally, naturally-occurring cholesterol in foods such as egg yolks or liver is protected by its chemical structure and coexisting antioxidants.

The primary oxidation concern lies within industrial processing of cholesterol-rich foods. Manufacturers often prefer to use eggs and dairy in powdered form because they easily incorporate into any processed product (powdered shakes and creamer, cheese flavoring, prepackaged cake mixes, seasoning packets, chocolate, etc).

To create food powders, extrusion and spray-drying processes force foods through tiny holes at *extremely* high temperature and pressure. This vastly increases the food's surface area while exposing it to intense heat. This instantly dehydrates the food, but easily oxidizes fat and cholesterol and completely denatures the final product.

> **Paleo Advantage:** The health term 'anti-oxidant' refers to specific nutrients that prevent and heal oxidative damage in the body. The abundant, colorful vegetables incorporated as Paleo staples are chock full of them! Additionally, naturally-sourced animal proteins and traditional fats are low in oxidized fats (remember, saturated fats are very stable). These foods reduce and heal oxidative damage, contributing to an overall vitalizing effect.

LDL and HDL – Freight Service for Fats and Cholesterol

Fat and water don't mix – that's a basic chemistry fact. Since blood is mostly water, effective transportation of fats in the blood requires that they are made water-soluble. This is done by wrapping fats in layers of protein; these structures are called lipoproteins (Latin for fat-proteins).

Since fats are lighter than water they float, so lipoproteins full of fat are buoyant with lower density. These "low density lipoproteins" are called LDL. As they travel through the body, LDL particles deliver their fats and shrink, becoming denser and less buoyant as they transition to "high density lipoprotein" or HDL.

1. LDL takes cholesterol *away* from the liver to deliver elsewhere for metabolic needs.
2. HDL picks up the same cholesterol particles after they have accomplished their tasks and returns them to the liver for recycling.

> **Key Point:** Every cholesterol molecule in the body is the same. HDL and LDL are *not* actual cholesterol, but merely vehicles for *all* fats in the blood (not just the bad, good fats too): HDL and LDL transport essential fats EPA and DHA, fat-soluble vitamins A, D, E and K, cholesterol, triglycerides and even trans fats.

LDL – Size Matters

LDL has been labeled *bad,* but the truth is that while some forms of LDL cause harm, others do not. It is critical to know what sub-type of LDL is present for accurate health assessment:

1. **Pattern-A LDL:** These large, billowy particles (imagine cotton balls) *do not* play a significant role in heart disease. They are 'fluffy' and bounce off arterial walls.
2. **Pattern-B LDL:** These small, dense particles (visualize a BB) can lodge in gaps between arterial cells causing damage which subsequently triggers inflammation and contributes to hardening of the arteries.

BE-ware of Pattern-B

In addition to the arterial damage it causes, pattern-B LDL itself is also more susceptible to oxidation. The more pattern-B LDL present in the blood, the higher the risk for cholesterol oxidation, inflammation and plaque development. Excessive levels of pattern-B LDL are linked to poor dietary habits:

- **Overeating Sugar/Starch** – This generates copious amounts of triglycerides from the surplus glucose.
- **Insufficient Antioxidant Intake** – Colorful vegetables and fruits provide antioxidants, but many people fail to consume adequate quantity or variety.
- **Oxidized Fat Consumption** – These fats are found in fried foods, processed foods, restaurant foods and any industrially processed oil (soybean, corn, vegetable, canola, cottonseed, sunflower, etc).

> **Paleo Advantage:** Eating Paleo eliminates the poor dietary habits associated with destructive pattern-B LDL and restores the prominence of pattern-A LDL: Paleo establishes a diet with much lower sugar/starch, much higher proportion of vegetables and elimination of unstable fats.

High Insulin Linked to High Cholesterol (Sugar and Grains are Guilty *Again*)

Even though cholesterol is necessary and healthy, elevated blood cholesterol levels can indicate imbalance of other metabolic processes. Additionally, high total cholesterol levels increase the odds that some of it becomes oxidized within the body, transitioning it from helpful into harmful.

When dietary cholesterol is restricted (as in a low-fat diet), the body will *naturally produce more* to compensate and maintain an adequate supply. Ironically, although the low-fat diet is promoted to reduce cholesterol, it actually guarantees steady *over*production of cholesterol. Of further consequence, the fat calories removed on a low-fat diet are commonly replaced with sugary or starchy foods which spike insulin. Excess insulin profoundly affects cholesterol levels:

1. Excess insulin causes inflammatory damage to arterial walls, *increasing need for cholesterol* to repair it
2. Excess insulin stimulates a key liver enzyme to produce *more* cholesterol (HMG-CoA reductase)

> **Paleo Advantage:** Excessive cholesterol production is generated *from excess sugar/starch* in the diet, not fat! A major, controllable way to extinguish cholesterol overproduction is to reduce sugar/starch intake, eliminating excess insulin's cholesterol-stimulating consequences.

A Case for Cholesterol-Rich Foods

If the body can produce the cholesterol it needs, is it still necessary to eat food rich in cholesterol? The answer is a resounding YES! Even though it's not crucial to consume cholesterol itself through diet, attaining the essential nutrients that naturally coexist with cholesterol is. This includes critical nutrients such as choline, zinc, iron and the fat-soluble vitamins (A, D, E, K). Not only do foods naturally high in cholesterol provide this nourishing package, but to properly assimilate these nutrients into our bodies, the accompanying cholesterol is required.

So, dig in to cholesterol-rich foods without guilt (from quality sources, of course): egg yolks, shellfish, seafood, fatty fish, fish eggs, bacon, liver, organ meats, butter, goose fat, duck fat, lard, a wide variety of meats such as beef, duck or wild game, and heavy cream (after the program). There are no plant sources of cholesterol.

> From the director of the Framingham Heart Study (ongoing since 1948):
> *We found that people who ate the most cholesterol, ate the most saturated fat and ate the most calories weighed the least and were the most physically active.* ~ William Castelli, MD

Eat that Yolk!

Even though the USDA Dietary Guidelines no longer limit cholesterol intake, years of marketing propaganda has created an entrenched fear of high cholesterol food which is challenging to unravel. One of the unfortunate targets has been egg yolks, a rich source of naturally-occurring cholesterol and its accompanying micronutrients.

The yolk contains almost half of the egg's protein, 80-90% of the egg's vitamins and minerals and all the *essential* fat. Include yolks when eating eggs – stop with the boring egg-white omelets!

Cholesterol Paradox

If high cholesterol truly caused heart disease, then countries documenting higher rates of elevated blood cholesterol should experience proportionately higher rates of heart disease. However, that's not the case. On the contrary, scientific studies reveal that countries with higher blood cholesterol levels are *least* susceptible to infection, have *lower* levels of cancer, have *better* recovery from disease and cardiac episodes, and overall *live the longest*!

These findings have received a 'paradox' label and have been discredited – they don't fit the original *hypothesis* that cholesterol damages health. It's time to reevaluate the data, accept the truth that cholesterol is a vital nutrient and disregard the negative propaganda about cholesterol.

Protective Effects of Higher Cholesterol Levels

It's understandable that after decades of demonizing cholesterol, its health benefits may be difficult to acknowledge and accept. Cholesterol is so vital to fundamental body structures and functions that a review is in order.

Sound and stable cholesterol presence protects from infectious disease, cellular damage and many metabolic dysfunctions (hormonal, digestive, neural transmission or vitamin deficiency). As we become older, *more, not less* cholesterol is necessary to assist with healthy and graceful aging.

Cholesterol Clarification - Q & A

1. **Aren't some forms of cholesterol bad?** Yes, avoid consuming or internally creating *oxidized* cholesterol. The Paleo diet and lifestyle is an effective strategy to do so.
2. **Don't high cholesterol levels predict heart disease?** Short answer, no. The next topic is Heart Disease which highlights its true origins as well as how to properly determine risk.
3. **What about "bad" LDL?** Lipid panels are further discussed in the next topic. For now, just know that not all LDL is bad.

Cholesterol Recap
Structures
• Cell membranes
• Brain and nerve tissue
Functions
• Fat digestion
• Vitamin D synthesis
• Hormone production
• Protect cells from free radical damage
• Assists immune system in disabling bacteria and bacterial toxins
• Aids in absorption of fat soluble vitamins A, D, E and K
• Contains anti-inflammatory properties
• Involved with healing mechanisms

We realize the above ideas are the exact opposite of the popular cholesterol narrative of recent decades. To assist in comprehending the real story about cholesterol, consider diving into more research about cholesterol-as-a-wholesome-nutrient (direct links available from ⌐ Paleovation):

- ⌐ MarksDailyApple The Definitive Guide to Cholesterol
- ⌐ Ravnskov Myth 9: The Benefits of High Cholesterol
- ⌐ BalancedBites Cholesterol Confusion, Clearing it Up
- ⌐ NerdFitness Is Cholesterol Killing Us? A Beginner's Guide to Cholesterol
- ⌐ DrSinatra Seven Must-Know Cholesterol Facts Your Doctor Won't Tell You
- 📖 *The Great Cholesterol Myth,* by Jonny Bowden, PhD, CNS and Stephen Sinatra, MD
- 📖 *The Big Fat Surprise,* by Nina Teicholz
- ⊛ YouTube Dr Jonny Bowden "The Great Cholesterol Myth"
- ⊛ YouTube The Cholesterol Hypothesis is Wrong – Malcolm Kendrick Part 1

Section II: Posture Check

Convenience and comforts of contemporary culture are great in many aspects – but the resulting sedentary lifestyle also comes with a cost. Just like the modern diet, human bodies aren't adapted to modern habits that encourage postural stresses like prolonged sitting, slouching at desks, sinking into soft furniture and endlessly rounding shoulders while dropping our heads to stare at phones.

All sorts of problems ensue when our bodies are mechanically stressed with repetitive, asymmetric postures and crammed into prolonged, unnatural configurations: back and neck pain, mobility issues and even less obvious digestive problems. Making a concerted effort to improve posture will positively affect many facets of health.

Benefits of Good Posture	
• Facilitates breathing	• Increases energy
• Improves circulation – decompresses blood vessels and stagnant lymph	• Enhances sleep quality
• Reduces back and neck pain	• Improves concentration and thinking ability
• Heightens confidence	• Boosts mood
	• Improves balance

Posture Affects Digestion

Slouched posture physically constricts, compresses and compromises digestive organs and processes, contributing to bloating, heartburn, belching, flatulence, ulcers, gall bladder disorders, diarrhea, constipation, etc. Additionally, restricted circulation impedes oxygen delivery and nutrient transport to and from the digestive system, creating consequences for every cell in the body.

Correcting the posture not only remedies mechanical compression of abdominal organs and circulatory system, but also encourages gentle, but constant, core muscle engagement. This core stability allows the diaphragm to fully retract into the bottom of the rib cage which further relieves digestive discomfort.

Point to Ponder: Another postural consideration involves the concept of 'rest and digest' because stress interferes with digestion through the action of cortisol. It's been shown that a calming posture employed after a meal (relaxed and upright or gently reclined) helps improve digestion by preventing cortisol's interference.

Posture Tips

Correcting posture may feel awkward at first, but practice and repetition will establish better postural habits and spinal strength. Of course, everyone's situation is different so there is no universal perfect posture; furthermore, corrections can be complicated by old injuries, surgeries, genetics and even emotions. Build your posture from the base up and use the following tips pertinent to your individual situation:

1. **Be Aware** – Remind yourself to pay attention to your physical position using timers, post-it notes, situational cues (first time standing in the morning, when sitting for a meal, lying down in bed) or your own method until correct posture becomes second nature.
2. **Balance the Weight** – Each foot (or butt bone when sitting) supports half the body weight.
3. **Feet** – Don't let the ankle collapse to the inside or roll outward. Evenly distribute the weight across the foot (ball, heel and outer edge) and line the ankle bones directly above the heel.
4. **Properly Tip the Pelvis** – When the pelvis has the correct rotation, the shoulders glide directly over the hips, allowing the spinal muscles to properly engage and support the backbone in its natural alignment.
   a. If your back is flat – untuck your tail; pretend you have a heavy, swaying tail as you walk.
   b. If you have a curved 'sway back' – tighten your abs and gently tuck your tail.
5. **Core Strength** – Many poor postures develop from weak core support musculature. Slightly pull the abdominal wall in and up.
6. **Be Symmetrical** – Hips, shoulders and ears should be symmetrical side-to-side and evenly stacked front-to-back (try looking in a mirror or examining photos of yourself).
7. **Pull/Retract Head Back** – Ears should align over the shoulders. Try the chin tuck stretch: give yourself a double chin while retracting your head back.
8. **Press Up Through the Crown** – Pretend you have a bucket of water balanced on the crown your head. This engages the small muscles around the spine and rib cage for proper support.
9. **Walk/Stand Deliberately** – Walk and stand tall. Imagine a rope pulling you up from the top of your head. Periodically walk/stand while pretending to be three times more confident than you are.
10. **Sit Up** – Balance comfortably on your sitz bones, the bumps at the base of the pelvis. When these butt bones support body weight, the vertebrae can naturally align. Try sitting on the edge of a chair with one leg dropped, rocking the pelvis forward on the sitz bones. Allow the shoulders to naturally retract.
11. **Move Symmetrically** – Keep body movements balanced and symmetrical. If you habitually do an activity on one side (cradle the phone, lean in a chair, carry a purse, etc), consciously engage the opposite side.
12. **Get Your Vision Checked** – Many postural compensations are due to visual impairment.

Emotional Postures: A classic example is an unhappy person who adopts a deflated, slouched posture…but what comes first? That discouraged posture may also *generate* depression – happy people who adopt a depressed posture actually start to feel sad! Conversely, sad people who consciously implement happy postures and expressions will feel better.

Helpful Posture Gadgets – Many postural support products are found online.

- Adjustable/standing desk
- Ergonomic chair
- Lumbar cushion/support
- Orthopedic pillow – and try using other pillows as props while sleeping
- Quality mattress
- Phone headset/Bluetooth
- Shoulder retractor brace or undergarment
- Shoe orthotics, inserts
- Foam roller
- Cushion, wedge or sitting cup for desk chair or car seat
- Glasses (specifically for computer, phone, etc)

Further Reading

- ᨒ ACAToday Spinal Health – American Chiropractic Association
- ᨒ Spine-Health Posture to Straighten your Back
- ⊕ YouTube Benefits of Good Posture - Murat Dalkılınç **(4 ½ min)** an excellent animated posture discussion
- 📖 *8 Steps to a Pain-Free Back,* by Esther Gohkale – details posture correction techniques. The book starts with simple lessons such as stretching the space between vertebrae while sitting or sleeping. Eventually she incorporates the complex lesson of changing the gait. Even if you do not have back pain, these exercises are an excellent tool to develop correct skeletal alignment.
  - ⊕ YouTube Find your Primal Posture and Sit without Back Pain: Esther Gohkale at TEDxStanford (6 min)
  - ᨒ GokahleMethod has more resources and traveling posture clinics

To-Do List:

- ☐ Day 19 is nearing, have you made jerky or granola yet? What can you get started today?
- ☐ Purchase and roast a chicken by Day 23
- ☐ Anything else (read a recommended article, work on your posture, take a walk)?

Coming Up Soon:

- ➤ Heart Disease is the next Paleo-Wise topic
- ➤ Breathing techniques to combine with good posture for stress relief

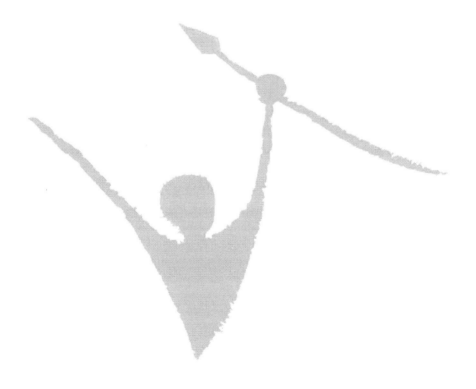

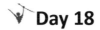 **Day 18**

> *We delight in the beauty of the butterfly, but rarely admit the changes it has gone through to achieve that beauty.* ~Maya Angelou

Today's Topics:
1. Paleo-Wise: Heart Disease
2. Belly Breathing

Fast Fare – Use Paleo Mayo
♥ Sautéed sausage and peppers
♥ Tri-color slaw mix with Paleo mayo

What homemade foods or grab-and-go items have you liked having on hand during this program?

_____

_____

What meals and routines are keeping you on track?

_____

_____

Of the cooking assignments, which one is your favorite (broth, mayo, veggie used as a grain, jerky, granola)?

_____

If your jerky or granola isn't finished, take the time to get that going today.

Section I – Paleo-Wise: Heart Disease

> *Cholesterol is no more a cause of heart disease than gray hair is the cause of old age.* ~ Nora Gedgaudas

Cholesterol-Heart Blame Game

In 2015, the US Dietary Council acknowledged that cholesterol is not linked to heart disease. It bears repeating: There is *no correlation* between cholesterol levels and heart disease (go ahead and Google "no correlation between cholesterol and heart disease"). In fact, this *theory* was always called the cholesterol-heart *hypothesis* because it was never proven. Cultures listed in the following table clearly do *not* fit the premise that high cholesterol and heart disease risk go hand in hand.

Well-Documented Paradoxes to the Cholesterol-Heart Hypothesis	
Population	**Contradiction**
Modern Aborigines	One of the highest rates of heart disease BUT lowest cholesterol consumption
Swiss / French	Some of the lowest rates of heart disease BUT high cholesterol consumption
Okinawans	Extremely low rates of heart disease BUT tendency for 'elevated' blood cholesterol

> **Good to Know:** Cholesterol does not cause heart disease which explains why, in more than half of new heart attacks, cholesterol levels are *normal* or *below*!

Inflammation – The Primary Factor in Heart Disease

The likelihood of a heart attack depends on factors including diet, lifestyle and genetics, but NOT cholesterol. By focusing solely on cholesterol, the real cause of heart disease has tragically been ignored: *Inflammation!*

Atherosclerosis is an *inflammatory* condition of the arterial lining. To heal the inflamed areas, the body deposits cholesterol on the inside of the arteries for repair purposes (discussed on Day 17). If inflammation is not alleviated, plaques eventually form over that damage. This process narrows and hardens the arteries, increasing the odds of heart attack and stroke.

Normally, non-oxidized cholesterol circulates freely in the blood and will not attach to healthy arterial walls. Plaque development occurs from either persistent inflammation or the presence of *oxidized* cholesterol and other *oxidized* fats. Cholesterol and plaque accumulation can therefore be a *symptom* of arterial inflammation but not the root cause of heart disease. The causes of inflammation have already been extensively discussed:

Factors that Contribute to Inflammation (and Heart Disease)		
(Note that high total cholesterol levels or eating a high-fat / high-cholesterol diet do not *cause inflammation)*		
Elevated blood sugar and insulin	Unmanaged stress	Smoking
Processed sugar/starch	Sleep deprivation	Excess alcohol consumption
Trans fats	Lack of exercise	Many medications
Oxidized fats (rancid oils)	Obesity (especially abdominal fat)	Chemicals (food and environment)
Oxidized cholesterol	Unhealthy gut flora balance	Genetics
Lack of antioxidants in diet	High triglycerides	Hypertension (high blood pressure)

Nearly all these factors are lifestyle related. That means changing diet and routine habits can vastly improve heart health at any age. Even for those with genetic predisposition, gene expression can be altered by reducing inflammation, increasing physical activity and consuming nutrients to support a healthy body.

"Heart-Healthy" Guidelines are Anything BUT

Heart disease has continued to escalate despite societal obsession with low-fat and low-cholesterol diets. Consider that popular "heart-healthy" low-fat diet recommendations actually endorse *heart-hurting* foods:

1. Low-fat translates to high carbohydrate consumption: starches, sugars and grains replace fat content
2. Low-cholesterol encourages consumption of butter alternatives and inflammatory polyunsaturated vegetable oils (PUFAs) rather than healthy traditional fats from animal sources

Ironically, this combination of increased sugar, starches and oxidized oils is the exact recipe to *create* chronic inflammation and heart disease!

> **Key Point:** The low-fat diet, overabundant with sugar/grains *and* reliance on low-cholesterol vegetable oils, is highly inflammatory – a significantly greater threat to heart health than saturated fat and cholesterol ever were!

Blood Markers of Inflammation (Real Heart Disease Risk)

There are significantly better tests for heart disease risk than total cholesterol or even LDL levels. The following blood tests assess inflammation as well as the risk of heart disease. Visit these sites for more explanation, ideal result ranges and additional tests such as calcium scans (remember, direct links available from ⌁ Paleovation):

- ⌁ DrSinatra Blood Inflammation Tests for Heart Disease Risk
- ⌁ MarksDailyApple Popular Blood Tests – The Facts, Ranges and Alternatives You Should Know
- ⌁ MarksDailyApple How to Interpret Advanced Cholesterol Test Results
- ◆ **C-Reactive Protein (CRP):** Determines level of inflammation, the primary risk factor for heart disease. The High Sensitivity CRP (hs-CRP) test score is ideally <0.8 mg/L.
- ◆ **Fasting Blood Sugar:** Levels > 100mg/dL have much higher risk of heart disease. <90 is desirable.
- ◆ **Triglycerides:** High levels indicate other problems such as insulin resistance (with risk of diabetes) or inflammation (and risk of heart disease). Ideally <100.
- ◆ **LDL-P:** Measures the number of LDL particles. A high count suggests excessive small, dense LDL particles (pattern-B LDL). Ideally <1000.
- ◆ **Useful Lipid Ratios:** The ratios below indicate a healthy lipid profile and lack of inflammation.
  - ○ **Total Cholesterol ÷ HDL** Ideally < 3.5
  - ○ **Triglycerides ÷ HDL** Some sources say <3, but ideally <2
- ◆ **LDL Particle Size:** Small, dense and aggressive pattern-B LDL particles are directly related to arterial inflammation. Multiple tests are available. The fluffy pattern-A LDL should be prominent.

Good to Know: High triglycerides, generated from excess sugar/starch consumption, are a far better predictor of heart disease than total cholesterol. C-reactive protein is an accurate indicator of inflammation (which is the primary risk factor with heart disease).

Fortunately, the anti-inflammatory Paleo diet combined with exercise improves all aspects of the blood profile:

Paleo Diet and Lifestyle	Improved Inflammatory Markers and Blood Profile
✓ Reduced sugar, grain/starch consumption ✓ Eliminate oxidized PUFA vegetable oils and hydrogenated fats ✓ Increased healthy natural fat consumption ✓ Increased EPA and DHA consumption ✓ Increased moderate-intense exercise or HIIT	● Lowers inflammatory blood markers like CRP ● Lowers blood glucose levels ● Lower triglycerides ● Lowers LDL numbers ● Increases LDL particle size (non-invasive pattern-A) ● Raises HDL numbers which improves cholesterol ratios

Cholesterol Concerns? High total cholesterol alone does not cause heart disease. However, there are other specific blood markers that *do* indicate increased heart disease risk (poor HDL ratios, high triglycerides, high CRP, high Pattern-B LDL count). The popular treatment is targeted solely at lowering cholesterol when realistically, a healthier approach is to correct the entire lipid profile – and that's accomplished with diet and exercise.

The Low-Down on Cholesterol-Lowering Drugs

Disclaimer: The following points critiquing statins (cholesterol-lowering drugs) can be substantiated with further reading – entire books have been written to dispel cholesterol's role in heart disease. Keep in mind, the authors of these books are highly criticized; also keep in mind, statins are a multi-billion dollar industry. Ultimately, the choice to take a cholesterol-lowering statin medication is up to the individual.

Statin drugs are prescription medications that effectively lower cholesterol levels by limiting its production. In fact, they do this so well that 1 out of 4 Americans over the age of 45 takes a statin medication to keep cholesterol levels down.

Reducing cholesterol levels is promoted as a prevention for heart attacks or bypass surgery. It's easy to sell this kind of linear thinking because people like numerical feedback. Lab numbers dropping provides positive reinforcement, especially when the assumption that lower cholesterol numbers translates into better heart health...except that reasoning is flawed.

Taking a statin does not address the root cause of heart disease – chronic inflammation! Confirmation of this is evidenced by the fact that, despite increasing statin use, heart disease rates continue to rise.

Faulty Statin Logic

There are major discrepancies in the statin logic:

➤ **Flaw #1:** Statins simply lower cholesterol levels, which are *not associated* with heart disease. Therefore, statins do not provide *prevention* or *treatment* for heart disease.
➤ **Flaw #2:** Cholesterol is *not associated* with heart disease risk, but inflammation is. Reducing cholesterol without addressing inflammation will neither treat nor prevent heart disease.
➤ **Flaw #3:** Artificially lowering an essential building block like cholesterol has dire consequences. Statins do not prolong life. Ironically, statins are associated with *higher risk of death from other causes*. The attempt to avoid heart disease by taking a statin isn't much of a victory if it means dying earlier from something else!

Statin Complications

Statin drugs *do* inhibit the natural production of cholesterol. However, cholesterol is crucial for survival! Restricting an essential nutrient like cholesterol will generate devastating side effects (listed in the table) which are often seriously under-reported because they get associated with normal aging.

Side Effects of Statin Medication	
● Diabetes	● Memory loss, amnesia, dementia
● Liver damage	● Impotence, sexual dysfunction
● Kidney failure	● Higher risk of developing breast and prostate cancers
● Lower IQ	
● Muscle pain or weakness	● Immune suppression, increased infection

Low Cholesterol Limbo: How Low Can You Go?

With fear revolving around cholesterol levels, cholesterol-rich foods and dietary restrictions, a too-low cholesterol disaster may be looming. Widespread obsession to reduce cholesterol numbers to improve heart health has overshadowed inquiry as to whether or not low levels really are healthy!

When total blood cholesterol drops too low, proper body function is compromised. A valid argument could be made that demonization of cholesterol has contributed to its deficiency. There are clear risks with total cholesterol numbers less than 150, though some speculate that even levels below 160 are detrimental:

LOW Cholesterol Impairments	
Compromised Function	**Increased Risk of Impairment**
Brain & Nervous System	• Memory loss, dementia • Nerve transmission • Brain function with age • Mental health disorders (depression, anxiety, bipolar, etc) • Hostile, violent, suicidal or aggressive behavior
Immune System	• Higher infectious disease risk • Higher risk of cancer
Vitamin D Production	• D3 deficiency linked to heart disease, osteoporosis, depression & cancer
Steroid Hormones	• Imbalances in estrogen, progesterone, testosterone and cortisone
Cell Membrane Integrity	• Weakened stability and function of ALL cells

Statin Stats

It's true: as statin use has increased, there has been a documentable decrease in *deaths* from heart attacks – a statistic selected to prove statins work (though also attributable to earlier symptom recognition and faster access to defibrillators and emergency cardiac care). A less-reported statistic however, is that despite higher prevalence of statins, the number of both *non-fatal heart attacks* and *heart disease diagnoses* continues to rise.

Statins do not address inflammation, the root cause of heart disease. Reducing cholesterol but ignoring the inflammation is like smashing the fire alarm but leaving the fire burning!

Statistical Magic – Relative Risk: Pharmaceutical drug benefits are often reported as an *X%* reduction in risk.

Hypothetical Example: Suppose a drug reduces the chance of a heart attack by 50% – pretty impressive. This drug clearly cuts the risk in half! Well, what if the risk wasn't that big to begin with?

Imagine the actual heart attack rate is 2 incidents per 100 'at-risk' individuals (a 2% actual risk). Administering the drug to all 100 people cuts that risk in half – now there is only 1 heart attack per 100 'at-risk' individuals. The *actual* improvement is only 1%.

This statistical maneuvering is highly profitable for the pharmaceutical industry. All 100 'at-risk' individuals need to take this drug to eliminate a 1% actual risk (continue reading to see who defines 'at risk'). Furthermore, the drug's side effects for the other 99% are often discounted.

🖐 ProteinPower Absolute Risk versus Relative Risk: Why You Need to Know the Difference

---

Statin Drugs Interfere with Critical Heart-Health Nutrients (CoQ10 and Vitamin K2)

- **Vitamin K2** – Statin drugs inhibit the synthesis of this vitamin. However, K2 is crucial for maintaining supple arteries because it regulates calcium balance. Vitamin K2 scans the body for inappropriate calcium deposits in soft tissue (like arteries), removes the calcium from those locations and redirects it into bones and teeth. Proper K2 levels can reverse arterial calcification (more K2 info on Days 7 and 16).
  - **Vitamin K2 deficiency** contributes to increased *arterial plaque levels*, blood calcium levels, osteoporosis, heart disease and calcification in soft tissues contributing to hardened arteries, kidney stones and stiff joints/muscles.

224

- **CoQ10** – A primary statin concern! In addition to blocking cholesterol production, statin drugs also block manufacture of CoQ10 (ubiquinol), an essential nutrient necessary *to supply energy to all cells*, especially heart, liver and kidney. Our bodies produce CoQ10 within the same metabolic pathway that's cut off by statins.
  - ○ **CoQ10 deficiency** symptoms include *heart failure*, high blood pressure, fatigue, chest pain, poor immune function and poor blood sugar regulation.

  Note: If taking a statin drug, supplementation with CoQ10 is absolutely necessary (search online "CoQ10 and statins")!

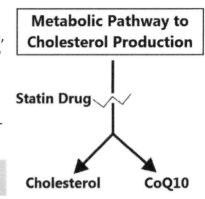

Metabolic Pathway to Cholesterol Production

Statin Drug

Cholesterol   CoQ10

| Conventional 'Wisdom' Sets the Stage for *Increased* Heart Disease Risk ||
Recommendation	**Detrimental Effects**
Low-Fat Diet	Overabundance of sugar/starch = excess insulin = *inflammation + overproduction of cholesterol*
Low-Cholesterol Diet	Encourages PUFA vegetable oil consumption = oxidized fats = *inflammation + plaque formation + internally-oxidized cholesterol*
Lowering Blood Cholesterol Levels	• Statin drugs = CoQ10 depletion = *less energy supplied to the heart* • Statin drugs = Vitamin K2 inhibition = *calcium deposited in soft tissues like arteries instead of bone/teeth*
The Kicker: There is *no correlation* between total cholesterol levels and heart disease!	

> **Irony:** Lowering cholesterol levels to prevent heart disease has produced unintentional health consequences that contradict the goal. Low-fat diet recommendations and pharmaceutical intervention actually create an environment ripe for heart disease: *Inflammation + oxidized fat/cholesterol + depleted heart nutrients!*

The Original Purpose of Statins

Statins were originally intended only for *secondary* prevention of cardiac episodes, meaning prevention of a *second* heart attack or stroke when there is clear evidence of pre-existing heart disease.

Primary prevention is not fully substantiated. Yet, the majority of current statin prescriptions are for *primary* prevention of cardiac events, even in healthy patients who only present with "certain risk factors." These risk factors are then defined by the pharmaceutical industry so statins can be used as preventative medicine.

For the majority of the population, including women, the elderly or *children*, statin benefits may not outweigh the risks. Complications of reducing cholesterol too low coupled with serious side effects, including *increased death by other cause(!),* may not offset a slight reduction in cardiac episodes (remember, cardiac episode survival rate is increasing due to better symptom recognition and faster access to emergency cardiac care).

Statin Exceptions: Groups that Benefit Most

Statin therapy for *secondary prevention* of heart disease may be beneficial, but surprisingly, it's not due to lower cholesterol levels. In certain populations, statins can act as an anti-inflammatory and reduce blood viscosity (making the blood thinner and improving circulation).

1. **Middle-aged Males *Who Have Had* Prior Cardiac Events:** Research shows this specific group, who *already have had a heart attack or stroke,* can improve odds against a second cardiac event or death. However, the risks may outweigh the benefits once the man exceeds ~70 years old because higher cholesterol levels actually become protective later in life.
2. **Individuals with Familial Hypercholesterolemia (FH):** Those with genetic FH tend *not* to respond to lifestyle interventions that correct the cholesterol blood profile, so heart disease risk remains high. **Interesting to Note:** Overall FH lifespan is still comparable to the general population because, even with specifically higher *cardiac* deaths, those with FH have significantly *less chance of a non-cardiac death* such as infection or cancer, displaying the protective benefits cholesterol.

3. **Individuals currently afflicted with very advanced cardiac conditions:** Again, for secondary prevention in existing and extremely aggressive cases.

Risk/Reward: There is a benefit/risk trade-off when taking a statin medication, even within specific groups with higher benefit potential. *Cardiac* death risk may decrease, but death risk from *non-cardiac* events increases. If you fall into one of these gray areas, consult your healthcare provider to determine whether statins are appropriate for your individual situation.

Reducing Heart Disease Risk Naturally

The most profound way to support heart health is through lifestyle change:

✓ **Change the Diet** – Eat anti-inflammatory by *increasing natural dietary sources of healthy fats* (coconut products, avocado products, olive products, wild-caught fish, pastured animals' fats and yolks and grass-fed butter) while *reducing carbohydrates and vegetable oils* – that's Paleo!

✓ **Reduce Stress** – Proper stress management reduces effects of cortisol and supports better digestion, brain function, sleep, healing and overall health (more about Stress and Cortisol on Days 11 and 12).

✓ **Incorporate Exercise** – This is so potent a strategy to lower heart disease risk that some researchers suggest drug companies be required to include it in clinical trials for comparison (more on Day 10)!

"LOVE YOUR HEART" LIFESTYLE RECOMMENDATIONS

INCREASE
- Physical Activity
- Healthy Fats
- Cholesterol-Rich Foods
- Antioxidant-Rich Foods

MAINTAIN
- Adequate Sleep
- Manageable Stress Levels
- Heart-Health Nutrient Intake

REDUCE
- Glucose Consumption (sugars, starches, grains)

ELIMINATE
- PUFA Oils
- Other Oxidized Fats
- Smoking
- Obesity

Detail of Heart Health Maintenance Strategies	
Heart-Support Nutrients*	**Healthy Fat- and Cholesterol-Rich Foods**

<ul><li>CoQ10*</li><li>Vitamin K2</li><li>EPA/DHA</li><li>Vitamin D3</li><li>Magnesium</li></ul>	1. Natural Saturated Fats
	  a. Grass-fed butter/ghee, lard, tallow, duck fat (select naturally-raised sources – commercially-raised are inflammatory)
	  b. Coconut oil and other coconut products
	  c. Palm oil

Antioxidant-Rich Foods	2. Monounsaturated Fats – olives, avocados, some nuts/seeds 3. Polyunsaturated Fats - EPA/DHA from fatty fish such as sardines or a supplement such as fish, krill or cod liver oils 4. Cholesterol-Rich Foods – egg yolks, liver and other organ meats, shellfish, fatty fish, fish eggs, seafood, heavy cream, butter and a wide variety of meats (sourcing matters)
<ul><li>Colorful veggies</li><li>Organ meats</li><li>Eggs</li><li>Meats</li><li>Berries</li><li>Red wine</li><li>Dark chocolate</li><li>Turmeric</li><li>Tea</li><li>Coffee</li></ul>	**Physical Activity**
	<ul><li>Increase non-sitting time (example: standing desk)</li><li>Increase low-level movement</li><li>Include occasional moderate-intense exercises and/or High-Intensity Interval Training (HIIT)</li></ul>

* Those taking statins *absolutely* need a high-quality CoQ10 supplement. More information on supplements in the Resource Section.

Bewildered or Befuddled?

Understandably, cholesterol and heart disease are confusing topics – even just the fact that cholesterol does not cause heart disease takes time to accept. Furthermore, it's challenging to apply this information to each individual case. If necessary, re-read the cholesterol and heart disease topics for better understanding.

Managing Cholesterol Naturally

If 'managing' cholesterol levels is a particular priority for you, here is a plan to naturally address that:

1. Employ *all* lifestyle changes noted above. These are the most profound ways to protect your heart.
2. Study the recommended reading in yesterday's and today's sections.
3. Study additional topics in this book including Stress (Days 11 and 12), Sleep (Day 13), Movement (Day 10) and Supplements (Resource Section).
4. Plan your lipid panel. Cholesterol tests are affected by dietary change (generally higher with high carb diet), weight loss/gain, infection, stress, pregnancy and season (higher in winter, lower in summer). If you are affected by any of these, allow your system some time to regulate and stabilize before a retest.
5. In the case your blood markers are still high for *inflammation*, consider Chris Kresser's 9-week program:
   - ChrisKresser High Cholesterol Action Plan

More Information
Online:
- PrimalBody-PrimalMind The Cholesterol Myth
- ChrisKresser The Diet-Heart Myth: Why Everyone Should Know Their LDL Particle Number
- MarksDailyApple The Definitive Guide to Cholesterol
- TheHealthyHomeEconomist The High Risks of Low Cholesterol
- Mercola Statins' Flawed Studies and False Advertising
- DrAxe Low Cholesterol Levels are Worse Than High
- THINCS.org (THe International Network of Cholesterol Skeptics)
- FunctionalMedicine Find a Functional Medicine Provider

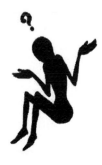

Documentaries – purchase on StatinNation.net or rent through NetFlix or Amazon
- ⌕ Statin Nation: The Great Cholesterol Cover Up
- ⌕ Statin Nation II: What Really Causes Heart Disease

Books
- 📖 *The Great Cholesterol Myth,* by Jonny Bowden, PhD and Stephen Sinatra, MD
- 📖 *The Great Cholesterol Con,* by Malcolm Kendrick, MD
- 📖 *Cholesterol Clarity: What the HDL is Wrong with My Numbers,* by Jimmy Moore & Eric Westman, MD
- 📖 *The Statin Damage Crisis,* by Duane Graveline, MD
- 📖 *Lipitor: Memory Thief,* by Duane Graveline, MD
- 📖 *Undoctored,* by William Davis, MD

Section II: Belly Breathing

The topics of cholesterol and heart disease are rather heavy, perhaps hard to grasp or accept. Take a moment to breathe deeply and tune into your body (do it now!) – breathing relieves stress.

Shallow or Chest Breaths

Breathing is an unconscious activity, obviously essential to life...and it seems like it should be easy and natural. However, most people breathe shallowly, only expanding their chest which has consequences:

- **Triggers Nervousness and Anxiety** – suggests a panic mode or hyperventilating
- **Over-Engages the Shoulder-Shrug Muscles** – induces chronic neck and/or shoulder pain

Take a shallow breath, only allowing your chest to expand and observe your shoulders lifting on the inhale and falling on the exhale. Believe it or not, this is not how we are supposed to breathe.

Deep Belly Breathing

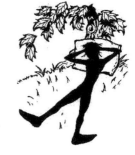

Watch a baby breathe – the belly expands, the chest does not, and the shoulders remain relatively stable. This is called belly or diaphragmatic breathing. Somewhere along our life journeys, most people lose this natural deep breathing technique and adopt shallow chest breathing.

Deep belly breathing can be relearned and there are marvelous health benefits from this simple change. Belly breathing reduces stress by turning off the release of cortisol (*fight or flight* mode) so all the negative effects of cortisol are diminished. At the same time, deep breathing activates the calming portion of the nervous system (*rest and digest* mode).

Benefits of Deep Breathing	
✓ **Regulates weight**	Reduces cortisol and blocks fat-preserving effects of cortisol
✓ **Increases vitality**	More oxygen, less stress, better sleep and detoxing benefits
✓ **Improves digestion**	Supplies oxygen to digestive tract; stimulates *rest and digest* response
✓ **Relieves pain**	Stops the body from tensing and exacerbating pain
✓ **Helps detoxify**	Rids the body of carbon dioxide and other waste products
✓ **Stimulates lymph**	Gently moves lymph to mobilize toxins and waste products
✓ **Improves posture**	Brings awareness to the body and naturally lengthens the spine
✓ **Increases lung capacity**	Restores full expansion of lung tissue over time
✓ **Improves sleep**	Calms the mind, relaxes the body, encourages onset of sleep
✓ **Lowers blood pressure**	Induces peacefulness, calms the nerves, reduces anxiety

How to Belly Breathe

Find a comfortable position (sit, stand or lie down). Put your hand over your belly button – this is the approximate level of your diaphragm, a flat muscle that acts like a platform under the lungs.

Gently inhale and expand your belly (chest and shoulders don't move), pushing out against your hand as you inhale through the nose – this draws the diaphragm down out of the rib cage and toward the abdomen as the lungs fill with air. Pause at the end of the inhale. Gently release as the belly returns to its normal position; some breathing techniques continue exhaling beyond neutral, retracting (hollowing) your belly to completely empty the lungs. The chest and shoulders are relatively stable through the whole cycle.

⊛ YouTube Learn the Diaphragmatic Breathing Technique uploaded by CioffrediPT (~4 min)

Practicing deep breathing a few times throughout the day releases stress and centers some focus on you, both of which reinforce healthy digestion and facilitate healing.

➢ Try these variations...and as you get better, increase the count and number of cycles
- **Box Breathing:** Inhale for the count of 4, hold for 4, exhale for 4, hold for 4, repeat
- **Double-Length Exhales:** Inhale for the count of 4, hold as you wish, exhale for 8
- **Alternate Nostril:** Close the left nostril on the inhale, close the right on the exhale, then switch

Are there any daily recurring moments you could implement belly breathing techniques to calm cortisol (during a commute, waiting for a download, putting children to bed, etc)?

1. _____

2. _____

To–Do List:
☐ Jerky / granola will be done by tomorrow
☐ Keep working toward getting those chickens roasted by Day 23 (info on Day 15)
☐ Anything else (scrutinize your use of Paleo crutches, go to bed early, add more foods to your lunch template from Day 7)?

Coming Up Soon:
- Day 19 has a Paleo-Wise "Free Day" to allow time to reread cholesterol and heart disease if desired
- Conventional wisdom has been wrong on more than one occasion – a review and wrap-up of common misconceptions appear tomorrow

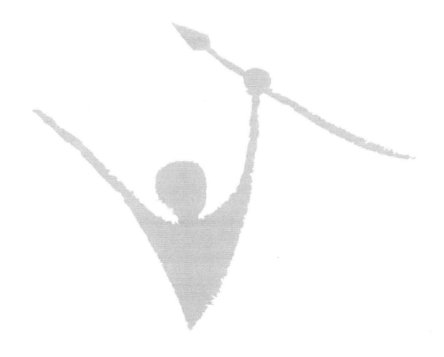

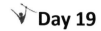

Day 19

Today's Topics:

1. Moving Forward and Releasing Old Dietary Habits
2. Paleo-Wise: FREE DAY
3. Movement Check-In
4. Cost Comparison: SAD versus Paleo

Fast Fare – Microwave Muffin
♥ Muffin in a mug
♥ Celery sticks and guacamole
♥ Jerky

Did you enjoy your homemade jerky or granola?   Yes   No

If not, consider a different recipe because both jerky and granola tend to be crowd pleasers.

Have you shared your jerky/granola with anyone? If so, what was their reaction? _____

Would you consider making the other option from Cooking Assignment #4 (granola or jerky)?   Yes   No

If so, go back to Day 11 for directions and recipes.

Section I: Moving Forward and Releasing Old Dietary Habits

It takes time to establish new Paleo habits. It's not just the foods and recipes – it's an entirely different *lifestyle approach.* You are just beginning to experience the countless positive health rewards of the Paleo Lifestyle!

Our goal is to offer a framework for building new effective habits for long-term health and healthy weight. Part of this process includes releasing old failed diet habits or rules that *don't work* (like eating "heart-healthy" grains and oils that have failed to prevent heart disease…and obesity and ill health).

Insanity is doing the same thing over and over again and expecting different results. ~Common cliché

Different results require a different approach…a change! The information in this book challenges the failed conventional wisdom surrounding diet, exercise and lifestyle habits. With an open mind, a little bit of research (including this book) and a "seeing-is-believing" experience (like your rejuvenated health from the Strict Paleo Protocol), you will be able to shed old beliefs and learn the most effective approaches for your body.

Complexity of Dietary Habits

Dietary change and be quite a challenge, mainly because our ingrained eating patterns are multifaceted:

- **Rituals** – daily or weekly dietary 'regulars' (taco Tuesday, candy bowl at work, pizza night)
- **Emotional Security** – sugary or starchy foods we gravitate towards for comfort
- **Sensory Triggers** – foods that make your mouth water with just the thought of them
- **Conventional Wisdom** – difficult to break away from widely-accepted dietary advice
- **Social Expectations** – gatherings with particular food expectations (like birthday cake or champagne)
- **Carbohydrate Cravings** – tough to manage certain trigger foods that intensify desire for more
- **Marketing** – bombardment from processed food advertisements specifically designed to induce cravings

Engineered to be Craved

Carbohydrate cravings listed above are inherent to human nature. Unfortunately, opportunistic food manufacturers design foods to specifically target these cravings so we'll eat more. Food engineering labs employ an army of chemists, physicists and even neuroscientists to develop enticing combinations of salt, sugar, fat, size, shape, crispiness, chewiness, crunch intensity, bite force, mouth feel, melt time and any other factor that can deliver the ultimate junk food goal: *Bliss point.*

Bliss Point: The term used in the food science industry to describe the exact combination of ingredients and textures to achieve maximum palatability, optimize the eating experience and create a strong desire for more.

Compound deeply ingrained dietary habits with managing carb cravings, plus resisting the constant temptations of unhealthy (but enticing) foods and it's no wonder that long-term diet success is so elusive. Forming new habits takes conscious effort – and consistency is the key!

Power of Choice

Regardless of how good you feel as you refine your personalized long-term diet, it's important to recognize that temptations will never cease. We're up against food engineers, cultural norms and the coworker with the candy bowl constantly tantalizing us with unhealthy choices. Therefore, long-term success resides in owning your power of choice. It's critical to *consciously choose* to let go of old habits and *choose* to have a positive outlook on your new life direction. In the words of Mahatma Gandhi:

☺ Keep your thoughts positive, because your thoughts become your words.
☺ Keep your words positive, because your words become your behavior.
☺ Keep your behavior positive, because your behaviors become your habits.
☺ Keep your habits positive, because your habits become your values.
☺ Keep your values positive, because your values become your destiny.

Old Dietary Dogma You *Won't* Miss

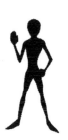

Part of long-term dietary success resides in realizing the negative aspects of prior habits, beliefs and behaviors. There are many tedious nuisances of the old, failed low-fat doctrine that feel great to shed! For example, no more fear of natural saturated fat or cholesterol (hello bacon and butter, good bye margarine)!

Additionally, some conventional wisdom health endorsements can cause more harm than good (for example, over-exercising in a manner that stimulates muscle wasting, or eating foods that provide damaged resources for your body to integrate – like any PUFA oil). Blind faith in conventional wisdom or believing you can "eat anything in moderation" becomes an excuse to stop paying attention to exactly what foods and lifestyle habits make us thrive (or sick)!

Old ways won't open new doors. ~Unknown

The more conscious we are about our choices, and their consequences, the easier it is build life-long healthy habits. What parts of the old conventional wisdom lifestyle are you thrilled to leave behind? Check all that apply:

Old Conventional Wisdom Rules: Habits, Hassles, Hype and "Healthy" Foods to Lose	
☐ Separating egg yolks	☐ Battling willpower to lose weight (as a sugar-burner)
☐ Salt restriction	☐ Bland oils like canola and vegetable oils
☐ Tediously counting calories*	☐ Eating only lean meats (dry chicken breast)
☐ Butter substitutes	☐ Tasteless foods such as tofu or rice cakes
☐ Weighing food portions	☐ Forcing down more water than you are comfortable drinking
☐ Chalky, high-fiber cereals	☐ Low-fat versions of naturally fatty foods
☐ Mid-morning energy crash	☐ Long hours of exercising or chronic cardio
☐ Fearing natural, saturated fats	☐ Failed weight-loss formula of "just eat less, exercise more"
☐ Fearing cholesterol-rich foods	☐ Basing a diet on foods that cause more harm than good
☐ Always hungry	(whole grains that contain gluten; cholesterol-free PUFA oils)
☐ Restricting caloric intake	☐ Defining success based on the number on the scale
☐ Turkey bacon (eat the real stuff!)	☐ Feeling helpless when it comes to controlling your health

* ⊛ YouTube Barry Groves - Why You Can't Count Calories

List any other parts of the old lifestyle paradigm (or consequences of which) you won't miss:

_____

When you change the way you look at things, the things you look at change. ~Wayne Dyer

The Strict Paleo Protocol is just a short-term diet reset; the rest of your success story is discovering what specific foods are right for your body long-term. This is accomplished via conscientious food reintroductions which we detail during the final week. Based on your personal sensitivities, you will learn how far you personally can deviate from the Paleo Template yet still maintain quality health.

Section II – Paleo-Wise: FREE DAY

Unfortunately, much of the conventional wisdom regarding healthy diet and lifestyle is difficult to shed, even though it's false. The topics in this book defy many deep-seated beliefs and may take some time to absorb and fully accept. Use this free day to review prior Paleo-Wise sections that you find challenging to believe.

Topics Worth Re-reading			
Day	Content	Day	Content
1	Fat Fraud	11	Stress and the Cortisol Response
2	Saturated Fats	12	Calming the Cortisol Response
3	Polyunsaturated Fats (PUFAs)	13	Importance of Sleep
7	Dairy and Calcium Sources	17	Cholesterol
10	Movement and Chronic Cardio	18	Heart Disease

Section III: Movement Check-In

Sedentary habits, smart exercise, good posture and breath work were discussed on Days 9, 10, 17 and 18. What suggestions have you incorporated into your current lifestyle?

Day 9: Sedentary Behavior	Day 10: Movement	Days 17 & 18: Posture & Breath
☐ Practice the Rising Test	☐ More causal, low-level activity	☐ Set reminders to check posture
☐ Replace sedentary behaviors	☐ Some activity to break a sweat	☐ Practice sitting upright
☐ Develop an 'omit the sit' plan	☐ A little HIIT interval training	☐ Try standing and walking tall
☐ Practice a flat-footed squat	☐ Some strength training	☐ Belly breathing
☐ Try balance postures	☐ Avoid chronic cardio	☐ Inhale/exhale to a count

You may already be experiencing increased energy levels (after the temporary slump of low-carb flu) and feel motivated to add more movement into your lifestyle. Below is a review of the four categories of movement for which our bodies are designed. Refer to the tables and descriptions on Day 10 for details.

The following activity is for those who are ready to devise an individualized exercise plan. For beginners wanting to incorporate categories 2, 3 or 4, an exercise class may be the best place to start (examples include CrossFit, Zumba, boot camp, yoga or circuit training). If you're not yet ready to add more movement, skip to Section IV.

1. **Low Intensity Activities** (*bare minimum* 2 hours per week)
   a. How many minutes of gentle movement are feasible per day? (A range is okay) _____
   b. What casual activities do you enjoy and intend to include?

   _____

2. **Moderate-to-High Intensity Activities** (2-3 times per week; more is fine if you recover and are uninjured)
   a. What is a feasible number of minutes to work out at your fitness level? (range is okay) _____
   b. What activities do you enjoy that cause you to break a sweat?

   _____

   c. How many days per week do you want to include the above activities? _____

3. **HIIT: High-Intensity Interval Training** (just 5-10 minutes per week)
   a. What activities are appropriate for your fitness level?

   _____

   b. Which day is most feasible for a HIIT workout if you must rest the next day? _____
   c. Do you want to overlap your HIIT workout with other activities planned in categories 2 or 4? If yes, how? (examples: elliptical machine on interval setting; interval calisthenics with a weighted vest)

   _____

4. **Strength or Resistance Training** (1-3 sessions per week)
   Which of the following resistance weights do you prefer to use? Check all that apply:

   ☐ Body weight   ☐ Weight machines   ☐ Free weights   ☐ Elastic bands   ☐ Other

   a. Select body movements you can use to incorporate all main muscle groups. It's okay that some motions engage more than one group. Aim for diversity and incorporate both pushing and pulling actions. Also, modifications for ability-level are perfectly acceptable (countertop plank, knees-down pushups):

Arms:	☐ Curls	☐ Pushups	☐ Dips	☐ Extensions
Shoulders/Chest:	☐ Overhead press	☐ Pec flys	☐ Lateral raises	☐ Chest press
Back/Core:	☐ Pullups	☐ Rows	☐ Plank	☐ Crunches
Legs:	☐ Squats	☐ Lunges	☐ Extensions	☐ Step ups

   Other ideas: _____

   b. Have you thought of ways to overlap strength training with cardio categories 2 and 3? If yes, how? (examples: CrossFit classes use HIIT movements incorporating free weights or body weight; Vinyasa Yoga postures move the body weight back and forth between the arms and legs)

   _____

Sample Week of Movement

The following example week shows how movement categories 2, 3 and 4 can be distributed through the week and how low-level movements (category 1) are incorporated daily. Weekly routines will naturally vary especially with strength-training muscle group exercises. Adjust activities to your own personal preferences and abilities.

Day	Category	Min	Activity [muscle groups worked]	Daily Low-Level (minutes)
Sun	4	20	Weight machines [arms/core]: curl, row, press, pullup, pulldown, triceps extension, etc	Stretch, foam roller (10) Walk a mile (17)
Mon	-	-	REST	Groceries/errands (60)
Tues	2	60	Tennis or golf or cardio machine	Garden (30)
Wed	2 & 4	75	Power yoga [arms/core/legs]	Play catch (15)
Thurs	2	30	Hike or tread water or bike ride or cardio class	Housework (40)
Fri	3 & 4	8	HIIT [legs/core] – burpees, squats, sprint up/walk down flight of stairs, lunge steps, crunches, etc	Wade, walk the dog (20)
Sat	-	-	REST	Gentle kayak or fish (120)

Using the personalized activities and time descriptions you recorded above, fill in the following chart. Remember to try to include some playtime, some outdoor activities when possible, and a couple rest days.

1. Select the HIIT day (category 3) followed by a REST day.
2. Choose a strength training day (category 4), also followed by a REST day.
3. Fill in the remaining days with some moderate/high intensity (category 2).
4. Finally, lay out the low intensity activities for each day along with minute estimates that would be appropriate to combine with the other activities on that day.

Day	Category	Min	Activity [muscle groups worked]	Daily Low-Level (minutes)
Sun				
Mon				
Tues				
Wed				
Thurs				
Fri				
Sat				

Section IV: What is the Cost of Paleo?

Many people feel that eating Paleo is more expensive than a Standard American Diet (SAD). However, when compared to restaurant fare, homemade high-quality Paleo delivers complete nutrition at the same price. Additionally it does not contribute to illness and inflammation: Paleo delivers vitality and health beyond monetary value (the lifetime cost savings from fewer prescriptions or medical interventions can be substantial!).

The following prices are rough estimates because cost varies by locale. Paleo cost savings could even be higher because the table does not consider any auxiliary budgeting strategies such as buying meats in bulk, growing a garden or home-brewing kombucha. Plus, there's the added economical (free!) and nutritional bonus of high quality bone broth when roasting an organic chicken at home.

What's the Real Cost?	
Restaurant Meal	**Organic and Homemade Paleo**
¼-Pound Burger Meal = $6.00 • ¼ lb hamburger • French fries • Large soda	**Grass-fed Burger with Organic Vegetables = $6.00** ✓ ¼ lb grass-fed beef = $2.00 ✓ Serving of organic greens = $0.50 ✓ Organic sweet potato for side = $2.00 ✓ Cup of purchased kombucha = $1.50
Foot-Long Sub Meal = $7.00 • 12" sub • Chips • Soda	**Lunchmeat Salad with Organic Veggies = $6.80** ✓ ¼-lb pasture-raised lunchmeat = $4.00 ✓ Serving of organic greens = $0.50 ✓ Assorted chopped organic veggies = $2.00 ✓ Cup of organic herbal tea = $0.30
Family-Size Chicken Meal = $20 • 8 pieces chicken • Mashed potatoes & gravy • Cole slaw • 4 Biscuits	**Organic Roasted Chicken Dinner w/sides = $22.00** ✓ 1 whole organic chicken = $12.00 ✓ 2 lbs organic potatoes = $4.00 ✓ ¼ lb grass fed butter = $1.50 ✓ 1 lb coleslaw mix = $2.00 ✓ 1 butternut squash = $2.50
Pasta Dinner = $9-12 + tip • Spaghetti and meatballs • Side salad • Garlic bread	**Organic Zoodles and Meatballs = $7.00** ✓ 1 organic zucchini = $1.50 ✓ Cup of organic marinara = $1.50 ✓ Grass-fed meatballs = $2.00 ✓ Organic greens & assorted veg salad = $2.00

Even when compared to cheap SAD *processed* foods eaten at home, high-quality Paleo wins again! When broken down into *cost-per-pound*, the Paleo foods deliver much more nutrition than SAD items.

SAD Item	$ / lb	Paleo Item	$ / lb
Potato chips	$4	Organic potatoes	$2
Salad mix	$4	Organic salad mix	$5
Beef jerky sticks	$11	Grass-fed ground beef	$8
Crackers	$12	Organic carrot slices	$2
Cereal, toaster pastry	$3 - 5	Pasture-raised eggs	$3 - 4
Popular candy bars	$12	Organic dark chocolate	$15
Canola or other PUFAs	$1	Traditional fats*	$6 - 15

High-quality grass-fed butter, olive oil, coconut oil, pastured lard, duck fat, tallow, etc

With the exception of traditional fats (compared to PUFA oils), the price per pound for high-quality organic produce or animal products is not outrageous. Admittedly, there is certainly a convenience factor to the SAD foods...but then again, *there is nothing convenient about repressed health and vitality.*

> *I would suggest that if you get in your kitchen and cook for yourself, you can eat like kings for a very low cost.* ~Joel Salatin, author of <u>Folks, This Ain't Normal</u>

Long-Term Budget Strategies

During the remainder of this Paleo diet reset and food reintroductions, you will be formulating personal long-term strategies. The biggest long-term budgetary commitment may be the traditional fats, but they tend to last a long time. Once you've accommodated for that, incorporate other high-quality foods when possible. If you have budget limitations, don't fret over including some conventional lean meats or produce – many of the Paleo health benefits are realized by simply removing detrimental foods (grains, added sugars, PUFAs, additives, etc).

Jot down any personal insights or other cost-per-pound comparisons you already noticed or plan to investigate:

_____

_____

To-Do List:

☐ Cooking Assignment #5: Purchase a whole chicken (or two) for roasting – finish by Day 23
☐ Anything else (join an online Paleo forum, read recommended articles on topics difficult to grasp, make the *other option* for Cooking Assignment #4 granola or jerky)?

_____

Coming Up Soon:

- Environmental toxins are an inevitable part of modern life. Tomorrow we'll discuss a few ways to reduce exposure (which will also reduce stress and hormonal disruption).

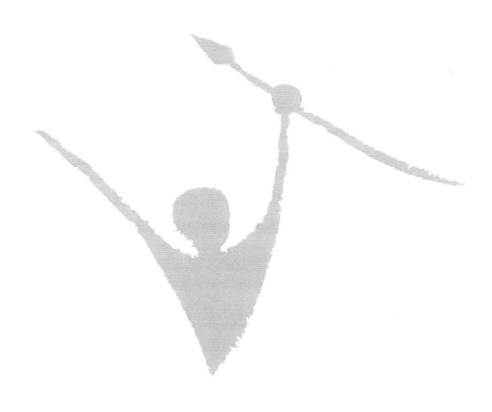

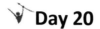

Day 20

> *There are two types of people who will tell you that you cannot make a difference in this world: those who are afraid to try and those who are afraid you will succeed.* ~Ray Goforth

Today's Topics:

1. Reflect and Be Proud
2. Paleo-Wise: Toxin Caution and Hormonal Imbalance

Fast Fare – Leftover Vegetables
♥ Omelet filled with leftover veggies
♥ Mixed olives from the olive bar

Care to note any special Paleo foods, food combos or new recipes you're eating today?

_____

_____

Have you had any difficulty in social situations during this program? If yes, what were the circumstances and what can you do differently next time to be better prepared (Prep D has ideas)?

_____

_____

Section I: Reflect and Be Proud

We expect that you've made some major changes during the last few weeks. What accomplishments make you the proudest at this point? Check all that apply

- ☐ Committing to my health
- ☐ Cooking my own meals
- ☐ Learning new recipes
- ☐ *Not* snacking between meals
- ☐ Taking off the blinders of conventional wisdom
- ☐ Tuning in with my body
- ☐ Eating consciously
- ☐ *Not* rewarding myself with food
- ☐ Developing new healthy habits
- ☐ Making time to nurture myself

Which of these has been the most difficult change so far? Why?

_____

_____

What strategies or attitudes have helped you maintain your commitment?

_____

_____

Section II – Paleo-Wise: Toxin Caution and Hormonal Imbalance

> *A great and decades-long experiment is being conducted, and we, the unsuspecting public, are the guinea pigs. Our living, working, and recreational environments are now loaded with toxins, more than 90,000 of which are registered with the Environmental Protection Agency (EPA).* ~Terry Wahls, MD

Subtract the Food Additives

The FDA has approved roughly 1000 food additives to improve stability, flavor, nutritional value, consistency, texture, color and eating experience. Some of these are as benign as salt or baking soda, but others are hazardous chemicals that have no business lurking in our food supply. Eating homemade Paleo is the best way to avoid additives but whenever selecting processed foods, choose wisely.

> ➢ **Excitotoxins: MSG and Aspartame (NutraSweet)**
> These flavor enhancers mimic neurotransmitters and over-stimulate brain cells to fire repeatedly, damaging both the nerve cells and nerve transmission. Despite the destruction, this heightened brain response makes the product taste extra delicious and instantly creates cravings for more.

MSG (monosodium glutamate) is highly correlated with obesity – in fact, obesity is regularly studied in MSG-induced obese rodents. Other concerns include headaches, heart palpitations, respiratory symptoms such as shortness of breath, behavior problems in children and long-term brain issues such as ADHD, learning disabilities, Alzheimer's, Parkinson's and Lou Gehrig's diseases.

Buyer Beware: Unfortunately, MSG has 40+ legal names including benign-sounding hydrolyzed or autolyzed yeast or protein. Furthermore, MSG bears a similar molecular structure to *natural* L-glutamate (a neurotransmitter which can be converted to L-glutamine, an amino acid) so the FDA code allows MSG to be labeled as a generic ingredient such as *natural* flavors, seasonings or spices.

*Any food that requires enhancing by the use of chemical substances
should in no way be considered a food.* ~John H. Tobe

➤ **Nitrates and Nitrites – Another Look**

These salts are used in small amounts to cure meats, retarding bacterial growth and giving them a fresh, pink color. They are present in processed meats like hot dogs, deli meats, sausages and bacon.

Surprisingly, the vast majority of our exposure to these compounds comes from our own saliva and vegetable consumption...so in and of themselves, nitrates are not dangerous. However, there are mixed reports about these chemicals morphing into carcinogens when heated at high temperatures. Therefore, cook cured meats "low and slow" (a lower temperature for a longer period).

Recently multiple nitrate- and nitrite-free preserved meat products have hit the market only to add confusion to the topic. These uncured products use naturally-occurring nitrates found in beet or celery extracts. Even though these extracts do the exact same job as commercial nitrate salts, the advertising claims have convinced the public that these 'uncured' meats are inherently healthier than cured meats. This is not the case.

⌁ ChrisKresser The Nitrate and Nitrite Myth

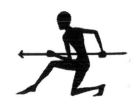

Precautions about cured meats revolve around the *quality* of the meat, not whether it has the sodium nitrate/nitrite. Pasture-raised bacon that has some added nitrates is a much healthier selection than factory-farmed, pork products that are uncured. Regardless, do not make processed meat a daily staple in your diet – limit it to a few times per week and cook it gently (no burned or charred meats).

Be aware, though, that some individuals are sensitive to nitrates and must be careful to select only high-quality uncured products or avoid them altogether.

➤ **Artificial Colors**

A majority of artificial colors are made from petroleum products or ammonia. They are linked to hyperactivity, asthma, allergies, impaired cognition, certain tumors, brain-nerve transmission interference and depression. Unfortunately, colorings lurk in the strangest of places like pickles, yogurt, toothpaste, farmed salmon, vitamins, medications, seaweed salad, vegetable juice, condiments and even *white* marshmallows.

*We are living in a world today where lemonade is made from artificial flavors
and furniture polish is made from real lemons.* ~MAD Magazine

Select products made with natural colorings such as beet juice, turmeric, saffron, paprika, annatto, chlorophyll, spinach, purple cabbage, fruit juice or another food you recognize. For a special occasion, there are food-based colorings available at natural grocers. And in a pinch, pulverized freeze-dried fruit can provide color.

➤ **Fructose: High Fructose Corn Syrup (HCFS) and Agave Nectar**
Fructose will be discussed in detail on Day 22 but it deserves a mention here because it infiltrates the food supply as a prevalent additive. When fructose is isolated into liquid form, the syrup is metabolized differently than fructose naturally found in whole fruit. Whole fruit sources gradually release fructose to the liver for proper digestion, whereas manipulated syrup forms create a large influx of unbound free fructose that overloads the liver. Additionally, fructose does not satisfy hunger because it bypasses the body's normal response to sugar intake, making overconsumption inevitable.

> **Buyer Beware:**
> 1. Agave nectar contains more fructose than high fructose corn syrup!
> 2. The Corn Refiners Association lobbied for legislation allowing HFCS to be labeled as plain *fructose*. Many yogurts, canned fruits, salad dressings and sauces now contain *fructose* in the ingredients.

Interrupt the Endocrine Disruptors (EDs)
Endocrine disruptors (EDs) are chemicals that imitate or interfere with the body's own hormonal signaling. They create problems with fertility, cognition, immunity, cell division and growth, behavior, obesity, diabetes, sexual development and function, thyroid health and cardiac health. Unfortunately, EDs play a major role in civilized life, with multiple cumulative exposures every day.

EDs include heavy metals, agricultural chemicals, plastics, air pollution and more. The list is a mile long but the major offenders are arsenic, atrazine, bisphenol-A (BPA), dioxin, fire retardants, glycol ethers, lead, mercury, organophosphate pesticides, perfluorinated chemicals (PFCs), perchlorate, phthalates, fluoride derivatives and bromide derivatives.

Due to their prevalence in modern society, reducing exposure to these compounds will not happen by chance. EDs are found in every household:

- Shampoo/conditioner
- Shaving products
- Cosmetics
- Deodorant/antiperspirant
- Toothpaste
- Nail polish
- Medications
- Birth control pills
- Household cleaners
- Air fresheners
- Plastics and vinyl
- Keyboard/mouse
- Cell phone cases
- Drinking water
- High-mercury fish
- CAFO animal products
- Pesticide residues
- Non-stick cookware
- CFL light bulbs
- Ink and toner cartridges
- Cash register receipts
- Fire extinguishers
- Flame-resistant carpeting
- Flame-resistant sleepwear
- Paint
- Brake fluid
- etc, etc, etc

Rather than fret about EDs (and cause a stress response), just be aware of where they exist in a typical household and gradually replace products containing these compounds with safer, more natural products (ideas in the following tables). Some sources of EDs are easily avoided while others have simple substitutes.

⌐ DrAxe How Endocrine Disruptors Destroy Your Body

Further Product Research
Please remember the skin is also an organ...a barrier between the body innards and the outside world. It can absorb chemicals directly into the body, so only put on your skin the same ingredients you are willing to put in your mouth. The tables on the next couple pages detail some toxin-limiting strategies. Also, the Environmental Working Group has multiple online guides to find the least objectionable products for your body and home (direct links available for all recommendations from ⌐ Paleovation):

Product Selection Guides
- ⌐ EWG Skin Deep
- ⌐ EWG Food News
- ⌐ EWG Cleaners
- ⌐ EWG Water Filter Buying Guide

Household and Personal Care Products
- ⌐ SlideShare Wellness Mama Natural Cleaning Guide
- ⌐ WellnessMama DIY Beauty Recipes
- ⌐ EarthEasy Natural Garden Pest Control
- ⌐ MarksDailyApple 19 Personal Care Products I Use or Like

Limiting Exposure to Endocrine Disruptors		
FOODS to Limit/Avoid	**Better Choice**	**Best Choice**
Canned goods lined with BPA	BPA-free canned goods	Purchase foods in glass bottles & jars
Processed, prepackaged foods in plastic packaging or treated with the preservatives BHA or BHT	Remove foods from plastic bags and store in stainless-steel or glass containers	Homemade, raw or fresh foods
High mercury fish (including marlin, shark, swordfish) and factory farmed fish	Select fish with a higher selenium content ThePaleoMom The Mercury Content of Seafood	Consume smaller wild-caught fish like sardines, anchovies and herring or supplement with purified fish oil or krill oil
Conventional produce	Use EWG Clean Fifteen and Dirty Dozen recommendations	Consume local, organic or homegrown produce
Conventional meat or dairy treated with rBGH or rBST	Select only lean meats from CAFO animals, buy antibiotic-free products	Consume organic, antibiotic-free, free-range, pastured, grass-fed and wild-caught products
Plant estrogens found in soy, flax		Choose animal protein sources including soy-free eggs

American consumers have no problem with carcinogens, but they will not purchase any product, including floor wax, that has fat in it. ~Dave Barry

KITCHEN ITEMS to Limit/Avoid	**Better Choice**	**Best Choice**
Tap water for drinking and bathing (the skin absorbs toxins)	Filter tap/bathing water	Reverse osmosis water, supplement with trace mineral drops
Plastic wrap, plastic food storage containers	Glass dishes with plastic lids	Stainless steel or glass storage containers with rubber seal
Non-stick cookware*, especially if scratched		Cast iron, stainless steel, enameled cast iron, glass or ceramics
Other plastic items (cutting boards, water bottles, strainers)	Reduce plastics' exposure to heat (hand wash, no microwave)	Use glass, ceramic, wooden, bamboo or stainless-steel items
Microwaving in plastics or with plastic wrap	Cover foods with a napkin when microwaving	Microwave only in microwave safe glass and ceramics, or reheat on stovetop

> ***How to Cook Eggs in Stainless Steel:** First, heat the *empty* pan for 3-5 minutes – yes, empty. When it's hot, add the oil/butter. Coat the entire pan to create a non-stick barrier. Finally add eggs, flip using a metal spatula.

BATHROOM ITEMS to Limit/Avoid	**Better Choice**	**Best Choice**
Dental products, body care products, sunscreens, shaving products, hair care and styling products, moisturizers, etc	Choose products free of dyes, petroleum, sulfates, fragrance, parabens and fluoride	Organic, green or homemade versions made from coconut oil, baking soda, castile soap, vinegar, lemon juice, borax or essential oils
Cosmetics, beauty products	Fragrance-free versions	Choose organic products
Feminine hygiene products	Use fragrance-free and chlorine-free products	Choose organic versions made from cotton and hemp, rubber and silicone (menstrual cups), sea sponges or THINX period panties
Conventional cleaners / detergents	Bleach alternatives	Organic or homemade versions

HOUSEHOLD ITEMS to Limit/Avoid	Better Choice	Best Choice
Synthetic fabrics/flooring including clothing, upholstery, mattresses and carpeting/padding	Choose natural textiles/flooring like cotton, linen, silk, wool, leather, wood, cork, bamboo	Choose organic natural fibers and products
Airborne particles from carpet padding or flame-retardant items	Open windows to air out the house	Use HEPA air filters and vacuums to contain the dust
Children's plastic toys, sippy cups	Wooden, metal, cloth, paper	Organic or non-treated versions
Products with VOCs (paint, vinyl shower curtains)	Low VOC paints	Natural milk paints, white wash, fabric shower curtains
Lead paint chips, lead from pipes or soldering leached into hot water	Replace old windows to reduce lead paint dust; replace lead pipes	Research how to remove lead paint without creating dust, use cold tap water for all cooking, soaking and drinking
Products containing anti-microbial Triclosan or its tradenames: Microban and Biofresh	Products without antimicrobial chemicals	Avoid inadvertent exposure by reading labels: Triclosan is present in everything from cutting boards to public hand railings to soft soap
Pesticides, fungicides, herbicides in lawn, garden, pet care and bug spray products		Natural repellants: garlic, soap, baking soda, vinegar, diatomaceous earth, cayenne, essential oil, mint

> *Someday we shall look back on this dark era of agriculture and shake our heads. How could we have ever believed that it was a good idea to grow our food with poisons?* ~Jane Goodall

Common Symptoms of Hormone Disruption

As evidenced by the extensive lists above (and these aren't complete), civilized human populations experience major exposure to endocrine disruptors. Widespread symptoms are materializing insidiously over time: thyroid problems, insulin resistance and diabetes, obesity, cognitive complications, ADHD, mood disorders, insomnia, pituitary and adrenal disorders, erectile dysfunction, low T, early onset of puberty, PCOS, infertility and menopause complications – essentially any hormone-sensitive condition could be linked to these chemicals.

Notice the prominence of reproductive conditions. Our discussion would not be complete without addressing the sex hormones, estrogen and testosterone.

Reproductive Health and Hormone Specifics

There are multiple factors that influence hormone expression and regulation throughout the body, but the best way to support hormone health comes from three main elements:

1. Providing proper building blocks and nutrients to create necessary hormones
2. Reducing exposure to endocrine disruptors
3. Regulating erratic hormonal fluctuations (stress-related cortisol, blood sugar-related insulin and leptin)

The Paleo Lifestyle addresses all these issues and creates the ideal environment for the body to reset hormonal interactions. Nutrient-dense and cholesterol-rich foods provide the base molecules for steroidal sex hormones (more about Cholesterol on Day 17). Eating homemade Paleo naturally reduces exposure to dietary endocrine disruptors as well as digestive stressors. Incorporating Paleo Lifestyle factors regulates other hormonal cycles by stabilizing and supporting blood sugar levels, stress response, sleep factors and exercise habits.

> *The power of healing is within you. All you need to do is give your body what it needs and remove what is poisoning it. You can restore your own health by what you do – not by the pills you take, but by how you choose to live.* ~Terry Wahls, MD

Irregular hormone levels are not resolved with hormone replacement therapy. However, combining dietary and lifestyle efforts normalizes all hormonal cycles and reduces consequences of reproductive hormonal disruption.

Low "T"?

Men as young as their 20's are reporting low testosterone and sexual dysfunction symptoms...but aren't men supposed to be capable of fathering children well into their 80's? Unfortunately, many of the environmental endocrine disruptors mimic estrogen and suppress testosterone production. This leads to another unfortunate detrimental hormonal cycle, one that softens or feminizes men's bodies. Excess estrogens promote fat gain – the enlarged fat tissue itself produces more estrogens which initiates even more fat production...

⫶⫶ MarksDailyApple A Primal Primer: Testosterone

> *To effectively support a healthy hormonal system, it is critically important to provide the body with sufficient amounts of estrogen-inhibiting phytonutrients [Paleo] to balance against the overwhelming surplus of estrogenic food substances and chemicals in the diet. ~Ori Hofmekler*

Uncomfortable Menstruation

Men, do NOT skip this section: This affects your wives/partners, mothers, sisters and daughters!

Unfortunately, painful periods, PMS and irregular cycles are widespread, but just because these symptoms are common does not mean they're normal. The anti-inflammatory effect of Paleo can alleviate uncomfortable menstrual symptoms, but be patient, it takes multiple cycles for these hormones to properly reset.

> **Lifelong Hormone Replacement?** The hormone-altering birth control pill has been prescribed to generations of women and young girls for painful periods, irregular cycles, pregnancy prevention and even headaches! We are now looking at an entire population of women taking hormones from adolescence through adulthood, only to begin estrogen therapy at menopause. Something is very wrong – nature did not make us hormone deficient!

Painless periods and stable moods are certainly attractive benefits of the Paleo Lifestyle, but what about pregnancy prevention? Is there a safe birth control alternative to artificial hormone medications?

⫶⫶ DrHyman How Do I Naturally Balance Female Sex Hormones?

Paleo-Friendly Birth Control – No pills, no IUDs, no hormones...only body awareness

It's difficult to trust a natural alternative to hormone-disrupting birth control methods because, unfortunately, the only well-known natural technique is the rhythm method which is *not* reliable! The rhythm method assumes ovulation will occur on the same day of the current cycle as it did in the previous cycle, yet ovulation day varies due to stress, poor diet, transitioning to menopause, nursing a baby, etc.

Fertility Awareness Method

This method, also known as FAM or natural family planning, pinpoints the days of highest fertility. In a typical cycle a woman has 18-21 *non*-fertile days...that's right, she is mostly NON-fertile! This assessment includes a generous "buffer" to make sure her body does not accidentally support any stray sperm.

FAM charts a woman's basal (resting) body temperature and observes changes in vaginal fluid. During ovulation, body temperature elevates slightly (literally goes 'into heat') and vaginal fluid becomes slipperier to aid in sperm travel and survival. Once fertility signals are understood, a couple can plan appropriate intercourse according to their desired outcome:

> ➤ A*void pregnancy*: Use a condom, diaphragm or abstinence method during the 7-10 *possible* fertile days
> ➤ *Achieve pregnancy*: Plan sex during the best chance for conception (the egg is only alive 6-12 hours)

FAM *does not* protect against STDs and is not recommended for those unwilling to diligently observe and record fertility signals. Correct interpretation of these indicators is vital for FAM success, but remember, *every* birth control method (the pill, IUD, condoms, injection, etc) has risk of failure.

Further Reading:

📖 *Taking Charge of Your Fertility,* by Toni Weschler
⫶⫶ Visit the accompanying website TCOYF to access the charting tools
⫶⫶ FertAware is another online resource

Rachel's FAM Experience: Since 2002 my husband and I have had three planned pregnancies and one nerve-wracking late period, but that is a heck of a track record! In fact, I do not know of any other method that would have worked better over 15+ years.

Strategies to Maintain Proper Hormone Levels

Healing from toxin exposure, reducing environmental hormone disruptors and rebalancing hormones will take time, but the Paleo Lifestyle is a valid approach to naturally support whole-body health including toxin purification/detoxification:

- Eat an **anti-inflammatory diet** – Paleo is perfect
- Consume sources of **EPA/DHA** (Day 3)
- Respond appropriately to **stress** (Day 12)
- Promote restful **sleep** (Day 13)
- Get the right kind of **exercise** (Day 10)
- Expose your skin to **sunshine** or supplement with **Vitamin D3**

To-Do List:

- ☐ Chicken roasting project is planned or already finished (complete by Day 23)
- ☐ Anything else (deep breathing exercise, reread stress relieving tips on Day 12, etc)?

Coming Up Soon:

- Toxin exposure can disrupt gut flora balance. Tomorrow we will discuss how to repopulate the good microbes, especially useful now that your gut has started to heal.
- Day 21 marks the 3-week point. There will be a short assessment of your current progress plus discussion about adding more fruit starting on Day 22.

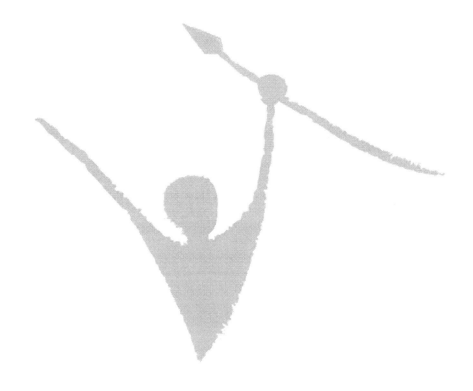

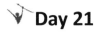 **Day 21**

Today's Topics:

1. 3-Week Look Back
2. Adding More Fruit
3. Paleo-Wise: Gut Health, Probiotics and Fermented Foods
4. How to Maintain a Healthy Gut Microbe Balance

Fast Fare – Use Paleo Mayo
♥ Green apples with coconut butter
♥ Deviled eggs
♥ Sugar snap peas

Are there any foods you had today that are worth noting? _____

What are your go-to foods, beverages or snacks?

1. _____
2. _____
3. _____

Is there a category in the Veggie + Protein + Fat template you need to incorporate more? How will you do that?

_____

Section I: 3-Week Look Back

By Day 21, your body is starting to buzz with new life...it has had enough time to acclimate to the influx of vital nutrients as well as the elimination of inflammatory foods. This is an ideal point for reflection. What changes are you witnessing in your body? Check all that apply:

Physical changes

☐ Sounder sleep   ☐ Clearer skin   ☐ Desire to be active
☐ Less achy   ☐ Lower blood pressure   ☐ Better performance
☐ Less pain with an old injury   ☐ Better stools   ☐ Quicker exercise recovery times
☐ Smoother joint movement   ☐ Easier digestion   ☐ Improved range of motion
☐ Fewer headaches   ☐ Thinking clearly   ☐ Feel stronger
☐ Steady energy levels   ☐ Less acid reflux   ☐ Clothing fits better

Any other physical changes not listed here?

_____

What do you still hope to improve? Many symptoms continue to heal and progress as time goes on.

_____

_____

Emotional Changes

The gut flora balance is shifting which can have a dramatic impact on mood. What sort of moods have you been experiencing? Check all that apply:

☐ Happy/joyful   ☐ Energetic   ☐ Alert   ☐ Confident
☐ Agreeable   ☐ Content/fulfilled   ☐ Full of wonder   ☐ Eager
☐ Interested/engaged   ☐ Calm/relaxed   ☐ Tranquil/peaceful   ☐ Clear-headed

The opposites are in this list. Are any of these still manifesting?

☐ Discontent/unhappy   ☐ Feisty   ☐ Troubled   ☐ Unstable
☐ Tense/edgy   ☐ Hostile/aggressive   ☐ Grumpy   ☐ Apathetic
☐ Alienated   ☐ Hesitant   ☐ Withdrawn   ☐ Anxious/worried

Stable emotions take time to develop. Has this been enough time for you? Thoughts?

_____

_____

The above lists also appeared on Days 9 and 13. Go back to compare your responses.

What differences surprise you?

_____

_____

Is there an aspect of your changing health that's not yet materializing or seems stagnant? Record your thoughts.

_____

_____

Section II: Adding More Fruit

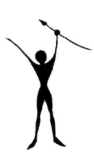

Tomorrow you are welcome to add more fruit if desired. From Day 22 through the end of the program, enjoy up to 3 servings of *whole fruit* per day (this does not include juice, dried or canned in syrup because those sugars are concentrated). Continue to use the Veggie + Protein + Fat template to ensure that fruit doesn't displace other nutrient-dense foods.

This is the perfect time to observe your body's reaction to some natural sugars as you're approaching the end of the program. Pay attention to your taste buds...some fruit is bred to be super sweet! You may find a preference for low-sugar varieties. Also pay attention to how your body responds to more whole fruit (might be positive, negative or neutral): digestive changes, energy levels, meal satisfaction, joint fluidity, sleep effectiveness, etc.

Is there a certain fruit you've been missing?

_____

Earlier in the program we mentioned a few recipes which include fruits. Browse back and see if this new fruit allowance inspires you to sample one of those ideas:
  ✓ Prep F has breakfast planning
  ✓ Day 12 has smoothies – feel free to add some fresh or frozen fruit if you enjoy smoothies

Applesauce is a common sweetener in Paleo cooking. Pork chops paired with applesauce or apple slices is a delicious combination. Any other ideas to refresh your recipes with some fruit?

_____

Section III – Paleo-Wise: Gut Health, Probiotics, Fermented Foods

All disease begins in the gut. ~Hippocrates

What's in the Gut?
Your body does not only belong to you...it houses *trillions* of microscopic digestive organisms in the small and large intestines to help evaluate and process every item that enters the mouth. How big is a trillion? Using time to put a trillion in perspective: a *million* seconds is 11 ½ days, a *billion* seconds is 32 years and a *trillion* seconds is 32,000 years!

This is an astronomical number of symbiotic beings living in our intestines and, it turns out, this has evolved into a very good thing. When working harmoniously, humans and the gut flora have a mutually beneficial relationship – we provide shelter and a safe habitat for these microbes and in return, they take care of some things that the human body cannot do on its own. Sufficient numbers and proper balance of the gut flora (primarily bacteria, but also includes yeasts and parasites) is crucial for nutrition, digestion, gut lining integrity, immune function and even stable moods.

Healthy Gut Flora Balance	
Body Function	**Role of Gut Flora**
Digestion	✓ Produce enzymes to break down phytates (anti-nutrients in grains/legumes) ✓ Ferment carbohydrates/fiber to make them digestible ✓ Metabolize bile acids to digest fat ✓ Create short-chain fatty acids to fuel cells in the colon lining
Vitamins & Minerals	✓ Synthesize K1, K2, B6, B12, biotin and folate ✓ Aide in absorption of magnesium, calcium and iron
Immunity	✓ Prevent growth of pathogenic bacteria ✓ Stimulate lymph to produce antibodies linked to allergy prevention
Emotional and Sleep Support	✓ Boost mood with feel good neurotransmitters – over 90% of serotonin and 50% of dopamine are produced and absorbed in the gut – microbes assist with production as well as keeping the gut healthy for proper neurotransmitter reception ✓ Establishing sleep/circadian cycles – melatonin is produced, in part, by gut microbes

It seems remarkable, but the little critters living inside of you have been linked to everything from autism to obesity, from allergy to autoimmunity, from fibromyalgia to restless leg syndrome, from delirium to eczema to asthma. In fact, the links between chronic illness and gut bacteria keep growing every day.
~Mark Hyman, MD, <u>Eat Fat Get Thin</u>, <u>The Blood Sugar Solution</u>

More Than a Gut Feeling

Have you ever experienced "butterflies" in the stomach, a "gut instinct" or the feeling of "gut-wrenching" agony? These are not just random clichés – the digestion-emotion connection is quite real: our guts truly help us *feel*. It's easy to link unbalanced gut flora with digestive trouble, but few consider the connection between gut flora, the nervous system and brain function.

The digestive tract is extensively packed with nerves, a network called the *Enteric Nervous System* (ENS) and often referred to as the 'second brain.' This 'gut brain' communicates with the actual brain as it monitors the internal environment, including ingested threats such as poisons or invasive bacteria. Digestive integrity greatly influences the quality of the *gut brain's* neural responses, including neurotransmitter production and reflexes.

Balancing Act: When Gut Flora is Out of Whack	
Complication	**Details**
Digestive Upset	Heartburn, bloating, constipation, diarrhea, excessive gas, complete lack of gas
Digestive Dysfunction	Inability to digest fiber, vitamin/mineral deficiencies due to poor assimilation, undigested food particles in stool, Crohn's disease, IBS or ulcerative colitis
Glucose Metabolism	Some strains of gut bacteria increase insulin resistance and cause sugar cravings (curiously, gut bacterial ratios are different in lean individuals versus obese; these ratios normalize with gut healing and weight loss)
Other Microbial Overgrowth	Small Intestine Bacterial Overgrowth (SIBO –bacteria populating the wrong intestinal areas), systemic candida, other pathogenic yeasts, fungi or parasites
Brain Function	Unfriendly microbes produce toxins, metabolic by-products and other inflammatory compounds that contribute to brain fog, mood disorders like anxiety or depression, autistic symptoms, reduced problem-solving skills and conditions such as Parkinson's, dementia, tremors or restless leg syndrome
Weakened Immune System	*Respiratory problems* such as asthma, allergies, sinus congestion, bronchitis, post-nasal drip, sinusitis *Skin issues* such as eczema, rosacea, psoriasis, acne *Autoimmune conditions* like Hashimoto's thyroiditis, lupus, MS, celiac disease, rheumatoid arthritis

Section IV: How to Maintain Healthy Gut Microbe Balance

There will always be some harmful microbes present in the intestines – it's impossible to completely eradicate them. However, pathogens can be controlled by a robust population of friendly probiotic microbes in the digestive tract. It's imperative to consciously and regularly repopulate the gut with sufficient quantities. Here are three steps to effectively discourage the bad bugs while supporting the good bugs:

A. Step 1: Starve Unfriendly Gut Microbes

Eliminate foods the bad bugs love: sugars and starches including all grains, legumes*, sweeteners, alcohol and spirits, high-sugar fruits, starchy vegetables like potatoes and dairy products (except grass-fed butter)

> **Great News:** Step 1 is already in full progress if you are actively implementing the strategies in this book!

*Legumes do provide fiber to support the good flora, but the high starch content can feed the bad flora. During the program, vegetables supply all required fiber. Reintroductions will determine legume tolerance for long-term inclusion.

B. Step 2: Create 'Enticing Intestines'

1. **Heal the Gut Lining** by consuming bone broth, fish oil or fatty fish rich in EPA/DHA, anti-inflammatory herbs and spices such as ginger or turmeric (more info in the Spice Guide on Day 2) and short- and medium-chain fatty acids found in coconut oil, MCT oil or grass-fed butter

2. **Feed *Prebiotics*** to the beneficial microbes – these foods encourage proliferation of the gut flora:

    a. <u>Fiber</u> – in some raw veggies especially asparagus, dandelion greens, Jerusalem artichokes, cruciferous family (broccoli, cabbage, cauliflower, Brussels sprouts), garlic and onion

    > **Note:** Some individuals with bowel disorders may need to start with cooked vegetables and gradually introduce raw veggies. If this describes you, read about FODMAPS on Day 8 and consider trying acacia fiber to feed the good bugs and comfort both diarrhea and constipation.

    b. <u>Resistant starch</u> (RS) – found in *green* plantains and bananas, raw starchy vegetables, or cooked and cooled potatoes (more about Fiber and RS on Day 15)

3. **Limit Exposure to Microbe-Killing Products** including hand sanitizer, antibacterial soap, antibiotics (unless necessary), animal products from factory farms (antibiotics are in the feed), chlorinated water, produce sprayed with pesticides/fungicides/herbicides, pet flea/tick treatments and shampoos, etc

4. **Reduce Stress and Get Plenty of Sleep** – switching metabolism from "fight or flight" to "rest and digest" maximizes digestion by limiting cortisol's interference on gut bacteria balance (more on Days 11 and 12)

C. Step 3: 'Belly Up' to Beneficial Bacteria

Many organisms in the gut have a very short lifespan so shifts in bacterial ratios can happen within a matter of days/weeks. However, long-term stabilization and maintenance of a hearty diverse probiotic population takes conscious effort, especially in modern germophobic cultures which encourage eradication of all microbes. Here are a few effective flora-sustaining strategies:

1. <u>**Probiotics**</u> – Most of these organisms function quickly then get excreted in the stool – therefore, a perpetual supply is necessary to maintain their presence. Probiotics can be resourced via foods and/or supplements. If you are new to fermented foods or drinks, start slowly to let your body adapt.

    a. **Probiotic-Rich Foods**: Fermented foods include homemade sauerkraut and kimchee, plain coconut milk yogurt or drinks like water kefir, kvass or kombucha. Homemade is best (*kraut recipe on next page). For a store-bought product to be fully effective, it must be refrigerated, non-pasteurized and free from carrageenan and added sugars. After the program, try including dairy-based kefir and yogurt if tolerated.

    b. **Probiotic Supplements**: Stomach acid can kill beneficial bacteria before they reach the desired destination in the intestines, so look for "enteric coating" on the capsules which ensures survival and protects microbial activity. Also, select refrigerated products (freeze-dried aren't as potent) with a large population, say 30-50 billion.

> **Good to Know:** Each manufacturer utilizes different strains of microbes. Consider rotating multiple probiotic products to gain exposure to a wider variety.

2. **Soil-Based Organisms (SBO's)** – These are probiotic spores naturally found in *healthy* dirt, but not in the depleted soil of chemically-laden commercial farmlands. SBO's tend to repopulate themselves in the gut so lower numbers are sufficient. Ingest SBOs through direct contact with healthy soil or via supplements.

   a. **SBO-Rich Behaviors**: Walk barefoot; do not peel organic root vegetables; spend time in the dirt or garden; eat unsprayed vegetables unwashed; spread compost in the flower beds; play with worms; visit a pick-your-own produce farm; jump in autumn leaf piles; etc.

   b. **SBO Supplements**: Start slowly with SBO supplements – the body must adjust to their presence and detoxifying effect. Spore-based organisms are very stable and do not require refrigeration or special coating to survive stomach acid. Prescript-Assist and MegaSpore are popular brands.

* DIY Fermented Foods – Reinvent the Ferment! A Natural Dietary Source of Probiotics

Lacto-fermentation is a traditional preservation method where foods are soaked in a salt water solution at room temperature. As probiotics grow during the fermentation, they produce enzymes, create vitamins and start to break down fiber, making foods more digestible. The highest quality ferments are homemade. To allow time for adaption to new microbes, start slowly with perhaps a spoonful a day and gradually increase over time.

Store-bought pickles and sauerkraut are not equivalent to lacto-fermented foods. Modern products destroy the beneficial bacteria with vinegar, heat processing or pasteurization. Any purchased fermented vegetable must be refrigerated and *un*pasteurized to retain the probiotics. A list of commercially available products is below.

Fermenting at Home

This is a terrific way to preserve vegetables! It does take initial time to prepare the vegetables and brine, but after that, there's little to do except periodically taste the ferment to monitor readiness. Search for lacto-fermented recipes online: pickles, kraut, ketchup, salsa, carrots or garlic as well as drinks such as kefir, kombucha or kvass. Recipes and techniques here:

  ⌂ SavoryLotus 85 Ways to Eat More Fermented Foods

Simple Cabbage Kraut

Makes two 1-quart jars. Variation: Add garlic cloves, herbs, caraway seed and other shredded vegetables like beet, carrot, turnip or onion.

Shred: (First reserve two full leaves) 1 medium head of cabbage; slice thinly with a knife or food processor.

Mix: In a large bowl, massage 2-3 Tbsp salt into the cabbage so the liquid is drawn out of it. It needs to be quite moist before jarring, so let it wilt up to 30 minutes before transferring to the jar.

Jar: Press each handful of cabbage tightly down in a clean jar, reserving at least 1 inch of air at the top.

Submerge: Place the reserved full cabbage leaf on top of the packed shredded cabbage. Press down until all cabbage is submerged and tuck the edges of the full leaf around the shredded cabbage – this prevents air contact with the vegetable. Weigh down the leaf with a small bowl, shot glass or rock to keep it under the brine.

[Optional] Extra liquid: If there's not enough liquid, dissolve ¾ tsp salt in ½ cup of purified water and top off.

Cover: Secure cheesecloth or a coffee filter over the top of the jars by tying a string or using a rubber band; or use an airlock if you have one. Do not use a tight-fitting lid as gasses produced during the ferment will build up.

Watch and Wait: Place on a plate to catch any bubble-over and set in a dark, room temperature environment. Check the kraut daily to make sure no vegetables are touching the air (sometimes they ride to the surface on a bubble – remove any with a clean spoon). If you notice small yeast/mold spots on the brine surface, it is normal but skim off with a clean spoon. Fermentation time depends on room temperature. Usually kraut takes 2-3 weeks to ferment, but start tasting it every day or two at 1 week old. When you like the flavor, put on the lid and store in the fridge.

Refrigerate Safely: Air exposure can cause mold growth, which we don't want. As you start to eat your ferment, repack into smaller jars and top off with brine. Without air exposure, kraut will last 3-12 months in the fridge!

Commercially-Available Ferments

If you're not interested in home-fermenting, there are fermented products in stores which provide probiotics. Look in the refrigerated section for sugar-free and raw items. Popular brands include Bubbies, Gold Mine, Farmhouse Cultures, as well as many online companies. Check local goods in stores and farmers' markets.

- Kraut
- Kimchi
- Pickles
- Pickled beets
- Pickled green tomatoes
- Kombucha
- Water kefir
- Coconut kefir
- Kvass

> **Good to Know:** *Do not heat* your fermented foods! Heat destroys the living microbes. Instead, add a small amount alongside an entrée or just eat directly out of the jar (snack idea!).

Consequences of Germophobic Culture

Your microbiome refers to the collective microorganisms living in and on your body including bacteria, protozoa, fungi and viruses. It is influenced by every living thing in your daily environment including people, pets and even houseplants. Sterile living conditions and depleted farmlands have consequently reduced the quantity and diversity of the microbiome. Additionally, it has been further assaulted by poor dietary practices – eating excess sugar/starch in recent generations has diminished the proportions of beneficial gut flora.

> **Sanitation and Sterilization:** Without a doubt, modern sanitation practices are crucial for a healthy living environment – imagine a city without sewers! However, just because soap and water are indispensable doesn't mean over-use of harsh disinfectants is better. Likewise, sterilization absolutely has its place, especially when dealing with open wounds or cutting boards tainted with raw meats; but excessive, habitual germ-killing behaviors and practices (haphazard antibiotic and hand sanitizer use) have dramatically altered the microbiome.

No One-Size-Fits-All Gut Flora Approach

Each individual has unique needs and sensitivities, so there's no perfect combination of resources to balance gut flora. Some people will need to further heal their gut and immune system before they are ready to comfortably incorporate raw vegetables, SBOs or ferments. Experiment with different strategies and combinations, but always listen to your body. If any particular strategy causes discomfort, discontinue and try another suggestion.

Further Reading (remember, direct links available from ᗡ Paleovation)

- ᗡ DrPerlmutter Brain Maker Foods
- ᗡ MarksDailyApple This is your Brain on Bugs
- ᗡ MarksDailyApple 7 Things You Had no Idea Gut Bacteria Could Do
- ᗡ KellyBroganMD Probiotics for the Brain
- 📖 *Brain Maker,* by David Perlmutter, MD
- 📖 *The Microbiome Diet,* by Raphael Kellman, MD
- 📖 *Happy Gut,* by Vincent Pedre, MD
- 📖 *Fermented: A Four-Season Approach to Paleo Probiotic Foods,* by Jill Ciciarelli

To-Do List:

- ☐ If you have not roasted a chicken, it's time...finish by Day 23!
- ☐ Browse Prep F and Day 12 for recipes that include fruit – anything you want to try?

_____

- ☐ What else (make sauerkraut, find a recommended book at the library, review crunchy snacks in Day 14)?

_____

Coming Up Soon:

- Tomorrow allows extra fruit into the dietary template. Fruit is still a cautionary food – keep your gut health in mind as you begin introducing more sugars.
- Next topic: Fructose, the Fruit Sugar...an appropriate discussion with the addition of fruit.

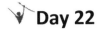 Day 22

Motivation is the single most important factor in any sort of success. ~Sir Edmund Hillary

Today's Topics:

1. Home Stretch – Preparation for Food Reintroductions
2. Introducing Long-Term Strategies
3. Paleo-Wise: Fructose

Fast Fare – Veggies + Protein + Fat
♥ Cherry tomatoes, olives, basil leaves
♥ Broccoli slaw w/mayo or olive oil
♥ Frozen burger with pat of butter

Notes on today's foods:

_____

Is it time to add in another foundation recipe (Prep B)? Which one?

_____

Review the Paleo substitute list on Day 6. Any new foods you would like to try?

_____

Have you made a 'veggie as a grain' recipe lately (Day 7)?   Yes   No

Is there another grain substitute you'd like to make during this last week? Which one? _____

Section I: Home Stretch – Preparation for Food Reintroductions

Congratulations...you have reached the final phase of the Strict Paleo Protocol! This last stage is often met with a variety of opposing emotions. Reactions range from unbridled anticipation of finally indulging in non-Paleo foods to the other extreme of hesitancy to reintroduce eliminated items for fear of jeopardizing new-found health and vitality (or finding a trigger food).

Information provided during this last week explains the reintroduction process to identify individual food tolerances. Additionally, you will learn how to incorporate that knowledge into a long-term maintenance plan compatible with your lifestyle. It may be tempting to start experimenting prematurely with maintenance mode strategies, but please remain diligent with the program rules through this last week. Focus on current goals and finish strong!

Healthy Baseline Chart (Page 344)

The keystone of food reintroduction is awareness of how good your body feels after a full month on the Strict Paleo Protocol. Therefore, each day for the next week, complete the Healthy Baseline Chart on page 344 to monitor multiple aspects of your current health and establish a record of Paleo improvements – this is your benchmark of comparison for gauging how each newly added food affects your body during reintroductions.

Section II: Introducing Long-Term Strategies

It's imperative to cultivate strategies to successfully support long-term goals. In addition to a 'safe foods' list determined during reintroductions, a maintenance mode plan also includes formulating a framework for future social situations, managing carb cravings, and even regaining control after diet deviations.

Many suggestions and ideas are interspersed through this final week. Begin by reflecting on your Paleo experience so far. Which portions of the program will you use as part of your maintenance mode strategies:

- ☐ Planning ahead for meals or batch-cooking
- ☐ Veggie + Protein + Fat template
- ☐ Keeping appropriate snacks handy
- ☐ Using the lunchbox template for quick ideas
- ☐ Including traditional, healthy fats
- ☐ Making Paleo-staple cooking assignment recipes
- ☐ Incorporating some pre- and pro-biotics
- ☐ Supplementing hard-to-attain nutrients

- ☐ Ensuring adequate low-level movement
- ☐ Exercising sensibly
- ☐ Prioritizing sleep
- ☐ Managing stress
- ☐ Connecting to the self and others
- ☐ Incorporating non-food rewards
- ☐ Listening to the body's responses
- ☐ Researching more about the Paleo Protocol

What other ideas will shape and structure your long-range lifestyle strategies?

_____

_____

What aspects of the Strict Paleo Protocol may not be important to your long-term goals?

_____

Maintenance Mode Variations

Maintenance mode can include a wide range of strategies and participation levels. The trial-and-error experimentation period following the Strict Paleo Protocol never truly ends because many influencing factors fluctuate over time (lifestyle changes, social opportunities, underlying stress, sleep allotment, exercise regimens, food tolerance levels, etc). Due to the wide variety of individual situations, no two long-term Paleo lifestyle plans look the same. To illustrate this variation, here are some of our personal hacks to maintain a healthy Paleo framework while accommodating to our unique lifestyles and periodically incorporating non-Paleo foods:

Variety is the Spice of Life!

Maintenance Mode: Paleo Strategies and Non-Paleo Foods

Rachel: With a family of five, our kids' sensitivities and ability to burn off carbohydrates influence the foods we have in our house. Though we don't eat grains on a daily basis, we do keep some gluten-free grains in the pantry. Each family member has different sensitivities so our meals are based on common well-tolerated foods with optional sides (like rice or grated cheese).

We love to cook so a large majority of our meals are at home and kids pack their school lunches, which is easier on the budget, too. If we go out to eat, each person orders based around their sensitivities (and we don't worry about ordering French fries because it's so seldom).

Here are examples of non-Paleo foods commonly found in my kitchen: Full-fat grass-fed cheese and yogurt, white and wild rice, rice paper wrappers, steel cut oats, canned beans, organic hummus, gluten-free non-GMO soy sauce, organic peanut butter, specific organic corn products (tortillas, grits and popcorn), a packaged mix for gluten-free pizza crust or dessert, wine.

Kelly: As a busy healthcare professional and gym junkie, I don't have much time to cook elaborate Paleo meals. Couple that with the fact that I really don't like cooking (but I prefer the taste and love the quality of home-prepared meals). My solution to stay mostly Paleo:

- <u>Batch Cook</u> – Almost everything I make includes sufficient leftovers to last a few days or for freezing.
- <u>Regular Roasted Veggies</u> – My favorites are tossed in melted coconut oil, salt, pepper and garlic. I reheat them for a side (half my plate is a 'side') or incorporate in a stir-fry, omelet or sauce.
- <u>Salad Bar, Hot Bar, Sushi</u> (occasionally with rice) – provided by a favorite local health-food grocer that I frequent 2-3x/week. While there, I often grab berries, red peppers (my fave go-to veggie), precut veggies for my next home cooking (cabbage slaw, sweet potato fries, zoodles) kombucha, salami, dark chocolate or an occasional dessert (single size only, and sometimes not Paleo!).

I can tolerate minor Paleo deviations several times per week without significant consequence. At a bar with friends, I usually compromise with hard cider or a vodka press and plain wings, sauce on the side.

Non-Paleo inclusions often in my kitchen: Stevia-sweetened soda, string cheese, ice cream, grass-fed whey protein, frozen spanakopita (weird, I know), whipped cream, chewing gum. When my grown sons were still at home, there were more cupboard deviations: chips/bread/grain products but gluten-free & non-GMO, conventional meats, rotisserie chicken, frozen meals, whey protein bars, pasta, white rice.

Section III – Paleo-Wise: Fructose

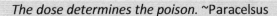

The dose determines the poison. ~Paracelsus

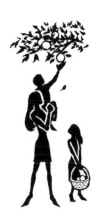

Fruit Sugar
Fructose is the sugar that naturally occurs in fruit. The form of fructose found in whole fruit is combined with fiber, vitamins, minerals, antioxidants, phytonutrients and enzymes. Generally speaking, whole fruit is a healthy *and anti-inflammatory* food.

Fruit During the Strict Paleo Protocol
The goal during this month of diet restriction has been to eliminate sugars, stabilize metabolism, calm the sweet tooth and minimize physical sugar cravings. The reality is that fruit is still sugar. Although generally a minor source, *excess* fruit consumption impedes sugar withdrawal efforts. That's why, for the first three weeks, fruit has been limited to one serving per day of the *low-sugar variety*:

Paleo Protocol Low-Sugar Fruits:
Most berries, green apples, grapefruit, lemon, lime, fresh figs

As of today, more fruit servings may be included per the guidelines below. Remember to pay attention to your body's reaction to increased fruit portions.
- Up to 3 fruit servings per day
- All *whole* fruits are now acceptable

Fructose Characteristics
When compared to glucose, fructose has some unique traits:
- **Does Not Trigger Insulin** – glucose is the primary sugar that stimulates an insulin response
- **Only Metabolized in the Liver** – whereas glucose is easily metabolized by every cell in the body
- **Does Not Increase Blood Sugar Levels** – fructose does not circulate in the blood for general use; therefore, it does not register on blood sugar measurements (lab tests only measure glucose)
- **Not Involved in the Satiety Pathway** – you won't get full eating fructose; consequently, consumption encourages overeating (more next on how an excess calorie load directs fructose to fat storage)
- **High Relative Sweetness** – fructose is sweeter than both glucose and sucrose (table sugar)
- **Its Sweetness is Perceived Faster** – reaches a higher peak and diminishes more quickly than that of sucrose or glucose, urging another quick bite/gulp to prevent an energy dip and satisfy the sweet reward

Increased Fructose Consumption
Fruit/fructose was once only a minor part of the human diet. Our ancestors only consumed fructose seasonally when fruit was ripe and occasionally when fruit was preserved.

Modern exposure to fructose from fruit alone has gradually increased in the past few decades. Sophisticated plant-breeding techniques have created larger and sweeter hybrids. As a result, fructose levels in fruit are significantly higher than just 30 years ago. Additionally, seedless varieties are faster to eat than their seeded cousins (think grapes, tangerines, watermelon) and lead to unintended extra consumption.

Reasons for Increased Fructose Consumption:
1. Year-round access to fruit with the advent of refrigeration and importation
2. Widely-available concentrated forms such as dried, freeze-dried or other processed fruit
3. Increased liquefied sweet sources such as high fructose corn syrup, fruit juice or agave nectar
4. Overeating any sweets (granulated sugar is 50% fructose)
5. Excess fructose consumption in one sitting (sodas, juices, liberal amounts of dried fruit)

> **50 Grams of Fructose:** This hefty dose of fructose is found in 4-5 medium apples or just 1 large soda

Good to Know: In the early 1900's, the average American fructose consumption was ~15 grams per day. Today it's easily 4-7 times that, mostly from quickly-absorbed, refined, concentrated, processed foods and beverages!

Primary Sources of Fructose

While many people associate fructose with fruit, most consumption of modern day fructose primarily comes from non-fruit sources:

1. **Table Sugar:** granulated, 50% fructose + 50% glucose, bound together to form the compound, *sucrose*
2. **High Fructose Corn Syrup:** liquid*, usually 55% fructose + 45% glucose, not bound together, just mixed

Other sources of fructose include: agave, honey, molasses, maple syrup, fruits, berries

*Liquid Nightmare: Naturally-occurring fructose in whole fruit is bound to fiber and other sugars. Digestive enzymes break apart these bonds and slowly release fructose into the system. By contrast, liquefied forms of fructose such as syrups, nectars and juices have unbound, free fructose that does not require the same enzymatic action – this fructose is instantly available and can easily overwhelm the liver.

> *Yes, from our long-term, huge studies in Singapore, Australia, the US and Europe, I think 100 percent fruit juice is as bad as sugar-sweetened beverages for its effects on our health.*
> ~Barry Popkin, PhD, author of The World is Fat

What, Exactly, is High Fructose Corn Syrup (HFCS)?

The word "fructose" in high-fructose corn syrup creates contradictory confusion:

- Fructose must be *healthy* because it's the sugar found in fruit
- Fructose must be *unhealthy* because it's in chemically-processed HFCS

There is no naturally-occurring fructose in regular corn syrup because corn is a grain, not a fruit – therefore, corn syrup is only glucose and not very sweet. To sweeten it, food scientists discovered a laboratory process to chemically convert some of the glucose into fructose. The resulting syrup is a blend of fructose and glucose.

The term "high fructose" relates only to corn, simply used to compare the fabricated, sweeter corn syrup to "regular" corn syrup. While some HFCS is no worse than table sugar with roughly the same concentration of fructose (50%), there are versions of HFCS that have much higher fructose concentrations.

Products that Typically Contain HCFS		
Liquids	**Sweets**	**Savory Items**
✓ Soft drinks	✓ Yogurt	✓ Condiments (BBQ, hot sauce,
✓ Sports/energy drinks	✓ Baked goods / desserts	ketchup, mayo, dressing)
✓ Fruit juice	✓ Canned fruit / applesauce	✓ Nut butters
✓ Flavored coffee creamer	✓ Granola / cereals	✓ Premade meals / fast food
✓ Sweet alcoholic mixers	✓ Nutrition bars	✓ Bread / crackers

Industrial Advantages of High Fructose Corn Syrup

HFCS consumption has increased by over 1000% since 1970! Our food supply is flooded with HFCS to such a degree that avoiding it is extremely difficult. For the food industry, it has been a miracle additive and is present in nearly every processed food due to the following advantages:

- **Improved Palatability** – enhances all flavors
- **Preservative** – extends shelf life
- **Lower Cost**– cheaper than other sweeteners, partly due to US government corn subsidies
- **Higher Solubility** – especially advantageous for sweetening liquids (sodas, condiments, creamers)

Marketing Magic: The Corn Refiners Association intentionally manipulates labeling of HFCS to confuse consumers. They petitioned the FDA to rename HFCS as *corn sugar*, which was denied. However, a corn syrup product comprised of 90% fructose is now legally labeled as plain *fructose* or *fructose syrup*.

Crystallized Fructose

Fructose is also available in crystallized form, sometimes touted as a 'safe' sugar alternative for diabetics and others seeking to control their carbs. Crystalline fructose has a low glycemic index and minimizes insulin surges (only glucose triggers insulin). However, this product is still fabricated from corn – it's essentially HFCS that has been further purified to 98-99% fructose. Though it doesn't contribute to spikes of blood glucose, crystalline fructose contributes to negative consequences of increased fructose load (keep reading).

Agave Nectar – Not a Sweet Deal

Though advertised as a natural sweetener, commercially-available agave products are nothing like traditionally-made agave nectar. Commercial agave is highly-processed with chemical enzymes, acids, resins and conditioners. Furthermore, the final product is devoid of nutrients, contains saponins (an antinutrient, read more on Day 8) and astonishingly, consists of 70-97% fructose!

> **Fun Fact:** Blue agave, the primary source of agave nectar, is an exotic yucca plant from Mexico that blooms only once in its lifetime. When fermented, the nectar becomes tequila.

Fructose Malabsorption

Some individuals are sensitive or intolerant to fructose digestion. This condition varies in intensity and is referred to as fructose malabsorption or sometimes irritable bowel syndrome (IBS). IBS is characterized by digestive interference in the small intestine that restricts the transport of fructose.

Ideally, fructose is absorbed within the small intestine. When its digestion is hindered, fructose travels to the colon where it disrupts gut flora and results in an assortment of symptoms including gas, belching, nausea, indigestion, bloating, constipation, diarrhea and abdominal pain or discomfort. This can be caused by an overly irritated gut, chronic inflammation or damage to the intestine from illness, infection or medication. Individuals with this condition may fare better on a special diet with reduced FODMAPs (discussed on Day 8).

> **Paleo Advantage:** By eliminating sugar and limiting fruit consumption, eating Paleo naturally reduces symptoms of fructose malabsorption. This smaller load of fructose is much easier to digest.

The Tipping Point – When Fructose Turns to Fat

The saying, "the dose makes the poison," fits perfectly here. Fructose metabolism changes significantly with *excess* calorie consumption when compared to calorie maintenance or calorie deficit. When total caloric intake is within reason, fructose is largely metabolized for energy production with minimal negative health consequences.

In a scenario of overeating, however, high dietary levels of fructose significantly increase triglyceride production. This encourages fat accumulation especially in vulnerable, health-compromising locations such as in the liver and around abdominal organs. Fructose contributes to fat production with other characteristics:

- Fructose disrupts appetite suppression signaling – no sense of feeling full leads to overeating
- Fructose stimulates the brain's sweet reward center – increases cravings for sugar

The point where fructose metabolism becomes detrimental is strongly dependent on individual circumstances: gender, athletic conditioning and health status (this metabolism also varies greatly between healthy individuals versus obese or diabetic).

> **Key Point:** When discussing fructose, a calorie is not a calorie. Fructose calories will be quickly directed to fat production *when total calories are in excess*.

Fructose-sweetened beverages like soft drinks and juice cause metabolic problems when calories are in excess, and studies have shown that people are not likely to compensate for the additional calories they get from such beverages. ~Chris Kresser MS, Lac, Unconventional Medicine, The Paleo Cure

Consequences of Excess Fructose + Excess Calorie Load	
✓ **Nonalcoholic Fatty Liver Disease** ✓ **Insulin Resistance** – leads to *obesity* and *type 2 diabetes* ✓ **Weight Gain**	✓ **High Blood Triglycerides** – including increased risk for *heart disease* ✓ **Uric Acid Production**, the culprit in *gout* ✓ **High Blood Pressure**

One way to direct fructose metabolism away from fat production is with exercise. Increasing the body's energy demands will naturally direct fructose conversion to glucose *for fuel* instead of fat *for storage* (more about Exercise on Day 10).

> **Good to Know:** Exercise is a powerful tool to prompt fructose metabolism in a healthy direction.

Minimize Detrimental Effects with a Paleo Diet

The negative consequences of fructose manifest with modern society's massive doses of fructose-laden foods, especially in conjunction with the following:

1. Unrestrained fructose consumption in one sitting (handfuls of dried fruit, sodas, juices)
2. A sudden influx of fructose, especially from liquefied forms (HFCS, agave nectar, fruit juice)
3. Uncontrolled total dietary calories, especially from carbohydrates

Those who follow a Paleo Diet rarely fall into any of those categories since the main source of fructose in a hunter-gatherer diet is fresh fruit.

Long-Term Fruit Recommendation

Source maters when it comes to fructose. *Whole, fresh* fruit is always a better source of fructose than concentrated or unbound sources. Tips to avoid the negative consequences of fructose:

➢ Discourage fructose metabolism from entering fat storage mode
- ✓ Eat a normal calorie load
- ✓ Limit *total* sugar consumption (remember table sugar is 50% fructose)
- ✓ Maintain a sensible exercise routine
➢ Most individuals can comfortably process 1-3 servings of *fresh* fruit per day
➢ Fruit juices and dried fruits typically contain high concentrations of fructose, as do agave syrup and honey. Consume these in moderation. After the program, *occasional* processed fruit or raw honey is fine as long as the rest of the diet and activity levels are within reason.

Further Information

- ⌐ ThePaleoMom Is Fructose a Key Player in the Rise of Chronic Health Problems?
- ⌐ MarksDailyApple The Definitive Guide to Sugar
- ⌐ ChrisKresser Will Eating a Paleo Diet Cause Gout?
- ✹ Ed.Ted Sugar Hiding in Plain Sight **(4 min video)**

To-Do List:

- ☐ Tomorrow is the deadline for chicken roasting
- ☐ Record today's values in the Healthy Baseline Chart
- ☐ What else (spend some time in nature, look up a recipe that uses whole fruit, reread a previous topic)?

Coming Up Soon:

- Do you eat offal? Day 23 highlights the benefits of nose-to-tail eating.
- Paleo is not the only diet based on traditional eating principles. Tomorrow we'll look at a few other ancestral approaches that may be useful in developing long-term strategies that work for you.

Day 23

People often say that motivation doesn't last. Well, neither does bathing - that's why we recommend it daily.
~Zig Ziglar

Today's Topics:
1. Paleo-Wise: Organ Meats
2. Incorporating Offal in the Diet
3. Long-Term Strategies: Building the Foundation

Fast Fare – Order Out
♥ Order bun-less burger w/bacon and extra tomato, onion and lettuce
♥ Side salad w/olive oil and vinegar

Recording Your Healthy Baseline

The most important step of reintroduction is awareness of how good your body feels following the Strict Paleo Protocol. Please record today's values in your Healthy Baseline Chart on page 344.

Did you eat more fruit today?   Yes   No

If yes, what was it and did you notice anything different about the taste after abstaining the past few weeks?

_____

By now you should have roasted a chicken, and for many people, that was the first time! Admittedly, it's more involved than picking up a rotisserie chicken on the way home (especially if you spatchcocked it), but the advantage is that you know what is going into your body. What were the best parts about roasting a chicken?

☐ Taste   ☐ Crispy chicken skin   ☐ Knowing the quality of the chicken
☐ Giblets   ☐ Having a new successful recipe   ☐ Knowing the exact spices and oils used
☐ Leftovers   ☐ Learned how to carve a chicken   ☐ Taking on an unfamiliar cooking project
☐ Bone broth   ☐ Easy way to feed a whole family ☐ Cheaper than boneless, skinless parts

Anything else good or bad (were you sad when the leftovers were gone)?

_____

Will you try this again in the future?   Yes   No

Section I – Paleo-Wise: Organ Meats

Nose-to-tail eating is not a bloodlust, testosterone-fueled offal hunt. It's common sense, and it's all good stuff.
~Fergus Henderson, chef, author of <u>The Whole Beast</u>

What is Offal?

Offal is the term given to the edible organs, entrails, miscellaneous trimmings and odd bits of a butchered animal. It essentially includes everything other than the muscle and bone. These cuts vary by region and cuisine and are also referred to as "variety meats," "organ meats" or the "fifth quarter" (the part left after a butcher divides an animal into four quarters).

Literally Offal: The term can be traced back to the words *off* + *fall* – imagine an animal prepared and hung for butchering. When the abdomen is sliced open, the innards "fall off" the carcass.

Traditional cultures never waste the gift of an animal sacrificed for food – every part is used, from bones to skin and nose to tail. This is a natural and nostalgic way of eating; it's the way people have eaten for centuries and continue to do so today in many international regions.

Examples of Offal				
• Liver	• Blood	• Cockscomb	• Gizzards	• Chicken feet
• Kidney	• Skin	• Intestines	• Testicles	• Sweetbreads (thymus/pancreas)
• Heart	• Lungs	• Bone marrow	• Tongue	• Pig feet (trotters)
• Brain	• Oxtail	• Spleen	• Pig ears	• Stomach (tripe, maws)

> **Fast Fact:** Bone broth is considered offal because of the use of bone marrow, tendons, skin and any other added organs such as the giblets!

Ounce per Ounce

Surprisingly, organ meats are some of the most nutritious foods on the planet. Because offal itself is organ and glandular tissue, these foods provide the exact nutrients needed to build and maintain our own organs and glands. These less familiar parts of the animal are literally nutritional life support.

Offal is a concentrated source of nearly every nutrient including unique vitamins, trace minerals, precursors to build DNA, antioxidants and quality proteins. *Plus,* all these nutrients exist in highly bioavailable forms.

Highly Nutrient-Dense Offal		
Fat-soluble vitamins: preformed and/or bioavailable versions of A, D, E and K (highest food sources for natural vitamin D)	**CoQ10:** essential for energy throughout the body but especially in the heart and liver	**Trace minerals:** chromium, copper, phosphorus, iodine, magnesium, selenium, zinc, calcium, potassium, manganese
B-complex vitamins: especially good source of B12 and choline	**Cholesterol:** a building block for our hormones and essential for arterial repair	**Omega-3 fats:** especially in wild-caught fish and pasture-raised animals
Iron: in its most bioavailable form	**Uncommon amino acids:** some offal contains hard-to-find glycine and proline	**Other:** an unidentified anti-fatigue nutrient and a bioavailable form of folate

How Did Offal Become Awful?

Some cultures shy away from incorporating offal, while other populations wouldn't dream of giving up favorite traditional meals (and even delicacies) made from the odd bits. Historically, organ meats were the most valued animal parts and saved for those with the highest societal status, which varied depending on the culture: elders, royalty, pregnant women, shamans, hunters, head of family, etc.

In just a few generations however, the narrative about organ meats in modern cultures has reversed:
1. Animal fats have supposedly become dangerous to health.
2. Steak and muscle meats (which historically were less valued than offal) are now extravagant foods while organ meats have morphed into cheap fillers for those with lower budgets.
3. Offal not used directly for human sustenance is earmarked for pet food, animal feed or fertilizer production, only solidifying the false premise that organ meats are not fit for human consumption.

Some people justify their aversion to offal in their diet based on false pretenses:

Awful Offal Myths	
Myth	**Truth**
Liver and kidneys filter the blood, so they must be chockfull of the toxins they remove.	These organs neutralize and expel toxins from the body; any non-excretable toxins are stored in the fat or nervous system tissue. Liver and kidneys *do not* directly store toxins – rather, they store the exact nutrients we need to neutralize toxins in our bodies.
Organ meats contain pre-formed vitamin A (retinol) which can be toxic in large amounts.	*Synthetic* vitamin A can be toxic in large amounts. However, natural sources of retinol do not pose a threat with the exceptions of polar bear liver, seal liver and dog liver – just go easy on those.
Organ meats cause gout.	Gout occurs when the kidneys cannot eliminate uric acid build up (usually from excess dietary fructose or disproportionate protein intake without enough fat). The vitamin A in organ meats protects the kidneys and supports the removal of uric acid.

Offal Cuisine – Eat on the Wild Side

Cooking with offal is frequently called "nose-to-tail eating" and refers to the practice of consuming as much of an animal as possible. For newcomers, this can be intimidating not only because the foodstuff is unfamiliar, but some offal flavors and textures are distinct and unlike any western fare. If this describes you, you are not alone.

Many westernized consumers exhibit a *yuck factor* when imagining organ meat consumption. Part of this is because the butchering process is removed from everyday life and prepackaged meats are the mainstay. Modern meat eaters have evolved into a "boneless, skinless, clueless" population when it comes to preparing anything other than pre-cut muscle meats.

However, remember offal foods are relished in other cultures. Fancy regional delicacies such as foie gras, pâté or terrines are designed to highlight the unique flavors and textures. Why not step out of the comfort zone?

Roasting a whole chicken is your gateway recipe for branching away from boneless, skinless or pre-ground meats. To start including offal, it is completely acceptable to begin with familiar items such as bone broth, liverwurst or quality sausage in natural casings before moving on to more exotic items. You may be pleasantly surprised to learn which offal products are easy to prepare or even some that may appeal to your taste buds.

> **Beef Tongue Taco Salad:** Tongue is an absolutely delicious meat. Boil it whole until cooked through. Then peel, chop and pan-fry until crispy. Mix with sautéed vegetables and taco seasonings. Serve on top of salad greens with salsa and guacamole. <u>Bonus</u>: Save the cooking liquid for the *very best ever* French onion soup base!

Offal on a Budget

It's easy to capitalize on others' squeamishness about offal: organ meat is more economical when compared to muscle meat (even offal from grass-fed animals with higher quality nutrition can be cheaper than conventional muscle meats). Not only do you get the healthiest parts of the animal, but you can save money doing it! Offal is a great way to include some pasture-raised animal products in your diet, especially for those on a tight budget.

Section II: Incorporating Offal in the Diet

For those who are new to nose-to-tail cooking, here are some simple ideas to overcome the initial apprehension of trying offal foods. As you become more familiar with the tastes and textures, there is no limit to the amazing, nutrient-dense meals you can prepare.

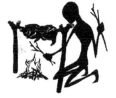

1. **Easiest Offal** – Shellfish such as clams, mussels, limpets or oysters are eaten whole, meaning all the internal organs are mixed right in - Bingo!
2. **Least Offensive Offal** – Bone broth, bone marrow, broth made from fish heads, sausage in natural casing, pork rinds, liverwurst, braunschweiger, foie gras or pâté
3. **Muscle Meat Offal** – Tongue, tail and heart are muscles, so their flavor and texture are closer to typical muscle meat and may appeal to an offal beginner
4. **Hidden Offal** – Most offal can be grated, ground or cut into small pieces to mix in with other ingredients making it less noticeable (meatballs, meatloaf, taco meat):
   - ThePaleoMom 50/50/50 Burgers
5. **Local Offal Foods** – Depending upon where you live, you may be able to find local offal dishes such as fried gizzards, liver and onions, menudo, chitterlings, blood sausage or rocky mountain oysters (though still beware of wheat or cornmeal breading and/or deep-fried versions)
6. **Reduce the Mineral Flavor** – Some organ meats have a strong metallic taste which can be reduced by soaking the organ in lemon water a few hours or overnight before cooking
7. **Seek Milder Cuts** – Some offal is strong-flavored or gamey (for example, beef or pork liver), this doesn't automatically mean other animals taste the same (chicken, calf, lamb and bison liver are milder)
8. **Use as a Supplement** – Try homemade liver pills, drink a liver shot or purchase a glandular supplement or desiccated liver capsule (more resources below)

Do not be too timid and squeamish about your actions. All life is an experiment. ~Ralph Waldo Emerson

Offal Resources

As you may suspect, sourcing matters. The best quality offal comes from pasture-raised and wild-caught animals, but do not discount factory-farmed organ meats. *All offal is incredibly nutritious* and can be included in your diet (direct links of the following are available from ⌐ Paleovation)

Recipes and Cookbooks
- ⌐ PhoenixHelix Link Love: Organ Meat Recipes
- ⌐ TheCuriousCoconut 100 Plus Ways to Eat More Organ Meats, Offal and Odd Bits
- 📖 *Beyond Bacon: Paleo Recipes that Respect the Whole Hog,* by Stacy Toth and Matthew McCarry
- 📖 *The Whole Beast: Nose to Tail Eating,* by Fergus Henderson [non-Paleo]
- 📖 *Odd Bits: How to Cook the Rest of the Animal,* by Jennifer McLagan [non-Paleo]

Need more Convincing?
- ⌐ WestonAPrice The Liver Files
- ⌐ MarksDailyApple It's Not so Offal
- ⌐ ThePaleoMom Tips and Tricks for Eating more Offal

Homemade Liver Supplements – If using raw liver, buy pasture-raised and freeze for 2 weeks before consuming (to kill pathogens). However, if your immune system is compromised, always cook the liver first.
- ⌐ RealFoodLiz The Raw Liver Smoothie Shot
- ⌐ PrimallyInspired Frozen Raw Liver Pills

Quality Organ Products
- ⌐ DrRons Organs and Glands
- ⌐ VitalProteins Beef Liver Capsules
- ⌐ EpicBar Beef Liver Bites
- ⌐ GrasslandBeef US Wellness Meats
  - Liverwurst containing liver, heart and kidney
  - Braunschweiger, dairy-free (one raw, one cooked)
  - Headcheese containing tongue and heart

"I Squeam, You Squeam, We All Squeam for Iced Spleen"

Overall, there is no need to squeam over offal. Maybe you already love it; perhaps you're willing to try it; or you definitely are not interested. Do what resonates for you, but also realize the dread about offal is cultural: if we had grown up eating and appreciating these foods, they wouldn't be unfamiliar. Regardless, it's okay to laugh at our cultural pretenses; offal does make for some interesting cooking (play along if you wish):

Your Secret Family Offal Recipe						
Your Initial (any one)			**Your Eye Color**		**Your Birth Month**	
A - Stewed	J - Grilled	S - Marinated	Amber – Goose		JAN - Livers	JUL - Tongue
B - Braised	K - Poached	T - Dehydrated	Hazel – Venison		FEB - Kidneys	AUG - Pancreas
C - Roasted	L - Stir Fried	U - Butterflied	Green – Lamb		MAR - Heart	SEPT - Feet
D - Minced	M - Leftover	V - Gelatinized	Brown – Bison		APR - Testicles	OCT - Spleen
E - Chopped	N - Fileted	W - Skewered	Blue – Pig		MAY - Eyeballs	NOV - Brains
F - Brined	O - Steamed	X - Barbequed	Black – Beef		JUN - Stomach	DEC - Tails
G - Raw	P - Curried	Y - Slow Cooker				
H - Pickled	Q - Sautéed	Z - Fermented				
I - Broiled	R - Tex Mex					

> *Do we really want to travel in hermetically sealed pope-mobiles through the rural provinces of France, Mexico and the Far East, eating only in Hard Rock Cafes and McDonalds? Or do we want to eat without fear, tearing into the local stew, the humble taqueria's mystery meat, the sincerely offered gift of a lightly grilled fish head? I know what I want. I want it all. I want to try everything once.*
> ~ Anthony Bourdain, Kitchen Confidential: Adventures in the Culinary Underbelly

What offal are you willing to try once? _____

Section III: Long-Term Strategies – Building the Foundation

> *The secret of change is to focus all your energy, **not** on fighting the old,*
> *but on building the new.* ~Socrates

After the reintroduction phase, you will evolve a diet that both maximizes health and fits into your personal lifestyle. The long-term guidelines are less strict, allowing more dietary freedom. However, please select foods responsibly – understand and acknowledge any personal tendencies that could sabotage your healthy baseline. Be creative about expanding foods and cuisine but rely primarily on nourishing foods that amplify health.

Because nurturing good health is a lifelong process, the following suggestions are offered to stimulate ongoing dietary refinement and help develop a personalized, lasting approach (dog-ear this page for future reference).

Ground Rules to Personalizing Your Long-term Plan

Ultimately, you know your dietary limits and weaknesses better than anyone else. Another person's successful dietary approach may not be the best option for you, especially if your willpower is tempted. Use the following ground rules as a guideline throughout dietary and lifestyle explorations (more details follow):

1. **Build a Solid Nutritional Base** by regularly consuming vegetables, animal proteins and healthy fats
2. **Acknowledge and Accept Your Personality Traits**, especially sugar/starch craving vulnerability
3. **Intentionally Modify and Revise Dietary Approaches, Patterns and Styles** via food variety, dining out strategies, varied adherence to the Paleo Protocol (Day 25), other ancestral eating patterns (more below), identifying carbohydrate craving triggers (Day 24), intermittent fasting (Day 27), etc.

Build a Dietary Base with Ancestral Eating Principles

Traditional diets from all over the world vary significantly in staple foods depending on climate and available resources. This natural diversity undeniably skews the ratios of carbohydrates, proteins and fats (each season often has its own proportions). Yet even with significant variance, all time-honored ancestral diets are incredibly nourishing and support the growth and development of the people from that region.

> *Nobody can go back and start a new beginning, but anyone can start today and make a new ending.* ~Unknown

Even though a nourishing healthy diet can be achieved in many ways, all traditional diets share several core principles. Use the following fundamentals as a base upon which to build, explore and expand your diet:

Traditional Diet Basics	
Principle	**Details**
Seasonal Produce	Utilize a large assortment of produce, especially local when available (emphasis on organic, grown in mineral-rich soil, not treated with harsh chemicals)
Humanely-Raised Animal Sources	Integrate a wide variety of animal-sourced foods from animals raised the way nature intended (eating their natural diet in a natural environment); incorporate nose-to-tail eating patterns by including bone broth, organ meats and odd bits
Balance of Raw and Cooked Foods	Consume both raw and cooked plant and animal sources (examples of raw animal foods: ceviche, pickled meats, sashimi, steak tartare, raw oysters)
Fermented Foods	Incorporate both plant and animal ferments such as sauerkraut, kombucha, apple cider vinegar with the mother, fish sauce (or grass-fed yogurt or cheese if dairy is tolerated)
Incorporate Bones	Cook meat *on the bones*, eat the bone marrow and use the bones again for bone broth
Exclude Processed Foods	Reject or strictly limit industrialized or highly-processed foods *and oils*

Beyond Paleo – Healthy Diet Variations in Modern Culture

The following nutritional platforms may be more *or* less successful for you than the Paleo Protocol. Each of these dietary philosophies offers valid strategies and tactics which may help narrow your search for an appropriate personalized diet. Basic details of these approaches can be found online.

Ancestral Dietary Explorations	
Diet and Description	**Who Benefits**
Low-Carb* or LCHF Diet* (Low Carb High Fat): Restrict carbs to <50g per day, might include full-fat dairy.	• Carb-sensitive individuals • Those interested in weight loss • Diabetics*
Ketogenic*: Restrict carbs to <30g daily; very high fat. We recommend Wahls Paleo Plus® for a carefully-crafted, nutrient-dense ketogenic template.	• Therapeutic diet for disorders including epilepsy, cancer, autism, Parkinson's, Alzheimer's, depression • Temporary diet for those needing to lose large amounts of weight
Bulletproof: Scientifically-backed, Paleo-esque program with further guidance for cooking techniques, fasting, supplementing, etc.	• Those interested in using their body as a science project; many trial-and-error approaches to find the best fit
FODMAP, SCD, GAPS, Low-Histamine: Each of these is a different approach to regulate foods to support gut function and boost digestibility.	• Those needing to heal leaky gut, build gut flora or improve digestion • Conditions such as ulcerative colitis, IBS, Crohn's Disease, autism
Perfect Health Diet: Includes higher ratio of carbohydrates from 'safe starches' such as white rice, taro or yucca.	• Individuals who use lots of energy such as athletes, children • Individuals with established insulin-sensitivity and fat-burning
Primal: Paleo plus some quality dairy.	• Those doing well on Paleo who are also dairy tolerant
Weston A. Price Foundation (WAPF): Emulates modern non-industrialized diets; includes raw dairy and traditionally-prepared grain.	• Those interested in incorporating other traditional foods
AIP (Auto-Immune Protocol): Further food restrictions to remove additional triggers such as eggs, nightshades, nuts and seeds.	• Anyone with an autoimmune condition not satisfied with their relief using a Paleo Protocol (details in the Resource Section)
Microbiome Diet: Incorporates specific foods and techniques to establish and maintain proper gut flora balance.	• Those interested in healing the gut, weight-loss, improving digestion or supporting gut health in general

*Diabetics must monitor blood ketone levels. Enlist the help of a licensed medical professional with knowledge of treating diabetics with low-carb or ketogenic diets to safely monitor the transition.

Refining Diet and Lifestyle Based on Personal Characteristics

Keep the following individual variances in mind while exploring your long-term diet development:

➢ **Metabolic Flexibility** – When fat-burning metabolism has been established (by eating Paleo), the body still easily burns carbohydrates and will preferentially switch to sugar-burning metabolism when sugar/starches are present. However, the body retains the memory of fat-burning to which it seamlessly reverts when glucose sources are depleted. Aim to preserve this flexible metabolism. The key is to not disrupt the underlying fat-burning action by consuming *too many* sugars/starches *too often.*

While this allows significant dietary freedom, the terms 'too many' and 'too often' are different for everybody. It's difficult to pinpoint when *your* unique body will lose metabolic flexibility and regress back to solely sugar-burning. In our experience, a single "off Paleo" day seldom impacts metabolic flexibility.

Even a couple consecutive "high starch" days can be manageable. Beyond that, cravings intensify and it becomes increasingly more difficult to *seamlessly* revert to fat-burning metabolism. Sensibly monitor hunger signals, energy levels, clothing fit, cravings, mood stability and other markers of health to indicate when carbohydrate consumption creeps beyond control.

> **Key Point:** Sugar-burning metabolism is easier than fat-burning metabolism, so the body preferentially stays in sugar-burning mode unless prompted to re-engage fat-burning by lack of sugar/starches in the diet. When the diet regularly includes higher amounts of sugars/starches, the body eventually 'forgets' how to switch on fat-burning mode (more about Fat-Burning in Prep G).

> ➢ **Carbohydrate/Starch Tolerance** – It is scientifically proven that carbohydrate tolerance varies between individuals for numerous reasons: ability to produce the enzyme *amylase* which breaks down starches, status of insulin sensitivity, types of carbs consumed, activity levels, current stress levels, tendency for addictive behaviors (including stress-eating), ongoing health conditions, etc.
>
> Some individuals are SO carb sensitive that just one higher starch meal starts an addictive binge that can last for days, weeks or even months: cravings erupt, hunger soars, willpower quickly fades! Others can regularly include one or two higher carb days per week without lingering consequences.
> Be careful! Until you *responsibly* test your personal carb sensitivity, there is no way to predict your ability to control starchy carb intake (more assistance determining Carb Sensitivity on Day 24).

> **Words of Wisdom:** In susceptible individuals, carbohydrate exposure can trigger heavy-duty cravings! These cravings can potentially start a downward, addictive spiral of incorporating perpetually more sugar and starch on a more frequent basis – eventually returning these individuals to exactly where they were before starting the program (read more about Identifying Triggers and Managing Cravings on Day 24).

> ➢ **Tendency for Addictive Eating** – Certain foods and beverages cause a release of dopamine, serotonin or endorphins; in susceptible individuals, consuming these items reinforces the brain's reward system. Take care in identifying personal triggers which may include grains, sweets, alcohol, dairy (especially cheese) or any item that is hyper-palatable for you. Though the Paleo Diet resets hormonal signaling to ease the cycle of food addiction, regular inclusion of a personally addictive food or beverage unravels that safeguard.
> ⏏ SaraGottfriedMD Food Addiction Part 1: The Science Behind the Syndrome

> ➢ **Digestive Sensitivity** – Dietary exploration revolves around *well-tolerated* foods (please do not regularly incorporate foods that trigger negative consequences). Some people need additional time to heal the gut and establish better digestive function. Several approaches highlighted in the Traditional Diet Basics Chart (previous) support gut health and gut flora balance by emphasizing well-cooked foods, low-allergy foods or prebiotic- and probiotic-rich foods. As healing progresses, more foods may be tolerated in the future.

What considerations do you personally need to address with your long-term lifestyle plan?

_____

_____

To-Do List:
- ☐ Record today's values in the Healthy Baseline Chart (page 344)
- ☐ What else (take a walk, make some spa water from Day 16, review the seasoning mixes on Day 2)?

Coming Up Soon:
- Tomorrow we discuss controversial foods (such as coffee) as well as review recipes so you're well-fed for the rest of the program and into the subsequent reintroduction phase.
- Managing carbohydrate cravings is critical to a successful long-term plan – tomorrow we'll give you a flowchart for determining how much of which carbs you can consume comfortably.

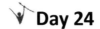

Day 24

> *Civilized man is the only animal clever enough to manufacture its own food...*
> *and the only animal stupid enough to eat it.* ~Barry Groves, PhD

Today's Topics:

1. Recipe Review
2. Paleo-Wise: Foods with Questions and Considerations (Coffee, Exogenous Ketones, GMOs)
3. Paleo-Wise: Wrap up
4. Long-Term Strategies: Managing Carbohydrate Cravings
5. Carbohydrate Tolerance Self-Test

Fast Fare – Incorporating Offal
♥ Liverwurst on cucumber slices
♥ Sautéed spinach + can of mushrooms

Recording Your Healthy Baseline

The most important step of reintroduction is to be aware of how good your body feels following a Strict Paleo Protocol. Please record today's values in your Healthy Baseline Chart on page 344.

Have you been incorporating more fruits?   Yes   No

If so, what did you notice about their flavor and texture? _____

Did anything surprise you with adding fruit back into your diet? Has it affected your digestion, mood, energy?

_____

Any other notes about today's food choices: _____

Section I: Recipe Review

Are you enjoying your current meals?   Yes   No   Have you fallen into a rut?   Yes   No

During food reintroductions, you will need to continue eating Paleo meals as you test reinstated food items. If you need some new inspiration, browse back through previously recommended recipes:

- Prep B: 28-Days of Paleo Meals
- Prep E: Quick Meal Ideas
- Prep F: Breakfast Ideas
- Day 1: 20-Minute Recipes
- Day 2: Snacks
- Day 5: Paleo Comfort Food
- Day 9: Lunchbox Template
- Day 10: Paleo Entertaining
- Day 13: Recipe Shake Up
- Day 16: Unsweetened Beverage Boredom

Which food and/or beverage recipes will keep you nourished and motivated as you approach reintroductions?

_____

Section II – Paleo-Wise: Foods with Questions and Considerations

Several foods, beverages and supplements create controversy when discussing whether they are part of a healthy diet. For the most part, tolerance will need to be determined by each individual, but do not include these particular items without a base understanding of why they can be problematic and how to reduce the odds of complications.

A. Coffee

Many studies have demonstrated significant health benefits from coffee consumption while others have shown coffee to be detrimental. Therein lays the confusion. There's no outright *good* or *bad* label for coffee – the reaction to coffee varies widely between individuals and is dependent on several factors starting with the type of coffee consumed.

Coffee Defined – Not a Sweet Deal

True coffee is black. However, contemporary coffee is often adulterated into clearly unhealthy concoctions that include copious amounts of sugar and processed additives. Typical ingredients include cream, powdered cream, sugar, artificial sweeteners, flavored syrups, whipped cream, even ice cream and sprinkles! As expected, sugar-laden milkshakes with a shot of espresso are *not* the coffees that offer health benefits.

Paleo Coffee Mixers: Coconut milk, nut milk, cinnamon, nutmeg, cocoa, vanilla, stevia (if sweetness is a must), honey or maple syrup (occasionally after the program) or even MCT oil and butter as in Bulletproof® coffee.

Coffee Pros and Cons

Most of the positive effects of coffee are attributed to coffee's antioxidants, polyphenols and bioactive compounds, some of which have insulin-sensitizing and anti-inflammatory properties. Other health benefits are directly attributable to caffeine – thus drinking caffeinated tea, likewise rich in antioxidants and polyphenols, is also associated with good health.

Benefits and Drawbacks of Coffee Consumption	
Pros	**Cons**
✓ High levels of antioxidants ✓ Improved brain function, cognitive performance and memory ✓ Increased metabolic rate ✓ Stimulates colon peristalsis (for efficient digestion) and reduces constipation ✓ Reduced risk of certain cancers (colon, prostate, liver), stroke, Parkinson's disease, Alzheimer's disease, cardiovascular disease, gout, gallstones and depression ✓ Improved workout performance ✓ Increased longevity – no matter the illness, coffee drinkers are less likely to die from it	✓ Caffeine can trigger the release of unhealthy levels of cortisol (especially when stressed) ✓ Tannins in coffee hinder iron absorption – can exacerbate iron deficiency ✓ Sleep disturbance ✓ Headaches ✓ Sluggishness (when the caffeine effect wears off) ✓ Irritates the tissues of the gastrointestinal tract and can exacerbate ulcers, IBS, gastritis or other gastrointestinal disorders ✓ Tends to be a diuretic – can be dehydrating (but less so with regular consumption) ✓ Dependency and withdrawal problems

Coffee Tolerance Considerations

In addition to the potential metabolic cons of coffee consumption, sometimes the coffee itself can be an irritant and hinder the body's ability to heal – in these cases it should obviously be avoided. This is true for people with hypersensitivity to any of the following: coffee, mold in the beans, caffeine or acidic foods. However, caution also applies to individuals who are enduring periods of significant stress, have adrenal fatigue or suffer from autoimmune disorders.

Tweaking any of the following factors can alter coffee tolerance:
- **Quantity** – How much is consumed in a day
- **Time of day** – Earlier in the day is best; sleep can be disrupted if consumed after noon
- **Quality** – Best if using filtered water and organic, mold-free beans
- **Intensity** – Caffeine content varies with preparation methods
- **How consumed** – Sometimes better tolerated with a meal versus on an empty stomach
- **Health considerations** – Generally not tolerated by those with autoimmune disorders, gallbladder problems, heartburn or in individuals who are slow caffeine metabolizers (effects are felt a long time)
- **Situational** – Not tolerated as well without proper sleep or during times of stress (increased cortisol)

Finding Quality Coffee

Coffee is susceptible to molding prior to roasting, thus, it's imperative to locate a quality source. Sometimes the symptoms of intolerance and drawbacks of coffee consumption arise from a poor-quality product.

To reap coffee's best benefits and reduce the chance it is contaminated with mold toxins or chemical residues, select *single-origin, organic beans* versus a 'blend.' When beans from multiple areas are blended, it increases the odds that some of the beans were not processed promptly and mold may have had an opportunity to grow. Additionally, artisanal coffee roasted in small batches is less prone to molding than large, mass-produced beans.

Doubting Decaf

Surprisingly, coffee's health-protective effects are not seen to the same extent with decaf. When selecting decaf coffee, a quality source is essential – higher risk of contaminants is a concern for the following reasons:

1. **Lack of Caffeine** – caffeine, in part, contributes to coffee's benefits but also protects against mold growth
2. **Decaffeination Process** – the most popular methods strip antioxidants and polyphenols but leave harmful residues of other substances (Swiss water process is the healthiest method to remove caffeine)
3. **Contaminated Beans** – most decaf is made with the lowest quality beans that were rejected for the caffeinated product; these beans often contain mold and toxins (regardless of the processing technique)

Bottom Line: How Much Coffee Can I Drink?

Short answer: it depends. For individuals with healthy digestive systems and stress response, two 8oz cups per day is reasonable. Some can handle more, some less. However, tolerance can change over time, especially with stress levels (coffee can compound cortisol's effects). And, just as with alcohol or bread, if you've never given up coffee, it may be worth a full elimination for 2-4 weeks to evaluate how your body feels without it (taper down to ease withdrawal symptoms if necessary).

> *I like coffee. It likes me back. I plan to keep drinking it.* ~Dave Asprey, founder of Bulletproof®

Further Reading

- ⌐ PaleoFlourish Is Coffee Paleo?
- ⌐ Bulletproof Benefits of Coffee: What Your Brain Does on Caffeine

B. Exogenous Ketones

Eating a lower sugar/starch diet stimulates generation of ketones for energy. Ketones are desirable because they encourage fat-burning metabolism and provide a reliable and steady source of energy. Additionally, ketones enhance efficient brain function, boost growth of neural connections and are the brain's preferred fuel.

Metabolic Benefits to Higher Blood Ketone Levels	
✓ Weight loss and muscle preservation	✓ Mental clarity and memory improvement
✓ Improved athletic performance	✓ Potential cancer prevention (cuts reliance on glucose)
✓ Anti-inflammatory effects	✓ Reduced insulin resistance

In addition to a lower-carb diet, higher ketone levels can also be produced by:

1. Fasting (more on Intermittent Fasting on Day 27)
2. Ingestion of MCT oils which are easily converted to ketones in the liver (more on MCT Oil on Day 2)
3. Supplementation with ketone salts, referred to as *exogenous ketones*

Note: Exogenous ketones tend to be used as an advanced supplement technique for specific athletic performance goals. However, some individuals are using these products daily as a method to boost ketone levels (or perhaps more likely, as an alternative to dietary change).

Not all Ketones are Created Equal

Exogenous ketones are those manufactured outside of the body (in supplement form), whereas *endogenous* ketones are the ones the body produces itself from ingested dietary fat or body fat stores. Both ketone forms provide alternative fuel for the body and brain.

Isolated Products Come with Risks

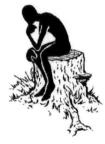

The above ketone benefits arise naturally when following a lower sugar/starch diet, but some individuals are prone to look for a shortcut. The controversial issue about *exogenous* ketones is not about the ketones but about the chemical structure in supplement form. Ketones themselves are harmless and only last a few hours in the system. However, in supplement form, some manufacturers include dangerously high quantities of minerals to stabilize ketones in the final product.

There are serious health risks with excessive potassium or calcium content – these can disrupt heart rhythms and increase the risk of cardiac death! Concerns about heart and kidney health compound if the products are taken frequently (which happens – some people take multiple doses because the effect only lasts a few hours).

> **Key Point:** If burning *body* fat is a goal, support your body's internal production of ketones with a lower sugar/starch Paleo Diet, HIIT exercise (Day 10) and intermittent fasting (Day 27).

Bottom Line: Is There a Place for Exogenous Ketone Supplements?

It depends on intention. A case can be made that exogenous ketones can effectively be used *occasionally as a tool* – perhaps as a boost to get back on track after dietary deviation, for a specific athletic performance goal or for improved mental clarity to complete an important task. However, do your research, find a product with safe mineral content, limit use and do not rely on supplements to provide ketones for your body – more fat will be burned when your body makes its own. As with all products, read labels and consult your healthcare provider.

- ᨏ Underlined <u>Undoctored</u> Beware Exogenous Ketones
- ᨏ <u>OptimizingNutrition</u> Are Exogenous Ketones Right for You?
- ᨏ <u>KetogenicSupplementReviews</u> Side Effects of the Ketogenic Diet: Are They Dangerous?

C. GMOs

Genetically-modified organisms (GMOs) are made by splicing genes from one organism into the DNA of a completely different species. This biochemical technique creates unique combinations of plant, animal, bacteria and virus genes that occur neither in nature nor through traditional crossbreeding or hybridization techniques. GMOs are brand new to the planet and unfamiliar to human digestive systems. Long-term implications have not been established; therefore, issues surrounding their safety are a source of ongoing debate.

GMO Purpose

The biotechnology industry introduced GMOs for a wide variety of applications:

Agriculture

- Create crops that are resistant to pests, diseases, temperatures, drought or herbicides
- Modify crops for vitamin enhancement (beta carotene in rice)
- Modify animal genetics for increased milk/egg production, disease resistance, higher meat proportions or modified growth hormones for faster maturation

Medicine

- Bacterial strains have been modified to produce medications (insulin was an early example)
- Vaccines are grown in modified chicken eggs
- GMO animals are used to grow transplant tissues and organs

Bioremediation

- Microorganisms used to remediate contaminated soil or water are modified to increase tolerance to temperature, pH and oxygen levels

GMO Risks

There are many unanswered questions and issues that arise and prevent full acceptance of GMOs. In the absence of credible independent long-term studies, the safety of GMOs is unknown.

- ✓ Potential problems if genetically-modified traits such as antibiotic resistance are unintentionally transferred to humans, livestock, wild animal populations, other crops or native plants
- ✓ Health concerns that human digestive bacteria may be vulnerable to modified traits (such as pesticide properties in GMO crops that could eradicate beneficial gut microbes)
- ✓ Chemical residues in foods due to higher pesticide and herbicide use on GMO crops
- ✓ Rise of super-weeds and super-bugs which require even more toxic herbicide/pesticide to control
- ✓ Mass destruction of non-target insect populations including bees and monarch butterflies
- ✓ Concern that GMO genes in farm-raised animals could be transferred to wild species (especially with fish)
- ✓ Offspring from GMO animals are less viable, risking extinction of both domestic and wild populations
- ✓ Ecological imbalances if previously non-invasive crops or animals grow out of control when modified

Labelling GMOs

To support transparency in food product labels, over sixty countries including European Union nations, Australia and Japan, require genetically-engineered foods to clearly be identified. In addition to that, there are over 300 regions worldwide that completely ban growing GMOs. Although labeling GMO foods is not mandatory in the US or Canada, GMOs are prohibited in organically-raised plant and animal products (organic label = GMO-free).

Common GMO Products	
Example	**Details**
Agricultural crops, including both food and textile	Soybean, corn, canola, sugar beets (table sugar), alfalfa, papaya, zucchini, yellow squash, cotton
Non-organic or non-wild animal products	Some have DNA modifications for growth; many are fed GMO feed: meats, dairy, eggs, honey, fish and seafood
Processed foods are infiltrated with GMO crop byproducts	Corn syrup, molasses, sucrose, hydrolyzed vegetable protein, textured vegetable protein, yeast products, flavorings, vitamins, enzymes, vegetable oils, fiber, etc

Effect on Farmers

Because genetically-engineered crops are entirely new life forms, the seeds can be patented to control use and distribution. Bioengineering companies that "own" GMO seeds can sue farmers if those seeds are found in unauthorized fields – this can happen if farmers collect and save seeds from a previous GMO harvest (to replant) or even if their non-GMO fields were contaminated as result of pollen drift from a neighboring farm. This raises issues over the cost and availability of seeds to farmers as well as long-term sustainability for small farms.

Bottom Line: Primary Concerns

There's a lot at stake for the big agriculture companies that develop these products so it's very difficult to find non-biased research regarding GMO safety. Long-term studies are not available because GMOs are a relatively new dietary and agricultural inclusion. Our main concerns fall into three categories:

1. When the plants are herbicide resistant, higher concentrations of chemicals can be used in those fields to control the weed population without harming the crop. This is not environmentally sustainable; additionally, higher concentrations of chemical residues will be present in the final product and the soil.
2. If plants produce a toxin that kills pests, what does it do in the human body? The ag companies report these products do not harm *humans*, but there are valid concerns regarding their effect on gut flora.
3. Because GMO crops are owned by the development company, farmers are no longer allowed to save seeds (it's technically stealing); therefore, new seeds must be purchased every year. Over time this creates giant monopolies controlling the food supply.

Steps to Limit Exposure to GMOs	
✓ **Eat Paleo**	Eliminates exposure to corn, soy, sugar and byproducts of GMO crops
✓ **Choose organic**	Foods are raised without GMO modifications in crops, animals or feed; especially relevant for meats & vegetables like zucchini, beets, yellow squash
✓ **Select wild animals**	Their DNA isn't modified, but they may forage in GMO corn or soybean fields
✓ ***Non-GMO Project* goods** ⇪ NonGMOProject	This third-party verification guarantees GMOs are only present in minimal amounts. The website contains info on the certification process, products that currently carry the label, their shopping app and GMO-free living tips.

Further Reading:

GMOs are a polarizing topic so it's challenging to find a non-biased source for GMO research. Try this:
⇪ Grist Panic-Free GMOs Series

No one will ever be more invested in your mental or physical health than you. ~Nora Gedgaudas

Section III – Paleo-Wise: WRAP UP

This is the last Paleo-Wise section of the program – the rest of the daily topics are dedicated to food reintroductions and long-term strategies. Now that the science side of the Paleo Diet and Lifestyle has been covered, take a moment to thumb back through the workbook. Notice how your thoughts about diet have changed throughout this program. If any of the Paleo-Wise topics continue to be difficult to absorb, please reread them and take time to research the further reading suggestions.

Paleo-Wise Sections Worth Reviewing	
Day 1 – Fat Fraud	**Day 11** – Stress and the Cortisol Response
Day 2 – Saturated Fats	**Day 12** – Calming the Cortisol Response
Day 3 – Polyunsaturated Fats (PUFAs)	**Day 13** – Importance of Sleep
Day 7 – Dairy and Calcium Sources	**Day 17** – Cholesterol
Day 10 – Movement and Chronic Cardio	**Day 18** – Heart Disease

Section IV: Managing Carbohydrate Cravings

This is major! Long term dietary success absolutely depends on understanding personal carbohydrate sensitivities, weaknesses and tendencies because sugar/carb cravings can quickly sabotage your efforts. It is necessary to test all sugars and carbs within a sensible framework – including Paleo-friendly sugars (fruits, honey, dates, maple syrup, molasses, etc) and starches (white potatoes). You *must* create a plan and develop strategies to manage your inner 'carb monster.'

Carb Control Strategies Review

Recollect the Sugar UNmerry-Go-Round from Prep F. The key to avoiding this perpetual cycle is to establish personal "too much" limits for sugar and starch.

Current health and metabolism levels factor into carb craving tendencies. Maintaining a Paleo dietary foundation undoubtedly helps to curb cravings; however, genetic, emotional and psychological factors come into play as well. For some, even small carbohydrate portions trigger long-range willpower battles. Maintaining a healthy lifestyle includes recognizing, minimizing, and sometimes avoiding, situations that challenge self-control.

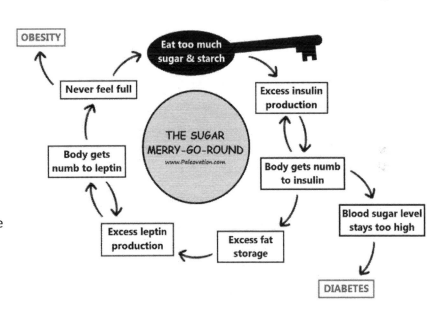

From past experience, how long does it take to regain control after sugar/starch overindulgence?

☐ Hours   ☐ Days   ☐ Weeks   ☐ Months   ☐ Years   ☐ Don't Know

It's up to you to strategically expand your diet by developing carb allowance rules. Step 1 is awareness of what may stimulate cravings. For you personally, what foods have typically triggered willpower battles in the past?

_____

_____

Food freedom means that when you fall off course, you don't let it ruin your day (or your week), physically or emotionally. It means you always have a plan for returning to a place of healthy balance, gracefully.
~Melissa Hartwig, Food Freedom Forever

Food reintroductions present an opportunity to consume higher-carb items (white rice, oatmeal, milk, hummus, refried beans, tortillas, bread, etc). Even while carefully following controlled food reintroductions, a highly carb-sensitive individual bears the potential risk that a single serving of a trigger food could cause diet management to spiral out of control. Each person must contemplate how to prepare for and survive an unintended ride on the Sugar UNmerry-Go-Round.

What non-Paleo food categories do you suspect may cause cravings or increased hunger for you?

☐ Whole grains   ☐ Refined grains   ☐ Dairy (cheese)   ☐ Sugar   ☐ More potatoes   ☐ Legumes

When trigger foods are encountered, you need a cravings plan. Good news: you already did this in Prep G! Go back and review your answers in Section IV on Managing Cravings and Creating a Distraction; write them here:

Craving Management Ideas	
Craving Strategies	**Activities to Create a 5-10 Minute Diversion**
1. _____	1. _____
2. _____	2. _____
3. _____	3. _____

Did these strategies work for you during the withdrawal and low-carb flu period?   Yes   No

Did you need to implement any of them after the initial sugar withdrawal period?   Yes   No

More Craving-Control Suggestions: Prep G details craving strategies, Prep E lays out low-carb flu relief tactics and Day 3 offers some Paleo crutches. All these suggestions are relevant to long-term dietary regulation. If carb cravings appear during reintroductions and/or intensify over time, what strategies will you employ to establish balance between indulging and regrouping?

☐ _____   ☐ _____
☐ _____   ☐ _____
☐ _____   ☐ _____

Carb Craving Supplements*
Just as a reminder, there are supplements that can help if cravings creep out of control (discussed in Prep G). Again, these are not required – they are just additional tools to assist with controlling carb cravings if desired. Read all product warnings for prescription drug interactions before purchasing.

✓ L-Glutamine   ✓ MCTs   ✓ 5-HTP   ✓ L-Tryptophan   ✓ Gymnema   ✓ Omega-3's

* All are available at ⌐ PureRXO.com/Paleovation – consider "CarbCrave Complex" for a comprehensive supplement

⌐ PrimalBody-PrimalMind Taming the Carb Craving Monster
⌐ BenGreenfieldFitness 12 Dietary Supplements That Massively Control Intense Carbohydrate Cravings

Section V: Carbohydrate Tolerance Self-Test

Tolerance to each specific carbohydrate source depends on 3 main factors:
1. Serving size
2. Combination with other high-carb foods during the day (overall glucose load can be a culprit)
3. Intensity of reaction, particularly worrisome if the carb triggers extreme willpower battles, additional splurging or an extended duration of uncomfortable cravings or hunger

Stress Mess – Cortisol and Cravings: Keep in mind that unmanaged stress can negatively affect carb tolerance levels (elevated cortisol by itself can stimulate sugar or starch cravings – read more on Day 11).

Use the flowchart below to create a conscientious inner dialogue to assess personal carbohydrate tolerance. You do not need to test foods that you already know create difficult-to-control consequences. Over time, this trial-and-error approach will categorize specific foods and amounts you personally can handle without lingering consequence. If cravings increase in intensity, frequency or duration at any time, use the strategies you outlined previously. Remember, a temporary lower-carb reset can be used to alleviate symptoms (forms are available in the Resource Section for up to a 14-day Strict Paleo reset).

Carb Tolerance Categories

Carbohydrate sources (both foods and beverages) can fall into any of the following tolerance categories. For susceptible individuals, both the Danger and Red Flag carbs can cause additional dietary digression.

- **Tolerated**: This food can be allowed *in that serving size or less* as long as cravings do not intensify or become unmanageable over time.
- **Conditional Tolerance:** This food can be included in that serving size or less on lower-carb days – may retest on a high-carb day to determine if it's truly tolerated.
- **Cautionary:** This food, eaten in that serving size or greater, challenges willpower and jeopardizes long-term dietary stability, especially when combined with other carbohydrate intake. Potentially retest a smaller amount on a low-carb day to better refine sensitivity and tolerance levels.
- **DANGER:** This food creates willpower battles and is detrimental to long-term dietary stability if eaten in that amount or greater. It's possible, but not necessary, to retest a smaller amount on a lower carb day to decide if this is a RED FLAG carb.
- **RED FLAG:** This food is hazardous to long-term craving control and dietary stability. List the pros/cons of eating this food and define the specific circumstances under which you would consider eating this again. It is best to completely avoid your RED FLAG foods.

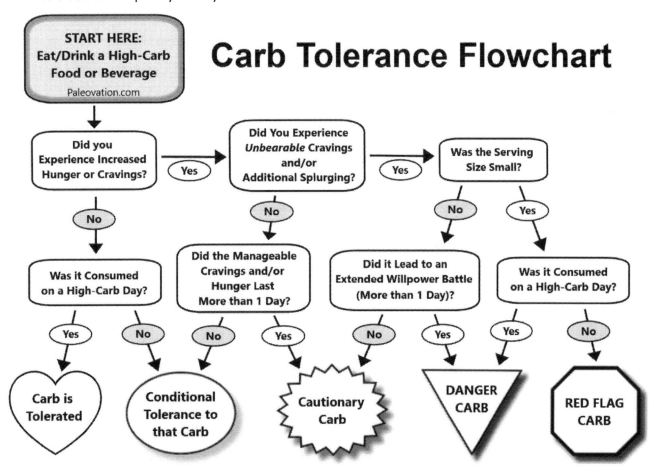

Regaining Dietary Control after Deviating

At some point, expect to stray a bit too far outside your personal tolerance zone. Long-term diet development is a trial-and-error process and note, *errors are to be expected*. Maybe it snuck up accidentally, maybe not. It doesn't matter. Use those incidents as learning experiences…but learn something from them! The first rule is to be gentle on yourself – there is no guilt involved while exploring your dietary boundaries.

> *Even a mistake may turn out to be the one thing necessary to a worthwhile achievement.* ~Henry Ford

1. **Do Not Beat Yourself Up** – Mishaps happen. It is not a failure unless you fail to learn from it.
2. **Review How the Lapse Started** – Was it gradual? Did it happen all at once? Examples:
   a. An unexpected stressful experience made it easy to rely on convenient carb-heavy meals.
   b. Sweets are abundant at work; now you eat them daily and want more when you get home.
   c. Over the holidays all diet rules were discarded and you feel back at square one.
3. **Formulate a *Comprehensive* Plan to Navigate These Scenarios in the Future:**
   a. Drink bone broth during stressful times to help unwind. Keep a list of your favorite Paleo comfort foods (Day 5), grab-and-go Paleo foods and fast recipe plans (Day 4). Always stock necessary ingredients (and/or leftovers) in the freezer, fridge and pantry.
   b. Keep Paleo snacks in your desk drawer and only allow one sweet treat at work per week. When you get home from work, immediately implement a destressing technique (cup of tea, workout to upbeat music, read a book, hot shower, etc). If a treat is still desirable after this, select a non-food reward (Day 15) or choose to make a single-serve treat from scratch (Day 28).
   c. Identify the worst offender(s) of the experience (example: holiday cookies or eggnog) then choose a suitable limitation – next time only allow gluten-free desserts or low-carb alcoholic beverages (alcohol options discussed on Day 26).
4. **Get Back on Track to Fat-Burning** – Sometimes you may need to reinstate the Strict Paleo Protocol for a reset (forms are available in the Resource Section for up to a 14-day reset). Other times it's sufficient to use the tools learned throughout this program:

   ✓ **Fasting** (Day 27)   ✓ **Destress** (Day 12)   ✓**Exercise** (Day 10)   ✓**Sleep** (Day 13)   ✓ **MCTs** (Day 2)

To-Do List:
- ☐ Record today's values in the Healthy Baseline Chart on page 344
- ☐ Research a fresh recipe for this final week, either from the recipe compilations posted in Section I today or review the cooking assignment ideas: Bone broth (Prep F), Mayo (Day 4), Veggie as a Grain (Day 7), Jerky or Granola (Day 11) or Roast a Chicken (Day 15)
- ☐ What else (review common Paleo adjustments on Day 14 or the non-sedentary action plan Day 9)?

_____

Coming Up Soon:
- Tomorrow we look at "Markers of Health" that develop with a healthy lifestyle. These traits help establish a point of good health and identify when you're ready for food reintroductions.
- Days 26 maps the reintroduction process, including common pitfalls to avoid.

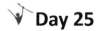 Day 25

Knowing yourself is the beginning of all wisdom. ~Aristotle

Today's Topics:
1. Food Reintroduction – Are You Ready?
2. Tweaking the Paleo Protocol
3. Long-Term Strategies: Author's Personal Approaches

Four days left of the Strict Paleo Protocol – what is keeping you on track?

Fast Fare – Finger Foods
♥ Coconut flakes
♥ Roasted pumpkin seeds
♥ Raspberries
♥ Pork Rinds

Recording Your Healthy Baseline
The most important step of long-term success is to be aware of how good your body feels while all the inflammatory foods are eliminated. Please record today's values in your Healthy Baseline Chart on page 344.

Section I: Food Reintroduction – Are You Ready?

Reintroducing some foods after your health has improved can be a big boost to quality of life for many people.
~Sarah Ballantyne, PhD, The Paleo Approach, Paleo Principles

Why Reintroduce Inflammatory Foods?
Most people feel amazing following a Strict Paleo Protocol and frankly, this is a healthy diet to enjoy indefinitely. Realistically though, it's *extremely stressful* to sustain 100% compliance 100% of the time. And as explained in the Cortisol topic (Day 11), extended stress of any kind (even with good intent) sabotages health.

Surprisingly, despite the full mental focus and discipline required to complete four weeks of strict Paleo, overall stress levels *decrease* due to the drastic *reduction of digestive stress* with the absence of inflammatory foods. In the next phase, strict compliance is eased to develop a manageable, *stress-free*, long-term maintenance plan.

> **Paleo Point:** The reintroduction process shapes a *safe foods list* to define *your personal* dietary boundaries.

The goal of the strict Paleo elimination phase is to establish a benchmark level of great health by adhering to defined rules. Once you know what 'feeling good' feels like, it's much easier to recognize which foods are tolerated well and which foods elicit a moderate reaction. Additionally, if any major negative reactions are experienced, that provides a clear motive to permanently avoid those offending foods.

Maintenance Mode = *Mostly-Paleo-Most-of-the-Time*
The long-term Paleo template is completely individual; no two maintenance modes look alike. What works for one person may be stressful to another. There's no pressure to be perfectly Paleo – it's okay to include some non-Paleo foods *as long as general wellness does not suffer*. Eventually a dietary pattern evolves that is primarily Paleo yet includes other well-tolerated foods.

Paleo Adherence: The 80/20 Rule or 90-90 Option
The following suggested templates are different approaches but result in the same amount of Paleo adherence:
1. **The 80/20 Rule:** Eat strict Paleo 80% of the time with 20% wiggle room. For example, 20% could be 2-4 non-Paleo meals per week (depending on how many meals are normally eaten). Or, an 80/20 individual may eat perfectly Paleo at home but order whatever they want at a restaurant once or twice a week.
2. **The 90-90 Option:** Eat 90% Paleo, 90% of the time. This person builds each meal with Paleo staples but typically includes a small (no more than 10%) portion of non-Paleo foods. A 90-90 person may prepare steak and veggie stir fry but include a small side of rice, quinoa, soy sauce or a Paleo-friendly dessert.
3. **Self-study:** Individualize it. It's okay to create your own template based on schedule, eating habits, preferences or health concerns. For example, a diabetic might adhere to primarily low-carb Paleo meals but include full-fat dairy. Another individual might fast every breakfast, eat salad bar lunch then enjoy a cocktail with a hearty Paleo dinner. You get to choose the most effective approach for your lifestyle.

> *Start by doing what's necessary; then do what's possible – and suddenly you are doing the impossible.*
> ~St. Francis of Assisi

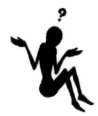

Are You Ready for Reintroduction?

Being 'addicted' to feeling wonderful is the foundation for food tolerance comparison, so achieving this blissful point is required before proceeding with food reintroductions. The eagerness and anticipation of eating restricted foods makes it tempting to skip this important self-evaluation step, but please take a moment to reflect. Be honest!

- ➤ Is your current level of health amazing to you?
- ➤ Are you satisfied with your progress?
- ➤ Have you been true to the Strict Paleo Protocol rules?
- ➤ Is there more room for improvement?

Check off the following health achievements you have already attained to help determine 'reintroduction readiness' or whether you could benefit from extending the program 2 more weeks:

Markers for Optimal Health	
☐ Excitement about your body's potential	☐ Clear skin
☐ Over the worst of the low-carb flu	☐ Stable energy levels
☐ Sound sleep	☐ Enjoying being active
☐ Noticeable relief of aches/pains	☐ Improved exercise recovery
☐ Increased range of motion	☐ Healthier food relationship (ex: no stress-eating)
☐ Comfortable stool consistency & frequency	☐ Mind/Body/Spirit feel balanced
☐ Improved digestion	☐ Improved ability to cope with stress
☐ Headache relief	☐ Better libido
☐ Hunger/cravings controlled	☐ Improved concentration and focus
☐ Better hormonal balance	☐ Mood stabilization
☐ Increased brain function	☐ Fat-adapted status

1. How do you feel about your current level of health? _____
   _____

2. What is your best improvement so far? _____

3. Are there any issues that are slow to improve or not improving at all? _____
   _____

4. Including today, you have 4 days left of the Strict Paleo Protocol. Do you suspect these final days will solidify any remaining, unchecked Markers of Optimal Health?   Yes   No   Maybe

5. Paleo crutches, described on Day 3, are designed to assist with compliance to the Paleo Protocol but extend the attainment of optimal health to a somewhat longer timeframe. Expect the best benefits to emerge after crutches are completely removed. How often did you use a crutch during the program?

   ☐ None   ☐ Seldom   ☐ Moderate   ☐ Frequent   ☐ Still using a crutch

6. During food reintroductions, you will be comparing how 'old' foods feel in your new body. Answer these questions to determine if your current body/health status is ready to test those old foods:

   a. If you employed dietary crutches, will you need more time on the Strict Paleo Protocol after Day 28:

      With crutches?   Yes   No   Maybe   *Without* crutches?   Yes   No   Maybe

   b. Have you seen improvement in your most-wanted health results (listed in Prep C)?   Yes   Not yet

   c. Are you satisfied and comfortable with your progress and current health status?   Yes   Not yet

   d. Are you well on your way toward your healthiest body?   Yes   No   Explain: _____
      _____

Section II: Tweaking Your Paleo Protocol

Food is information, not a math equation. ~JJ Virgin, <u>The Virgin Diet</u>

Each body equalizes at its own rate. If 28 days of Strict Paleo Protocol has not brought the expected returns, extend the program another 14 days.

Do you suspect you'll need an extension to reap more benefits?   Yes   No   Maybe

Tips for Improving Results

Whether or not you plan an extension, read through the following adaptations that can make the Strict Paleo Protocol more productive. Consider incorporating some of these in your final days and/or long-term plan.

1. Remove or reduce all dietary crutches (discussed on Day 3)
2. Add supplements such as probiotics or digestive enzymes to support a leaky gut (see other supplement suggestions in the Resource Section)
3. Implement other digestion strategies discussed in Healthy Bowel Habits (Day 8)
4. Consume more nutrient-dense and anti-inflammatory powerhouses:
   ➢ Bone broth
   ➢ Liver and other organ meats (Day 23)...but if you cannot stomach it:
      ● Cut raw or cooked liver into tiny pieces and freeze – swallow 5-10 pill-style daily
      ● Purchase a high quality desiccated liver pill or glandular supplement
   ➢ Ginger and turmeric (curcumin) – fresh or ground, mixed in foods, made into a tea, in a capsule, etc
   ➢ More fatty fish or an EPA/DHA supplement (Day 3)
   ➢ Gelatin or collagen (Days 6 and 16)
5. Incorporate more healthy sleep recommendations (Day 13)
6. Review stress topics – elevated cortisol is *extremely counterproductive* to overall health (Days 11 and 12)
7. Eliminate eggs for the next 2-3 weeks (some programs eliminate eggs from the start)
8. Remove dairy proteins by eliminating butter (even grass-fed) or switching to ghee or clarified butter

---

How to Clarify Butter: Gently melt grass-fed butter in a saucepan – do NOT stir. Some white particles (milk proteins) will separate and float to the top, others sink to the bottom. Skim off the top ones with a spoon. When the rest have settled, carefully pour the yellow butter oil into a container, discarding all particles. This is clarified butter. For ghee, let the bottom particles toast a while before pouring off the golden liquid.

Extending the Strict Paleo Protocol

If continuing with a 2-week extension, please use the included 14-Day Extension Log and Food Diary charts in the Resource Section to document how your meals satisfy the Veggie + Protein + Fat template. At the end of the additional time, reassess your Markers of Optimal Health in the previous chart to determine your next step:

A. **Begin Food Reintroductions** – if you are satisfied with your health improvements
B. **Try the Autoimmune Protocol (AIP)** – if health complications have not reduced to a comfortable level

Should I Skip the Extension and Just Start the AIP (Autoimmune Protocol) Now?

The AIP is more rigid than the Strict Paleo Protocol so it tends to be a dietary discipline that is approached in phases. Those with known autoimmune conditions are welcome to begin the AIP at any point. For others with borderline symptoms, continue the Strict Paleo Protocol and monitor the following for the next two weeks:

Continued Health Complications		
Fatigue	Inability to lose weight	Memory issues
Muscle weakness	Yeast infections	Allergies
Low immune system	Bowel issues	Rashes
Swollen glands	Anxiety/depression	PMS
Poor sleep	Migraines	Thyroid problems
Low blood sugar	Absence of any of the optimal health markers listed above	

The more issues persisting after the extension, the better you may respond following the stricter AIP Guidelines detailed in the Resource Section. Additional online information:

- 🖰 ThePaleoMom The Autoimmune Protocol
- 🖰 ThePaleoMom You May Have an Autoimmune Disease but Don't Know It

> **Healthy Baseline:** We want you to feel exceptional before you reintroduce any foods...this is the only way you can compare potential reactions to how good you *know you feel* without those foods.

This is your *opportunity to develop a personalized optimal diet!*

Reintro Limbo

Reintroduction guidelines, detailed tomorrow, are carefully designed to prevent an old favorite non-Paleo food (like pizza's barrage of wheat + cheese) from sabotaging the hard work you've already completed.

Most *single* food items are safe to add – except for those containing gluten (wheat, barley, rye). Gluten attaches to the intestinal lining and interferes with symptom assessment from *any* foods reintroduced afterwards. If you want to assess gluten tolerance (you don't have to), make it your *final* reintroduction.

At this point, which foods are you missing the most?

1. _____
2. _____
3. _____

Which foods do you suspect had negative impacts on your body prior to this program?

1. _____
2. _____
3. _____

Name two foods that you think might be the gentlest first reintroductions for your body:

1. _____
2. _____

Are there any foods that you do not miss and would just as well not reintroduce anytime soon?

1. _____
2. _____

> **Rachel's Story:** After being vegetarian for 10+ years, I hesitated to reintroduce legumes for two reasons: I did not miss them and I felt they led to my initial health decline. It was nearly 1½ years after beginning Paleo that I slowly started testing chili beans, hummus and peanut butter and realized I tolerate them quite well. The extra elimination period could have facilitated thorough healing, so I did not mind that time without legumes in my diet.
>
> **Kelly's Story:** Early in my Paleo journey, I was at a grocer getting frustrated reading labels of refrigerated almond and coconut milks – all contained additives, including carrageenan. Due to time limitations, I simply grabbed organic half & half since I wasn't obviously sensitive to dairy. After including dairy cream in my tea the next 3 days, I woke on day 4 with notable edema, especially around my eyes and fingers. I learned that I tolerate a single exposure to cream but not on consecutive days.

Section III: Authors' Personal Long-Term Lifestyle Strategies

Each individual will develop personalized long-term lifestyle strategies to maintain an overall anti-inflammatory diet and good health. Through the remainder of the program, we highlight multiple ways to find balance between expanding lifestyle horizons while still upholding the pillars of health: diet, exercise, stress-reduction and sleep. As examples, we've listed some of our personal strategies and mindsets that keep us on track while following a Paleo Template. Honor what works for you but change it when necessary.

Authors' Long-Term Diet and Lifestyle Strategies		
We both estimate ~80% compliance with the Paleo Diet		
Topic	**Kelly**	**Rachel**
Healthy Food	• Always have "grab-&-go" veggies available – my favorite is red peppers which I eat like an apple. It's also easy to fill those with quick tuna salad. • Accept the fact that I'll be eating more often with a fork (finger foods typically involve bread, grains and/or they're fried in inflammatory oils). • Use coconut milk in tea or coffee. • Crunchy snacks are pork rinds or sunflower seeds in the shell instead of chips or popcorn. • Enjoy a high fruit day periodically • I use only coconut or avocado oils for cooking (occasional sesame oil for flavor) • I buy precut veggies (often from a salad bar) for coleslaw, stir-fries or large salad • I always cook enough for leftovers to last another day or two. • No grains with my meals at home; I'll *occasionally* indulge in *limited* grains when eating out.	• Learn to cook well: Our meals at home are often more delicious (and way more nutritious) than ordering at a restaurant. When my kids help with cooking they are more likely to eat healthy foods. • Avoid bread: I eat bread a handful of times per year. Gluten-free products are relatively expensive, so those are occasional. • Strictly monitor foods that contain canola oil: By staying cognizant and limiting just canola oil I can cut out a horde of processed foods (chips, crackers, hummus, pre-made foods). It doesn't mean I never eat them, I just watch how often. • Avoid foods that do not bring pleasure: pasta, donuts, milk chocolate, sweetened drinks, anything with FD&C Red #40. It's not to deprive myself, I just lost my taste for them and I'd rather save my indulgence for ice cream. • Properly prepare grains: We occasionally include white rice, steel cut oats and organic grits. Before cooking, I rinse and soak grains (sometimes overnight) to reduce phytates.
Sweet/Starch Cravings	• When sweet cravings hit, I buy or make single servings (search 'Paleo Mug Cake') • Chew gum until craving subsides • 80+% dark chocolate • Stevia-sweetened soda • Make cocoa tea with coconut milk and stevia (tastes like hot chocolate!)	• Know my carb triggers: If I choose to eat tortilla chips, I know I'll pay with ~3 days of *intense* carb cravings. Popcorn or grits (even though they are corn-based) do not provoke the same consequence. • I keep chocolate on hand: I often have 70+% dark chocolate in my fridge (for emergencies).
Indulgence Days	• Personal rule: 1 day of non-Paleo indulgence is fine; 2 consecutive days OK; I'm careful not to go 3 consecutive days as that will incite cravings and symptoms • Allow *limited* deviation from strict Paleo a couple times per week (but not in a row). My weakness: chocolate! • Eat clean a couple days before and after a known 'off-Paleo' day (like holidays or social gatherings)	• Give myself permission to indulge (especially high-quality foods): Grass-fed cheese, ice cream, dark chocolate, Paleo baked good like cookie or muffin, wine, potato chips cooked in coconut oil. As long as I don't go overboard, my body tolerates these very well and I really enjoy eating them. • Bake freezable Paleo treats for kids: Keep them in the school's freezer so they have something special for celebrations at school.

Topic	Kelly	Rachel
Lower Calorie Days (Intermittent fasting)	• Skip breakfast – only use coconut milk in tea or coffee • Eat soup to feel more full • Make stir fry with loads of veggies • Drink more tea through the day • Remind myself how good I feel after a day of restricted calories!	• Skip a meal: I often skip breakfast, I drink coffee, tea or bone broth until lunch. • Bone broth: I don't do it often enough, but every time I drink a mug I'm surprised by how nourished I feel. • Limit starch servings: If I have a grain, it's a small serving…much less than pre-Paleo
Long Term Diet Management	• No up-sizing my clothes! (I rarely get on a scale). When my pants get tight, I reduce higher calorie foods for a week. • Occasionally keep a food journal to force accountability (🖑 MyFitnessPal). • Partake in a project/craft that keeps my hands busy (like writing this book!) • Intermittent fasting – I regularly skip breakfast 2-3 days per week. • Known fact: If it's in my house, I'll eat it. When grocery shopping, I won't put tempting foods in my cart, especially if I recently indulged. • To 'allow' for extra indulgence, I'll partake in and extended exercise activity. My favorite is a long bike ride followed by an alcoholic beverage or ice cream.	• Keep junk out of the house: If my family eats super clean at home it gives us more freedom to eat worry-free at special occasions and outings. • Keep health on track with random resets: Commit to one alcohol-free month each year. Use a random 7-21 day strict Paleo reset when I stray too far. • Beware of which strategies work for me: I used to do a weekly 36-hour fast and even though I felt great afterward I realized I highly disliked missing family dinner. So I changed my strategy to several skipped meals during the week. • Reduce sugar in baking: By rule, when I bake a treat I use 2/3rds of the sugar called for without sacrificing flavor. If chocolate chips are part of the recipe (I like Enjoy Life® mini-chips) I can easily cut the sugar in half and let the chocolate carry the recipe.
Exercise	• Exercise 4-5x/week, rotating between weights and cardio. • Weight workouts I alternate between push and pull muscle groups • Interval setting when on cardio machine • listening to my favorite music during exercise augments my stress relief.	• Work out in a fasted state: I usually get my workout done in the morning. • Tailor the workout to my needs: Rotate between different styles of yoga depending on my energy levels (total of 2-5 classes/week). • Get daily exercise: Even if I don't work out I incorporate some form of movement daily.
Social Strategies	• Bring something Paleo-friendly: shrimp cocktail, deviled eggs, grain-free salad • As an alcohol alternative, I'll drink sparkling water with lime. • When at bar, I order plain wings (sauce on side) and choose hard cider instead of beer to limit gluten exposure.	• Request "half the pumps" for a flavored coffee: Periodically I enjoy a café mocha. I ask for half the syrup to get the chocolate flavor without over-the-top sweetness. • Skip the extra glass of wine: Have a cup of tea instead, but sometimes I take the wine. • Bring Paleo food: Offer to bring a dish to pass.
Travel	• I try to stay low carb when traveling; in mixed company or at someone's home, I'll allow some dietary latitude • I plan for travel dietary deviations by being stricter before and after travelling	• Fast on travel days: If there isn't good food available (especially at airports), I stick to beverages.

Topic	Kelly	Rachel
Sleep	• Excess sugar will trigger insomnia • If sleep is slipping, I'll take a power nap • A very dark room is a must • *Occasional* sleep aids: melatonin, magnesium supplement or Epsom salt bath (caution is required: for me, these often trigger 'rebound insomnia' in the middle of the night)	• Prioritize sleep: I'm almost always *asleep* by 10pm. • Sleep environment: I follow many of the sleep suggestions and recently added a red lightbulb to my bedside lamp, I love it! • If I develop insomnia in the wee hours (1-3am), it's my cue to cut back on wine to reset my sleep.
Stress Management	• Listen to upbeat music • Participate in upbeat music (I play trombone with UW Alumni Band and a local college jazz band) • Exercise – go to the gym, bike ride • Read a book • Take a nap • Take a bath, sauna or whirlpool • Laugh!	• Manage stress-levels: My personal dietary tolerance is highly correlated with stress. If a period of high stress is unavoidable, I must rein in my diet or I become puffy, moody & unwell. • Monitor my mood when fasting: Sometimes fasts become overly stressful for me so I give myself permission to stop early. • Yoga: I practice yoga every day, even if it's just a breathing or mindfulness exercise.
Attitude	• I consciously focus on positive things. • Gratitude – I especially try to be thankful for what I have rather than focusing on negatives of what I'm lacking. • I try to laugh every day • Smile!!! • I choose not to hold anger, resentment, or other negative emotions as I've learned that will make me sick. • I don't ask "why me" questions. I consciously rephrase questions surrounding difficult circumstances to "what" or "how" questions: "What do I need to learn?" "How do I proceed?" • By allowing some Paleo deviations, I remain happy and stress-free...and harbor no dietary guilt. Cheers to that!	• Keep an open mind: Because I research diet and lifestyle modifications to improve health, I find fascinating reasons to make peculiar changes (chicken feet broth, cricket flour, eating offal, meditating, occasional sprinting, fasting, handstands, etc). I'll just try it – some strategies have served me well. • Give up the quest of being perfect: I've learned to comfortably stray throughout my entire lifestyle. I buy organic cleaners but use Cascade in my dishwasher. I am healthy but don't need to fit into a certain pant size to be happy. I prioritize some organic produce (apples, lettuce) but still buy others conventional. I don't eat full Paleo but incorporate principles from many ancestral diets. I used to CrossFit, but I really like yoga better. Sometimes, I order fish & chips (gasp!).

Practice, Practice, Practice

Many of these lifestyle hacks are unique to our individual bodies and circumstances. We've learned to notice subtle physical and functional disruptions as biofeedback and modify accordingly. Please realize that self-centric knowledge takes time, like putting a puzzle together. Be curious. Experiment. Observe. It's a natural progression.

To-Do List:

☐ Record your Healthy Baseline Chart values for today (page 344)
☐ Anything else (review bowel support on Day 8 or sleep strategies on Days 13, stock up veggies)?

Coming Up Soon:

• Tomorrow specifically outlines the reintroduction process including food suggestions, tips, how to recognize a negative reaction and common pitfalls
• Day 27 details how to adjust your long-term, healthy lifestyle plan for periods of plateau

Day 26

Today's Topics:

1. Food Reintroduction Guidelines
2. List of Food Groups to Reintroduce
3. Additional Considerations

Fast Fare – Canned Seafood
♥ Salmon cakes fried in coconut oil
♥ Cabbage leaf wrap
♥ Mini bell peppers

Recording your Healthy Baseline and Favorite Paleo Foods

The most important step of reintroduction is to be aware of how good your body feels following a Strict Paleo Protocol. Please record today's values in your Healthy Baseline Chart on page 344.

Favorite Recipes from the Program:

Meal (Prep B): _____   Breakfast (Prep F): _____

Snack (Day 2): _____   Paleo Substitute (Day 6): _____

Lunch (Day 9): _____   Entertaining Idea (Day 10): _____

Section I: Food Reintroduction Guidelines

The Paleo Protocol is a well-balanced diet and safe to follow long-term. It is NOT required to reintroduce any of the restricted foods. Remember, these non-Paleo foods are technically "less healthy" than Paleo choices so they should never displace nutrient-dense foods like vegetables, meats, fish and seafood, traditional fats, whole fruits or nuts.

> *They say you should know your limits and work within them. But how can you really know your limits unless you try to expand them?* ~Jonathan Cainer

Realistically, most individuals are curious about their tolerance levels. Before you test any of the following foods, please reread the information on why these were eliminated in the first place (chapter references are provided). Each food topic contains tips to improve digestibility and further reading resources.

Reintroduction Precautions

- You are determining food intolerances, not allergies. Do NOT reintroduce known allergens.
- If you are sick, stressed or otherwise unwell, postpone reintroduction until you are feeling your best (return to the Strict Paleo Protocol to reduce digestive stress and give your body a rest).
- If an immediate negative response occurs (vomiting, stomach cramps) promptly discontinue that food.

Steps for Reintroduction: 4-Day Cycle (or if completely symptom-free, 3-day cycle)

Some food reaction symptoms may not manifest for several days; therefore, you need a full 4-day cycle to test and observe each reintroduced food. Some experts shorten the cycle to 3 days *but only if you're feeling exceptionally well*. Reintroduction can start with any food group that interests you *except* gluten-containing grains. Save gluten for last – it takes considerably longer to return to a healthy baseline after gluten exposure.

1. **Day 1:** Choose a food to reintroduce. Consume that food several times throughout the day.
2. **Days 2, 3 (and 4):** Return to the Strict Paleo Protocol to avoid any other stimuli.
3. Record all meals, snacks and symptoms of the cycle in the Reintroduction Diary (Resource Section).
4. After the 3rd day, review your notes to determine how well that food is tolerated. If not certain after 3 days, be sure to add a 4th day for further observations.
5. If experiencing symptoms, continue the Strict Paleo Protocol until you feel better. *Only when you've returned to your healthy baseline*, start a fresh food to reintroduce.

> **Take Notes, Take your Time!** The reintroduction process requires diligence, but upon completion, you will know exactly which foods are vitalizing for you and which foods compromise your health.

The Key: Do Not Rush Food Reintroduction!

This is your personal experiment. Do not sabotage the hard work of this program by reintroducing too many foods too quickly...if a negative reaction occurs after multiple foods are hastily or haphazardly reintroduced, there is no way to identify the specific trigger.

- ✓ Do NOT combine multiple food categories
- ✓ Carefully monitor your health and *write it down* in the Reintroduction Diary
- ✓ Do NOT add sugar to any of the reintroductions (sugar alone could trigger a response)
- ✓ If you have no interest in reintroducing a certain group, skip it and move on
- ✓ After a negative reaction, restrict your diet; consider reintroducing again later for a 'second opinion'
- ✓ Pizza is a loaded weapon comprised of too many potential triggers: cheese, grains, gluten and chemicals. We recommend first reintroducing these foods individually to test tolerance. Fortunately, there are combinations of dairy-free, grain-free or gluten-free frozen pizza versions available.

> **Example of a Poor Food Reintroduction:** An individual reintroduces yogurt on Day 1 and feels great, so the following day they try rice. Later that evening, terrible diarrhea develops and immediately the rice is blamed (forgetting about the yogurt eaten the day before). However, it is entirely possible that the yogurt, not the rice, triggered the reaction.

Common Reactions During Reintroduction

Trigger foods can affect any aspect of wellness: the body, mind, spirit, emotions, energy, attitude. If something doesn't feel right, make note in your Reintroduction Diary. Even if the connection is not immediately clear, a trend may develop over time.

Common Negative Reactions During Reintroduction		
Digestion	**Appetite**	**Sleep**
Nausea	Unexplained hunger	Insomnia
Vomiting	Cravings develop	Excessive sleepiness or fatigue
Acid reflux / heartburn	**Skin**	Snoring
Stomach cramping	Mouth ulcers / canker sores	**Energy**
Bloating / gas	Skin rashes	Racing heartbeat
Changes in stool consistency	Itchy skin	Buzzing energy
Changes in stool frequency	Acne, blemishes	**Focus**
Musculoskeletal	Face flush	Difficulty concentrating
Muscle pain	Crusty eyes, corners of mouth	Memory issues
Inflamed joints / joint aches	**Edema**	**Mood**
Stiff body	Sinus change – stuffy, drippy, etc.	Anxiety
Old injury flares up	Fluid retention	Depression / loss of happiness
Headache	Puffiness	Cranky / irritable / short temper

Food "Tolerance" is Subjective

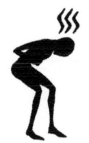

Depending on the person, a small zit may be intolerable but two hours of intense stomach cramping may be worth the indulgence! Only *you* can choose the comfort level of a food reaction.

> **Beware:** It's easy to disregard a food reaction. A particular food might cause tiredness, yet that symptom could be blamed on interrupted sleep, a difficult work project or a strenuous workout. For now, assume the tiredness is a reaction to the reinstated food. This is especially important to prevent justifying a negative reaction from an old favorite food by blaming symptoms on something else.

Can I Reintroduce any Faster? You have the option to test foods individually or within a related group:

1. **Individual Item Reintroduction:** Choose a single food to reintroduce several times during the day. For example, eat plain yogurt for breakfast, yogurt dressing on a lunch salad, beef curry with yogurt sauce at dinner and unsweetened yogurt/berries blended (consider frozen version) for dessert.
2. **Reintroduction by Group:** Choose multiple related foods to eat throughout the day. For the dairy group, try yogurt at breakfast, add cheese at lunch and cream of broccoli soup (made with real cream) later in the day. If you experience a negative reaction during a group reintroduction:
    1. Return to the Strict Paleo Protocol to recover your healthy baseline
    2. Separate the individual items to identify which caused the reaction (in this example yogurt, cheese, cream) and dedicate a full 4-day independent cycle for each food
    3. You can do these consecutively or return to the troublesome group at a later date

> *It took me about eight years to put together the program that I have been living for twenty years.*
> ~Marilu Henner, Total Health Makeover

Words of Wisdom: Be Aware of Tolerance Fluctuations

Just because adding a food now causes a reaction doesn't mean it'll stay that way forever. Our bodies are constantly changing; stress levels are constantly changing; life is constantly changing. If you experience a negative reaction to a food, put it on hold and consider reintroducing again at a later date. When you give your digestion and gut flora further time to restore, tolerance can improve.

Regardless of tolerance, there may be certain foods that are best to avoid long-term, gluten for example *(and, there's no point in ever adding processed junk food back into your diet!)*.

1. One or two successful exposures does not guarantee a food is completely 'safe'
    a. A reaction may develop if the food is consumed on several consecutive days
    b. Leaky gut, hormonal disruption and inflammation creep up over time (that is how they got there in the first place!); pay attention to developing symptoms
2. Tolerance levels vary over time
    a. Increased healing of the digestive tract and gut flora improves tolerance
    b. Experiencing a stressful event, trauma or illness decreases tolerance
    c. Hormonal fluctuations can affect tolerance either way
3. Some foods are *insulinogenic* (dairy products) or *carbohydrate-rich* (grains and legumes). These affect both insulin and blood glucose levels, so carefully consider how much to include in your daily lifestyle.
4. The mind can influence tolerance levels. Expecting that a food will make you sick can actually make you sick (like a placebo effect). Therefore, reintroduce foods with a calm mindset to instill 'rest-and-digest.'

Sugar Seduction: Do not be seduced by an old favorite sweet food; *taste it again for the first time*. Notice that frosting might have the mouthfeel of sweetened vegetable shortening; donuts might be insanely sweet or too greasy; soda may taste metallic and syrupy. If you recognize a new dislike to a sweetened food, please...stop eating it. Otherwise you risk becoming numb to the sweetness, requiring continually higher amounts of sugar to satisfy cravings and the brain's sweet-reward system.

Section II: List of Food Groups to Reintroduce

The following list of foods can be reintroduced in any order (with the exception of gluten-containing grains – save those for last, if at all). Begin with whichever food you've been craving the most while on the Strict Paleo Protocol!

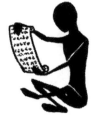

A. Dairy (Day 7)
B. Non-Gluten Grains / Pseudo-Cereals (Prep D and E)
C. Legumes (Day 8)
D. Concentrated Natural Sweeteners (Prep C and F, Day 22)
E. Gluten-Containing Grains (Prep E)

A. Dairy (Day 7)

Dairy contains lactose, casein and whey – any of which can provoke a reaction (most commonly lactose). **Always choose *full-fat dairy*, preferably grass-fed (pasture-raised) plus organic or raw if available.**

- **Lactose**: The milk sugar found in most dairy products, highest concentrations in milk, buttermilk
- **Casein**: A protein in moderate- to high-protein dairy products like cheese, yogurt, kefir, low-fat milk
- **Whey**: Another milk protein, high concentrations in ricotta/cottage cheeses, whey protein powder

Reintro Example: Paleo granola with milk in morning, sour cream on a salad for lunch and cheese in the evening. Do NOT introduce ice cream to determine dairy sensitivities due to the high sugar content.

Special Dairy Considerations:

- Adding a probiotic during dairy introduction assists with digestion
- Fermented dairy products such as yogurt and kefir may be tolerated better than other dairy
- If cow dairy elicits symptoms, try goat, sheep, yak or camel products which are more digestible
- For athletes interested in testing tolerance to whey protein powders, select quality sources from grass-fed, pastured cows that are *cold-processed* without added chemicals. More information:
    - ⟡ MarksDailyApple Whey Protein
        - o Quality sources include: ⟡ Bulletproof Upgraded Whey
            - ⟡ Opportuniteas Grass-fed Whey
- To determine if a dairy reaction is from the lactose, casein or whey:
    - ⟡ MarksDailyApple Dairy Intolerance: What It Is and How to Determine if You Have It

B. Non-Gluten Grains and Pseudo-Cereals (seeds that act like grains) (Prep D and E)

There are no nutrients in grains that cannot easily be obtained through Paleo-eating. These grains are not a replacement for Paleo foods but can be added to an otherwise well-balanced meal. Surprisingly, white rice is generally well-tolerated because the bran/husk has been removed. Soaking, sprouting, fermenting, pounding, mashing and roasting will reduce plant toxins and improve digestibility.

In This Category: white rice, brown rice, wild rice, oats/oatmeal, corn (non-GMO preferred), polenta, corn nuts, grits, buckwheat, amaranth, millet, quinoa, sorghum, teff, chia

Reintro Example: Omelet with side of oatmeal at breakfast, corn tortilla tacos for lunch, rice noodles with shrimp stir fry for dinner and gluten-free crackers with bacon guacamole for snack.

C. Legumes (Day 8)

All beans contain phytic acid which can be reduced with proper preparation. If you are healthy, without digestive issues and willing to properly prepare beans, 1-2 servings per week are unlikely to cause issues.

In This Category: beans (any kind), black-eyed peas, chickpeas (garbanzo), edamame/soy (non-GMO preferred), lentils, green peas, peanuts or natural peanut butter (organic preferred), refried beans, tofu and other organic soy products (tempeh, soy sauce, soy lecithin, soy nuts, etc)

Reintro Example: Tofu stir fry with gluten-free soy sauce for breakfast, lentil salad for lunch, celery with natural peanut butter or hummus for snack and ham and bean soup for dinner.

D. Concentrated Natural Sweeteners (Prep C and F, Day 22)

Be particularly conscientious with this reintroduction because *sugar is sugar*. Even natural sugars significantly alter the gut flora and disrupt the insulin-leptin balance. Yes, some natural sweeteners are higher in nutrients than processed sugar, but not enough to make a significant contribution to diet, improve health or justify overindulgence.

In This Category: coconut sugar, maple syrup, molasses, evaporated cane juice, raw honey, date sugar, date paste, stevia, dextrose, dried fruit

Reintro Examples: Honey in your tea/coffee, chicken with molasses barbecue sauce at lunch, Paleo cookie sweetened with coconut sugar for snack and maple syrup sweet potatoes at dinner.

> **Paleo Advantage:** After completing a month of sugar elimination with the Paleo Protocol, you will discover that not nearly as much sugar is necessary to satisfy your sweet tooth!

E. Gluten-Containing Grains – Save for Your Last Reintroduction, if at all (Prep E)

We repeat, save for last! Gluten takes significant time to clear from the system (ranging anywhere from 3 weeks to 6 months!). Remember, it's sticky like glue and attaches to the inside of the intestines. Some people find that fermented products such as sourdough or ancient grains such as einkorn, red fife, triticale, kamut, spelt and emmer are easier to digest. Others just cannot consume gluten at all.

> **In This Category**: wheat (bulgur, durum, semolina), barley and rye. Gluten-containing foods include bread, bagels, muffins, baked goods, pasta, couscous, pizza, pretzels, crackers, breaded foods, beer, tabbouleh, pie crust, bleu cheese (gluten is often present in the mold), soy sauce, malt vinegar, licorice, foods fried at a restaurant unless they have a dedicated gluten-free fryer, etc
>
> <u>Reintro Example</u>: Bagel for breakfast, sourdough sandwich at lunch, pretzel snack and pasta dinner.

Section III: Additional Considerations

Accidental Overindulgence

Take care to consume non-Paleo food in normal portion sizes. It doesn't matter how healthy someone is, an entire pound of cheese or box of gluten-free pasta will definitely disrupt hormonal balance, upset the digestive system and cause an inflammatory response. The reintroduction process is designed to uncover what foods can be repeatedly included in the long-term diet, not determine what foods can be overeaten.

> <u>Note</u>: If overeating does happen, observe how uncomfortable your body feels. Sometimes triggering an extreme reaction is all that's necessary to avoid overindulging in those foods again.

Beware of Industrial Oils (Days 3 and 4)

We do *not* recommend ever reintroducing industrial PUFA oils restricted during the program. Oils such as canola, corn, vegetable, soybean, safflower, sunflower, cottonseed, grapeseed, etc, are undeniably detrimental to health. They are highly vulnerable to rancidity, inherently contain trans fats as a byproduct of industrial processing and produce even more toxic compounds when heated (*plus* the body incorporates these damaged molecules into cells!). Continue to use traditional Paleo fats.

Dark Chocolate

If you choose to consume chocolate, varieties with the lowest sugar and highest cocoa content are preferred. Read ingredient labels – select chocolate that has at least 70% cocoa and does not contain soy-lecithin.

> *My soul's had enough chicken soup...now it wants dark chocolate!* ~Anonymous

Alcohol

If you suffer from serious health issues or if weight loss is a goal, it's not recommended to include any form of alcohol in your diet. Alcohol causes dehydration and electrolyte imbalances and it's a toxin that can lead to liver damage and more dangerous health diseases. Addiction is a very real concern that has further health and social implications.

Yet, alcohol can be a relaxing and enjoyable luxury when consumed *in moderation* and, realistically, there are many opportunities to partake. Because Paleo is a lifestyle to be molded into a maintainable long-term template, the following information is provided to assist in making the best choices when considering alcohol options. Each body is different so pay attention to how various alcohols make you react.

> **Good to Know:** The distillation methods to produce hard liquor remove all traces of gluten from sourced grains. However, those with celiac disease must still be cautious. The final product may contain traces of gluten due to either poor facility practices that introduce cross-contamination or the inclusion of gluten-containing colorings and flavorings added after distillation. ⌐ Celiac Gluten-Free Alcoholic Beverages

The following strategies can limit health complications of alcohol; organic options are always preferred:

1. Drink with a meal *and* early in the evening to avoid sleep interruption.
2. Most alcohol products are very high in carbohydrates; select dry and unsweetened varieties.
3. White wine is generally better tolerated than red.
4. Clear, distilled spirits (no flavors or coloring) are also better tolerated, including tequila, gin, vodka.
5. Hard ciders are gluten-free but do contain sugar; select a dry version to lower the carbohydrate load.
6. Beer is not gluten-free. Most gluten-free beers are sorghum-based and don't necessarily taste like beer. Omission® beer out of Oregon makes a great-tasting beer then removes gluten after brewing (this "gluten-removed" beer is okay for gluten-sensitive individuals, but caution is advised for celiac disease).
7. Be wary of mixers which contain all sorts of sweeteners and additives.

Further Reading:
- Bulletproof Alcohol Infographic and Hangover Cures
- PaleoGirlsKitchen Paleo Drinking Cheat Sheet

Alcohol Source Chart
Made from Fruit
• **Red Wine** – Fermented grapes; skin provides tannins (dry taste) and resveratrol (antioxidant)
• **White Wine** – Fermented grapes, skin is removed
• **Champagne** – Fermented grapes; fermented a second time by adding yeast and sugar
• **Brandy** – Distilled wine (careful of caramel coloring)
• **Cognac** – A more specific type of brandy; distilled wine
• **Hard Cider** – Fermented apples, sometimes other fruit is added; yeast may also be added
Grain-Free Sources
• **Tequila** – Distilled from the agave plant
• **Rum** – Distilled from fermented sugarcane or molasses
Brand Dependent
• **Vodka** – Distilled potatoes, grains or sometimes fruits and/or sugar
• **Hard Soda (very high sugar)** – Fermented vanilla, ginger or other extract; may include barley
Made from Gluten-Free Grains
• **Sake** – Japanese rice wine; fermented rice (careful of added barley)
• **Sorghum Beer** – Fermented sorghum
Made from Gluten-Containing Grains
• **Beer** – Fermented wheat, barley and hops with yeast
• **Whiskey** – Distilled fermented grain mash, including barley, rye, wheat and corn
• **Bourbon** – More specific type of whiskey. Distilled from primarily corn, but also wheat, rye and barley
• **Scotch** – More specific type of whiskey; distilled from primarily barley, but also wheat and rye
• **Gin** – Distilled from grain mash including barley, corn, wheat, infused with extracts

A Low-Stress Masterplan

Make it a priority to cultivate a low-stress version of your long-term Paleo Template. It's understandable to be cautious during reintroductions to preserve the heathy baseline and monitor carb cravings, but meet these challenges with a positive mindset. Negative judgments or constant fretting over minor dietary deviations simply magnify stress and are counterproductive to realizing the extent of your compatible foods. Loosen the Paleo reigns reasonably and nourish your entire body with gratitude, joy and worry-free eating.

> **Power of Positive Thinking:** Positive affirmations can soothe reintroduction worries. Examples include: My body is healing. My digestive system is healthy. My choices support my health. The food I reintroduce nourishes my body. I am knowledgeable about lifestyle strategies. I am adept in managing my long-term plan.

Further Reading:
- ✍ <u>BalancedBites</u> My Nutrition Challenge Is Over…Now What?
- ✍ <u>RealFoodWithDana</u> Whole30 Reintroduction Tips & Mistakes
- ✍ <u>EmpoweredSustenance</u> 3 Ways to Successfully Re-Introduce Foods after Elimination Diets

---

Paleo Bag-of-Tricks: After finishing this program, a shorter 7- to 21-day Paleo Reset can be done any time. Many individuals recommit to the Strict Paleo Protocol a couple times per year to keep tabs on health. Subsequent resets rarely compare to the intensity of the initial transition yet the results are just as valuable. Forms for up to a 14-day Paleo reset are available in the Resource Section.

To-Do List:
- ☐ Record today's values in your Healthy Baseline Chart page 344
- ☐ Anything else to stay strong as you finish the program (revisit stress relief strategies on Day 12, choose your first reintroduction and reread the section on why it was eliminated during the program, roast some bacon as described in Prep E)?

_____

Coming Up Soon:
- Tomorrow explores weight-loss and fat-burning strategies to preserve and build upon your new habits
- Day 28 begins the "check-out" procedure to evaluate your health and compare it with your responses during the preparation days

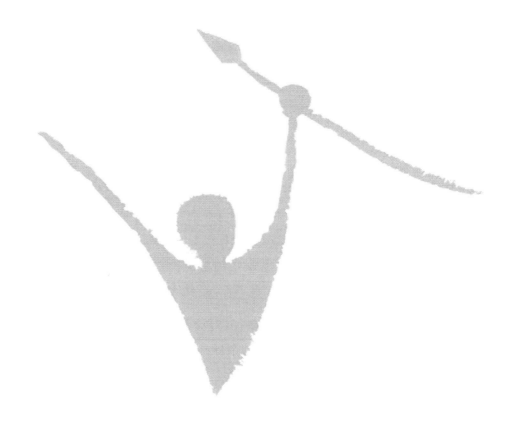

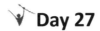 **Day 27**

People are under the illusion this is a journey of perfection. It is not. Paleo is about changing our relationship with failure. ~Dean Dwyer, <u>Make Shift Happen</u>

Today's Topics:
1. Weight-Loss Plateau
2. Intermittent Fasting
3. Long-Term Strategies: Planning a Getaway

Fast Fare – Use Paleo Mayo
♥ Tuna salad in cucumber boat
♥ Pistachios
♥ Seaweed Snax

Which Paleo habits will help you maintain a healthy diet long-term?

☐ Vegetables covering half the plate
☐ Cooking with traditional, healthy fats
☐ Using the Veggie + Protein + Fat template
☐ Eating a wide variety of colorful foods

☐ Keeping a list of Paleo go-to recipes
☐ Having fresh cut veggies on hand
☐ Avoid PUFA oils like canola or soybean
☐ Sourcing quality animal products

What else? _____

Record your Healthy Baseline

The most important step of reintroduction is to be aware of how good your body feels following the Strict Paleo Protocol. Please record today's values in your Healthy Baseline Chart on page 344.

Section I: Weight-Loss Plateau

Dietary change has the power to revive the entire body. Yet sometimes despite careful attention to diet, progress slows or stops (whether in terms of weight-loss or health-gain). It takes time for the body to fine-tune after dietary change. Do not be surprised by a plateau period. Until the body is acclimated to the new 'normal,' it may temporarily resist progress, needing a gentle nudge to continue growing healthier.

Weight Loss Plateau – Don't Focus on the Scale

Weight loss certainly is a motivating factor to adopt dietary and lifestyle modifications. However, now is not the time to focus on the scale. Although losing weight is a welcomed side effect of the Paleo Diet, the primary focus is truly on nourishing the body and improving health.

The scale simply shows a snippet of what is happening in the body, measuring only the pull of gravity on all the bones, fat, muscles, fluids and organs. It does not measure health *or* success *or* lean body mass *or* self-worth.

Body Composition

The Paleo Diet naturally encourages fat-burning metabolism which results in *size loss*, not necessarily weight loss. The scale doesn't determine how you'll look – your size and weight are determined by your body composition, particularly the percent of muscle versus body fat. Two people may weigh the exact same but a highly athletic person with a high percentage of muscle can be several sizes smaller than a sedentary person who has a high percentage of fat (more on Day 10).

MUSCLE versus FAT: A Space Case
Focus on Size Loss, Not Weight Loss: We discussed "Muscle weighs more than fat" details on Day 10. Visualize these parameters:

- **Volume** – a 1 x 1 x 1 foot cube filled with muscle will, indeed, weigh more than the same cube filled with fat
- **Weight** – a 20-lb bag filled with fat will be almost three times larger than a 20-lb bag filled with muscle:

Muscle takes up 1/3rd the space of fat!

Muscle is dense, active tissue that burns more energy than fat and is the foundation of a leaner, stronger and more energetic physique. If you're going to weigh a certain amount, isn't it preferable to be made of compact muscle rather than jiggly fat?

Don't be distracted by the number on the scale, especially when health is improving. Resistance to weight loss while in fat-burning mode may indicate cells are absorbing more nutrients, bones are growing denser, muscle mass is increasing, tendons or joint padding are thickening, or many other subtle improvements.

> **Better Ways to Track Progress:** use body metrics and health quiz questions (Prep C), before and after photos, Markers of Health (Day 25), a progress journal or the old-fashioned How-Do-Your-Clothes-Fit-and-Feel method

Section II: Intermittent Fasting

Historically, the next meal was never guaranteed. Since the beginning of time, people have gone hungry now and then. The human body has evolved to flourish with irregularity and randomness, not predictability. Unfortunately, modern culture is obsessed with eating regularly which puts the body in a state of auto-pilot.

Intermittent fasting (IF) is a dietary pattern that cycles between periods of eating and not-eating, capitalizing on the body's responsiveness to randomness. *Short* phases of not-eating (including sleep time) have powerful positive effects on health, including fat loss and even increased longevity.

Amazing Health Benefits of Intermittent Fasting:
- **Weight Loss** – Stored body fat becomes more accessible. Additionally, the body selectively burns fat while preserving muscle.
- **Improved Insulin Response** – The body does not release much insulin during a fast. This lull recalibrates insulin sensitivity and protects against type 2 diabetes (more on Insulin in Prep F).
- **Reduced Inflammation** – The free radical damage within cells decreases during a fast; therefore, markers of inflammation decline (more on Inflammation in Prep A).
- **Improved Brain Health – Fasting** reduces inflammation within the neural pathways, promotes mental clarity **and** boosts a protein in the brain that activates growth of new nerve cells, thus protecting **brain** cells from changes associated with Alzheimer's and Parkinson's disease.
- **Anti-Aging Effects** – The body removes or regenerates damaged structures to maintain quality and conserve energy, thereby preserving youthful cells and extending cell lifespan (more below).
- **Reinforced Fat-Burning Metabolism** – The more frequently the body must burn fat for fuel, the easier it is to switch back and forth between sugar *or* fat burning metabolism for energy needs.
- **Lowered Blood Triglycerides** – Triglycerides are periodically burned for fuel which improves cholesterol profiles and lowers cardiac disease risk factors.
- **Other Notable Benefits** – Ability to influence gene expression, regulate hormones throughout the body, initiate the body's repair and rebuilding mechanisms, raise human growth hormone (HGH), give the digestive system a chance to reset, boost the immune system, etc.

Anti-Aging Autophagy
For survival purposes, our bodies will naturally preserve energy and nutrients when food intake is irregular or scarce. It does this by scanning the body for damaged or aging cells via a revitalizing process called *autophagy*.

1. **Repair Existing Cells:** Certain cells are identified for restoration. Because it takes less energy to repair a cell than to create a new one, this procedure conserves energy.
2. **Remove Inefficient Cells:** Damaged cells are selected for removal. The body then recycles vital nutrients from these cells for other body needs, providing nourishment.

Food irregularity stimulates this revitalizing process to clear aging cells and preserve youthful, efficient cells. Unfortunately, the three-meals-per-day pattern of modern cultures puts the body into a state of predictable food consumption where it anticipates and relies on consistent nutrient intake. Because survival risk has been eliminated, the need to conserve energy goes dormant and the body stops scanning for damaged cells. The unpredictability of intermittent fasting is a way to encourage and keep the anti-aging autophagy process active.

> **Key Point:** Unless the body's preferred pattern of unpredictable food intake is intentionally replicated (by intermittent fasting), there is little reason for the body to remove old, weakened tissue and salvage useful nutrients. Old cells will be left intact, contributing to premature aging.

Calorie Restriction is 'Natural'
Fasting has been prevalent throughout evolution…sometimes because food was not available, other times as spiritual practice. Even just a century ago, there were no supermarkets, refrigerators or easy access to food year-round – the unpredictability of meal frequency and portion size was naturally maintained. Fasting from time to time is actually more 'natural' than regularly eating three square meals per day with snacks between!

Intermittent fasting is not about extreme or extended calorie restriction – it's more about varying the timing of meals. The key word is 'intermittent' to encourage randomness. Periodic bursts of food deprivation force the body to remain alert and versatile, prompting systems to reset. Ultimately this improves cell function, hormone activity, gene expression, youthfulness and normal body weight!

> **Fasting and Fat-Burning:** It takes 12-14 hours for the body to empty its reserve glucose stores and begin tapping into fat reserves. To stimulate full intermittent fasting benefits, food restriction must exceed that time window.

Examples of Intermittent Fasting*	
Category	**Description**
Shortened Eating Window	An easy method for beginners: Create a 16-18 hour fast including sleep time by skipping breakfast or dinner. This restricts food intake to a 6-8 hour window.
5-2 Fasting	Eat normally 5 days per week. Semi-fast any 2 days per week by restricting food intake to 1/4th the regular calorie-load (consume 500-600 calories on those days). Semi-fast days are not consecutive, but can be to preserve randomness.
Single Day Fast	Fast a full day about once per week. This method creates a 36+ hour fast depending on when the "break-fast" meal is eaten following the fasting day.
24 On / 24 Off	Eat normally for 24 hours, fast the next 24 hours, repeat. Day 1 eat breakfast, lunch and dinner, finish by 6pm. Day 2 fast all day until 6pm and then eat a dinner. Day 3 eat normally until 6pm, begin a 2nd fast to end at 6pm on Day 4.
One Hearty-Meal Fast	Fast most of the day. Eat a single, hearty meal anytime during the day but at least 3 hours before bedtime.
Spontaneous Meal Skipping	Skip meals when convenient several times per week. Note: Depending which meal is skipped, this method may not provide a long enough time interval between meals to stimulate full fasting benefits.
Protein Fasting	Intentionally add one day per week of high carbohydrate intake but low fat/protein ratios. This encourages the body to recycle proteins from aging cells.

*People who are underweight, have a history of eating disorders or certain medical conditions should not fast without consulting a knowledgeable medical provider first.

> **Skipping Breakfast:** "Breakfast is the most important meal of the day." This common advice is severely misinterpreted and not just in terms of proper foods, but timing too. Look at the word: **Breakfast = break + fast** *Breakfast is simply the first meal eaten after a fast* – it 'breaks the fast.' Agreed, this meal is very important because it sends the first dietary messages to your body after a rest. Breakfast shapes the direction of metabolism (sugar-burning versus fat-burning) and digestive stress (inflammatory versus anti-inflammatory); but no one said it had to be at 7 o'clock in the morning! Enjoy your 'break-fast' any time during the day!

Tips for Successful Intermittent Fasting

Keep an open mind about fasting. There are easy ways to incorporate occasional fasts in a long-term plan:

- **Start Small** – Skipping a meal or condensing the eating window is a simple method to experiment with fasting. One successful fast often paves the way for longer fasts in the future.
- **Personalize It** – There is no single, correct way to fast. Feel free to plan one or let a fast happen spontaneously (travel days, busy day full of errands, etc). Start with planning a shorter fast, then extend it if not hungry. Make fasting compatible with other lifestyle factors – for example, skip breakfast to have coffee with a friend or fast most of the day and break it for a family dinner.
- **Stress-Free** – The body might interpret a fast as a stressful event. If this is coupled with unmanaged daily stress, cortisol spikes and subsequent insulin releases will undermine the benefits of fasting. Fast on your least stressful days and *actively manage stress throughout the non-eating period* (more about Cortisol on Days 11 and 12 – if fasting creates stress-related cravings, use craving strategies from Day 24).

- **Hydrate with *Low-Sugar* Beverages** – Fasting means different things to different people. Some fast on water alone. Others consume tea, coffee, bone broth, green vegetable juice, coconut milk, Bulletproof™ coffee, lemon water or other low-sugar liquids.
- **Stay Busy/Active** – Incorporate a variety of low-level activities during the fast. Additionally, it is possible to exercise in a fasted state *if you're feeling energetic*. If you choose to exercise, don't push it. Allow energy levels to guide the intensity of the workout and pay attention to hydration (Movement and Electrolyte topics on Day 10). Consider breaking the fast right after the workout when the body is naturally more efficient with nutrient placement.
- **Sugar-Burners** – Fasting is easier for those already accustomed to fat-burning. A sugar-burner typically struggles against willpower and withdrawal symptoms. Though a fat-burner can feel physical hunger, it is not the same driving hunger of a sugar-burner. Hunger of a fat-burner is more easily ignored and tends to dissipate with stress-managing distractions (gardening, walking the dog, enjoying music, cup of tea, etc).
- **Breaking the Fast** – Let hunger levels determine how much to eat following a fast. There is no need to increase food intake to make up for missed calories. Replenish your body with nutrient-dense foods in amounts to satisfy hunger. *Caution:* A fast is not an excuse to binge on unhealthy food as a reward.
- **Eventually, Try an Extended Fast** – At some point in the future, try a longer fast of 36+ hours (including sleep time) to observe how the body responds. Of course, this may create uncomfortable or persistent hunger before bedtime, but try distracting yourself or going to bed early. Mental and physical benefits are often revealed upon waking the following morning. Try it once – you may love the results.

Mindset Matters: Intermittent fasting is a viable tool to reset metabolism and full-body function. When used within the right mindset, fasting is part of a healthy regimen. However, there are a few things fasting is *not*:
1. Fasting is *not* a green light for consuming copious amounts of unhealthy foods before or after. Continue to base your diet on well-tolerated, wholesome foods.
2. Fasting is *not* a punishment. Use the technique to accelerate the body's fat-burning metabolism but *only because you want to*, not because you are paying penance for poor food choices.

Special Considerations for Intermittent Fasting
Generally speaking, a short break from eating is an excellent tool to fine-tune the body, encourage fat-burning metabolism and even age more gracefully. Most respond well, but there are a few special cases to note:
1. **Fertile Women** (pregnant, lactating or actively trying to conceive) – Fasting is not recommended for women in these specific categories. If weight loss is necessary, consult with a qualified nutritionist or knowledgeable healthcare provider to implement a personalized program.
2. **Underweight or Undernourished** – First establish a nutrient-dense diet to which the body responds. Do not limit nutrient intake until these issues are corrected.
3. **History of Eating Disorders** – Enlist direct, professional supervision for any fasting regimen, if at all.
4. **Blood Sugar Imbalances** – Those who monitor blood sugar levels need professional supervision through a few initial fasts before they are ready to fast on their own.

Read More About Intermittent Fasting:
- ChrisKresser Could You Benefit from Intermittent Fasting
- UltimatePaleoGuide Intermittent Fasting 101
- MarksDailyApple Why Fast? Note: This is a complete 7-part series, read sections relevant to you.
- *The Complete Guide to Fasting,* by Jason Fung, MD, with Jimmy Moore

Fasting + Interval Training (WOW! Encourages even *more* fat-burning)

Caution: This technique is more advanced. Wait until healthy diet and exercise routines are well-established before incorporating this in your lifestyle strategies (more on Movement, Strength Training and HIIT on Day 10).

 Fasting is one method to reinforce fat-burning metabolism. Interval exercise training is another. To supercharge fat-burning, merge these techniques by exercising in a fasted state (especially HIIT). This combination manipulates the adrenaline/cortisol response to burn even higher percentages of fat.

The most popular approach is to exercise in the morning before eating (the body will have had roughly 12 hours of overnight fasting prior the workout). Not only is fat burned specifically to fuel the workout, it also encourages the body to *burn a higher percentage of fat for the next 72 hours*!

🖐 Mercola Interval Training and Intermittent Fasting

Workout Fuel for Fat-Burners: For those who need to provide some energy before a workout yet want to remain in a fat-burning state, consider supplementing with MCT oil. After the workout, replenish nutrients with a protein + healthy carb recovery snack (this replaces depleted glycogen stores; healthy carb options on Day 10).

Supplement with MCT Oils: The medium-chain fats in coconut oil (or concentrated MCT oil) are easily-absorbed and burned quickly as energy. Use MCTs to swiftly boost fat-burning mode, particularly useful to fuel a fat-burning workout or for recovery after a carb-heavy day (more about using MCTs on Day 2).

Section III: Long-Term Strategies – Planning a Getaway

Prior to starting this program, you created specific guidelines to use outside of the home (Prep D, Section III). Many of them can be applied toward your long-term lifestyle plan with modifications.

A Getaway Plan

Remaining compliant with a dietary regimen during some real life 'deviations' (like a vacation or time visiting relatives) may appear daunting. It doesn't have to be. Surprisingly, food tolerance often improves during these times because regular daily stress levels tend to be lower! So relax, enjoy the trip and loosely structure your getaway within a few dietary parameters:

1. **Establish Personal "No-Exceptions" Rules** – Examples include:
    a. Eat a high-protein breakfast every day
    b. Always eat a green vegetable at lunch and dinner
    c. Avoid all trigger foods that cause stomach cramping (or your worst symptom)
    d. Fast during part of the trip (on the way there or back – details on Intermittent Fasting above)
2. **Consider Specific Allowances Ahead of Time** – Examples include:
    a. When invited to someone's house, eat what they serve unless it violates a no-exception rule
    b. For dessert options, choose one with the least gluten
    c. Try the local food and beverages regardless if they qualify for your regular diet
3. **Be Your Own Advocate** – Examples include:
    a. If staying at someone's house, ask to stock a few personal groceries
    b. Present an allergy card to the chef at a restaurant: 🖐 SafeFARE has a free printable template to list allergens; other sites can translate for a fee
4. **Know the Local Foods and Rules** – Examples include:
    a. In general, European food products are much higher quality than the US (less pesticides, less adulterated, better growing conditions). Many people report the ability to eat bread in France or sausage in Germany even if US versions cause digestive upset.
    b. Local specialties tend to be high quality foods. Research ahead of time and seek them out.

After the getaway, you may feel fine or you may want to return to the Strict Paleo Protocol for a week or two to reset. Use any of the long-term strategies to get back on track and restore fat-burning metabolism (Days 22- 27).

To-Do List:

☐ Record today's values in the Healthy Baseline Chart on page 344
☐ Anything else (check the veggie guide for more colorful produce ideas on Day 1, select the first food to reintroduce and put it on your grocery list, look into a non-food reward from Day 15, etc)?

Coming Up:

- Paleo treats
- Re-evaluate your health and compare to your pre-Paleo status

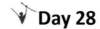

Day 28

Motivation is what gets you started. Habit is what keeps you going. ~Jim Ryun, athlete and politician

Today's Topics:
1. Revisit Measurements
2. Fill out Post-Paleo Check Out Form
3. Paleo Treats

Fast Fare – Grocery Store
♥ Rotisserie chicken
♥ Salad bar vegetables fried in butter

For your final day on the Strict Paleo Protocol, imagine a talented chef was cooking all your Strict Paleo Protocol meals...*and* you have an unlimited budget. What would you request?

Breakfast: _____

Lunch: _____

Dinner: _____

Snacks: _____

Beverages: _____

Have you eaten any of these foods before?   Yes   No

Are you willing to make one of these recipes as a celebratory meal to use during reintroductions?   Yes   No

Record Your Healthy Baseline

The most important step of reintroduction is to be aware of how good your body feels following a Strict Paleo Protocol. Please record today's values in your Healthy Baseline Chart on page 344.

Section I: Revisit Measurements (Compare to Prep C)

Body Metrics Chart

Again, you do not need to share these values with anyone...this is just for you! Record your current results or measurements in the following table and compare to Prep C. It's okay to delay the blood work for a while – some tests require time for the body to stabilize before the reading will be accurate: A1C is roughly a 3-month snapshot of blood glucose levels and cholesterol tests fluctuate during times of weight gain/loss.

Body Metric Benchmarks				
Suggested Blood Work			**Physical Measurements** (Measure at the fullest point)	
Test	**Ideal**	**Test Result**		
HDL	> 50		Chest	
Triglycerides	< 100		Waist	
Total ÷ HDL	< 3.5		Hips	
Triglycerides ÷ HDL	< 2		Arm	
LDL-P	< 1000		Thigh	
Fasting glucose	< 90		Neck	
A1C	< 5.0		Weight	
CRP	< 0.8		Blood	_____
25-OHD (vit D)	40-60		Pressure	

Though we discourage using the scale as the *sole* source of health feedback, monitoring weight helps with accountability and is an element of the big health picture. Remember, body composition improvements may not be revealed by weight change alone (Day 27), so also compare physical measurements.

For those who noted initial weight, what was your weight *change* since beginning the program? _____

For those who took physical measurements, how many inches were gained/lost? _____

Blood Work Options

If you intend to revisit these blood work values in the future, mark this page for when your body stabilizes enough for testing. After 4 weeks of Paleo, you may already observe lower fasting glucose and lower CRP, and though there is probably improvement in the cholesterol profile, wait until weight gain/loss stabilizes to retest.

⤴ MayoClinic Tests and Procedures for standard bloodwork ranges

🔹 **Lipid Panel**: Cholesterol is a necessary component in a healthy body and brain. High *total cholesterol* does not necessarily indicate poor health (just as *too low* total cholesterol does not indicate good health; levels below 150 or 160 are problematic for brain health). General recommendations for a healthy cholesterol panel:

- **HDL:** >50 but in general, more is better
- **Triglycerides:** <150, but the lower the better; some sources recommend below 100.
- **Useful Lipid Ratios:** The ratios below indicate a healthy lipid panel and lack of inflammation:
  - **Total Cholesterol ÷ HDL** Ideally < 3.5
  - **Triglycerides ÷ HDL** Some sources say <3, but ideally <2
- **LDL-P (particle count):** LDL comes in different sizes so particle size matters: large, fluffy LDL particles are healthy and desirable, but the small dense ones are not. The LDL-P test measures the total number of LDL particles and a high count suggests excessive, unhealthy, small LDL particles and is ideally <1000.
  Note: The LDL-C number on a typical cholesterol test is an estimate of how much LDL is present, it does not correlate with the particle size.
      ⤴ DocsOpinion The Difference between LDL-C and LDL-P
      📖 *Grain Brain*, by David Perlmutter, MD
      📖 *The Great Cholesterol Myth,* by Jonny Bowden, PhD, CNS, and Stephen Sinatra, MD, FACC
      📖 *Cholesterol Clarity,* by Jimmy Moore and Eric C. Westman, MD
      ⤳ Re-read topics on Cholesterol and Heart Disease on Days 17 and 18

🔹 **Fasting Blood Glucose Level**: Best to keep this less than 100; over 100 indicates pre-diabetes and over 120 indicates diabetes. <90 is desirable.

🔹 **A1C:** This measures blood sugar level over time and is a more accurate picture than the Fasting Blood Glucose which is just a one-moment snapshot. The A1C measurement averages ~3 months of blood sugar levels, so do not retest this until after you have been eating Paleo-style for at least three months. A 'normal' score is between 4.5 and 5.6 percent; 5.7 - 6.4 percent indicates pre-diabetes and two separate test results of 6.5 or higher indicates diabetes. Optimal levels are 5.0 and below.

🔹 **CRP:** C-Reactive Protein measures the amount of inflammation currently in the body. Some drugs can affect levels (birth control pills, NSAIDS like ibuprofen, Tylenol, etc) so advise your healthcare provider accordingly. The higher the score, the more systemic inflammation present. Ideal results are < 0.8 mg/L.

🔹 **Vitamin D Levels:** Ideal scores for the 25-OHD test range from 40-60mg/mL. Vitamin D fluctuates with sunshine exposure. It's common to take a supplement in the winter.

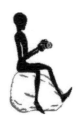

Picture Time

Everyone gets to take an after picture (or at least look in a mirror). Wear the same attire as your "before" photo if you took one. If you don't have a specific "before" image, just find a recent photograph to compare and contrast: Gaze into your eyes. Study your expression. Inspect your skin tone. Observe your posture. Notice your demeanor.

Note changes: Has puffiness reduced? Is muscle tone or bone structure (like cheekbones) more defined? Can you see more vibrancy, more enthusiasm, more confidence? What do these pictures illustrate that you already knew?

What surprised you about the photos?

Consider how a photo taken 1 month from now will compare to these two images.

Section II: Post-Paleo Check-Out   Date: _____

Please record any specific observations or clarifications in the notes below.	Strongly Disagree -2	Disagree -1	Neutral 0	Agree +1	Strongly Agree +2	Blown Away +3
I have even energy levels throughout the day.	☐	☐	☐	☐	☐	☐
I fall asleep easily and sleep soundly.	☐	☐	☐	☐	☐	☐
I rarely have food cravings.	☐	☐	☐	☐	☐	☐
I'm satisfied with both my hunger levels and my response to hunger.	☐	☐	☐	☐	☐	☐
My joints and tendons are comfortable and work smoothly.	☐	☐	☐	☐	☐	☐
I am satisfied with my range of motion (flexibility) throughout my body.	☐	☐	☐	☐	☐	☐
I have relatively few aches or pains (including neck, back, headache, joint, muscle, etc).	☐	☐	☐	☐	☐	☐
I am satisfied with my athletic performance and body's response to physical activity.	☐	☐	☐	☐	☐	☐
My body heals quickly from overuse or injury.	☐	☐	☐	☐	☐	☐
My immune system functions properly (rarely catch a cold, recover from illness well, etc).	☐	☐	☐	☐	☐	☐
My skin, complexion, hair, nails, teeth and gums are all healthy and strong.	☐	☐	☐	☐	☐	☐
My moods are stable and easy to control.	☐	☐	☐	☐	☐	☐
I am satisfied with my mental clarity and ability to focus.	☐	☐	☐	☐	☐	☐
In general, I am able to calmly respond to stressful situations.	☐	☐	☐	☐	☐	☐
My digestion functions properly (no stomach cramps, heartburn, bloating, painful gas, etc).	☐	☐	☐	☐	☐	☐
My elimination function is normal and comfortable (no diarrhea, constipation, etc).	☐	☐	☐	☐	☐	☐

*This category is provided for improvements that truly were above and beyond expectations

Notes:

Score and Compare

To score this form, a "strongly agree" response scores +2 points, "strongly disagree" is -2, and neutral is zero. And just in case you were really surprised by your improvement, the "blown away" category scores +3!

Post-Paleo Check-Out Score: _____

Go back to Prep C and compare your responses with the Pre-Paleo Check-In Form.

Pre-Paleo Check-In Score: _____

Where are your biggest gains?

1. _____
2. _____
3. _____

What has surprised you the most?

1. _____
2. _____
3. _____

How will you actively support your good health improvements?

1. _____
2. _____
3. _____

Section III: Paleo Treats

There are a wide variety of tantalizing and satisfying foods that fall into Paleo guidelines, including desserts. Although it takes time to settle into a long-term Paleo groove, eventually there will be room for some Paleo-friendly sweets. Please note that experimenting with Paleo treats should be deferred until *after food reintroductions are complete*.

Disclaimers:
1. Before adding any treats, please finish food reintroductions to learn personal tolerance levels
2. Paleo sugars are from natural sources, but *sugar is still sugar* – monitor portion sizes and frequency
3. We're addressing Paleo treats because it's handy to have special occasion strategies for indulgences that won't upset the stomach, but that doesn't make these foods healthy
4. Review how to assess your carbohydrate and starch tolerance (Day 24)

Eating strict Paleo for 28 days definitely impacts the sweet-reward system in the brain and it's common to develop a heightened sense of sweetness: you will be satisfied by less sweetness. Use this to your advantage. When the time is right to make some sweet choices, do your best to preserve your new taste buds.
1. **Cut Back on Sweetener When Possible:** It's possible a lightly-sweetened treat will be just as satisfying as the fully-sweetened old version. For example: when baking, reduce the sweetener by a third; when sweetening a beverage, start with half the normal amount (including when ordering at a café).
2. **Reduce Portion Sizes:** Slow down and savor smaller portions of sweets (especially those that are fully-sweetened) to prevent falling back into old patterns or cravings.

Let's face it: Life happens, cravings happen, special occasions happen.
You don't have to feel guilty about going a bit off-plan; just make the best choice possible and move on.
~Tammy Credicott, Paleo Indulgences

Types of Sugars

There is ongoing Paleo debate between choosing calorie-free sweeteners versus other natural sweeteners like honey, but the main point is this: If you do not consume sugar very often and do not have blood glucose or insulin resistance issues, then select a sweetener with a taste you enjoy from a company you trust.

Sweetener Options to Try		Sweeteners to Avoid
Very Low Calorie	**Regular Calorie Load**	
Stevia, sugar alcohols (erythritol, hardwood xylitol, maltitol, sorbitol), yacon syrup, inulin powder, monk fruit extract	Raw honey, maple syrup, date paste, evaporated cane juice, coconut sugar, homemade jam, dried fruit, organic molasses, organic sugar & brown sugar	Table sugar, agave nectar, corn syrup, fructose, high fructose corn syrup, sucralose (Splenda), aspartame (NutraSweet, Equal), saccharin (Sweet'N Low)

Some individuals are sensitive to certain alternative sweeteners (for example: tasting a bitter aftertaste; or digestive upset from sugar alcohols). Most Paleo blogs have their own take on sweeteners, and no one agrees. Do some research and experiment until you find your sweet success:

- ⌐ <u>Bulletproof</u> Kick Your Sugar Habit with these Bulletproof Alternative Sweeteners
- ⌐ <u>PaleoPlan</u> Paleo Sweeteners 101

Homemade Paleo Treats

There's no lack of Paleo treat recipes. If you crave something, there will be a Paleo version of that recipe online! In addition to innumerable baked goods, you'll also find: fudge, gummies, coconut milk ice cream, energy balls, chocolate sauce, waffles, crepes, milkshakes, peppermint bark, sorbet, pudding, caramel, donuts, truffles, marshmallows, parfaits, sundaes, candied nuts, candied bacon, etc.

> **Watch the Carbs:** If you are especially carb sensitive, any sweets can catapult carb cravings. If that's your case, look for ***ketogenic*** recipes – they use less starchy flours and lower calorie sweeteners to keep net carbs low.

- ➢ **Gluten-Free Flours** – Due to the huge surge in gluten awareness, commercial gluten-free flour mixes are widely available but are often made from other grains like rice, corn or oats. This may be fine for some individuals, but there are plenty of grain-free options for those who need/want to limit grains.
- ➢ **Grain-Free Flours** – These rarely bake like wheat flour and likely *do not* substitute 1-to-1 for wheat. Most recipes call for a combination of flours to create the desired texture. Start by using highly-rated recipes or cookbooks since experimenting requires some trial-and-error.

Grain-Free Flour Options	
Starchier (More Glucose)	**Less Starchy**
Plantain flour, cassava flour, arrowroot flour/starch, tapioca starch, potato *starch* (potato *flour* tastes like potatoes), taro flour/powder, sweet potato flour/starch, green banana flour	Almond meal/flour, ground nuts, ground seeds, coconut flour, cricket flour, tigernut flour

Grain-Free Baking Tips:

1. Coconut flour is very high in fiber which requires a lot of eggs, oil and other liquids to soften it. For best texture, let the batter rest before cooking – this gives the fiber time to absorb the liquid.
2. Plantains and green bananas create a texture similar to wheat flour. They make an excellent batter base for pancakes, breads, cookies, hush puppies, tortillas, etc. Using a food processer, blend chunks of plantain or banana with eggs until smooth. It's also possible to purchase plantain and banana flours.
   ⌐ <u>PaleoHacks</u> 5-Ingredient Paleo Bread Recipe, ⌐ <u>PurelyTwins</u> Plantain Bread. Paleo. 3 Ingredients.

> **Resistant Starch (RS) in Baking:** Some starches such as raw potato starch or plantain flour are high in RS, meaning the starch resists digestion and does not break down into glucose (Day 15). However, before getting excited about baking a cake with minimal carb impact, recall that this type of RS reverts back to digestible starch when cooked. Go ahead and enjoy the cake, but the final product does not offer resistant starch benefits.

High-Quality Pre-Made Treats, Baked Goods and Mixes*

Many Paleo-friendly treats can be found at local health food stores or natural foods sections in large grocers and sometimes overlap with organic treats or vegan treats. *Be careful to read labels* since most treats are not Paleo compliant (may contain gluten-free grains, agave nectar, cheese flavoring, etc). Paleo treats can include:

- Chocolates
- Cookies
- Brownies

- Pudding
- Pancakes
- Candies/mints

- Chips
- Cupcakes
- Crackers

- Shakes
- Gummies
- Cereal

- Pizza Crust
- Pasta
- Muffins

* One online source of products is Thrive Market which can be accessed from a link at ⌐ Paleovation

There are many sources of Paleo treats found at online retailers (just search "paleo+_____" – for example, paleo cookies, paleo pizza crust, paleo bread mix, paleo brownies, paleo cake mix, etc). Continue to watch ingredients because many companies include *some* Paleo products, but it doesn't guarantee the entire product line is Paleo-friendly. Additionally, dairy is a common ingredient in flavorings (example: cheddar crackers).

⌐ PaleoBakingCompany*	⌐ PaleoFoodMall*‡	⌐ SimpleMills	⌐ CavemanCookies
⌐ WellnessBakeries*	⌐ PaleoPrimeFoods*	⌐ PaleoTreats*	⌐ NamasteFoods
⌐ OneStopPaleoShop*‡	⌐ StevesPaleoGoods*	⌐ ThriveMarket‡	⌐ BirchBenders
⌐ WildMountainPaleo*‡	⌐ PureTraditionsFoods*	⌐ GoRaw	⌐ JacksonsHonest
⌐ BarefootProvisions*‡	⌐ WhiteLionBaking*	⌐ Capellos	⌐ HailMerry

* exclusively Paleo products   ‡ Paleo shopping networks

> **Emerging Paleo Products:** These lists are only the beginning. Continue to watch for new brands and products at sources like Etsy, local Paleo startups, Amazon, the protein bar companies listed in the Snacks topic (Day 2) or the ⌐ PaleoFoundation, which maintains a list of certified Paleo products.

Monitor Treats, BUT *Enjoy* When the Time is Right

Long-term diet and lifestyle development is an ongoing process. Enjoy treats now and then, especially low-sugar or low-starch items that you tolerate well. And, if there is something really special (for example, wedding cake or a bakery in Paris) and it's worth the consequence, enjoy every bite to minimize cortisol interference!

Section V: Keep Reading. Keep Researching. Keep Learning.

> *You're on your own. You know what you know. And you are the one who'll decide where to go.* ~Dr. Seuss

Long-term dietary success does not happen accidentally. It comes with practice, being mindful, staying curious and using trial-and-error techniques to uncover the right personalized approach. The following books written from the Paleo perspective are valuable for ideas and real-life applications:

Post-Elimination Diet Guidance	
📖 *Food Freedom Forever,* **by Melissa Hartwig**	A guide to help individuals gracefully navigate long-term food choice. Readers learn how to gain control over their food habits in a guilt-free, judgment-free, fear-free manner. Recommended for those needing additional guidance to overcome a poor relationship with food or for those just curious about additional strategies.
📖 *Wired to Eat,* **by Robb Wolf**	This program lays out a scientific approach for determining carbohydrate tolerance. Learn to use a blood glucose monitor to illustrate how your body reacts to different carb sources. Recommended for those who need to monitor blood glucose or anyone willing to deeply explore personal carb tolerance.

To-Do List:

- ☐ Finish the Healthy Baseline Chart
- ☐ Start your carefully-planned food reintroductions
- ☐ **Enjoy your new health and vitality!**

> *The recipe is simple: Eat Clean. Play Often. Crush Life.* ~Mary Shenouda, PaleoChef.com

~ This page intentionally left blank ~

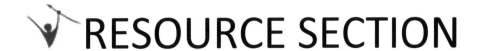# RESOURCE SECTION

Downloadable / printable copies of select forms, charts and graphics are available online: ⌐ Paleovation

~ This page intentionally left blank ~

⚡ *Paleovation Workbook* Group Manual

Success as a Group

The Paleovation Workbook is perfect for groups to complete together. Fitness clubs, health and wellness centers, sports teams, employee wellness programs, church groups, social clubs, therapy groups, community centers or even just a few friends can use this book to guide their collective Paleo experience.

For most groups, it's best to designate a group leader to facilitate. This can be anyone interested in coordinating the group – the leader does *not* need to be a professional. For casual groups, it is possible to alternate leaders; for example, rotate host and leader each meeting.

Five weekly meetings are necessary to span the entire program, the 6th meeting is optional. This manual will guide the entire group process. The layout for each meeting consists of two parts:
   A.   **Group Leader Preparation** – to be completed prior to the meeting
   B.   **Meeting Agenda** – a group discussion and activity guide for pertinent book topics

Meeting Topics	Material Covered
#1: Preparing for Success	Introduction, Prep A and B
#2: Low-Carb Flu	Prep C-G, Days 1-4
#3: Establishing Paleo Habits	Days 5-10
#4: Stress and Sleep Support	Days 11-18
#5: Long-term Strategies and Guidance	Days 19-27
#6: [Optional] Discuss Reintroduction Trials	Day 28, Resource Section

Getting Started

The following outline is provided to organize and maximize a successful group experience.
   1.   **Meeting Duration:** 60-90 minutes depending on group dynamics and enrichment activity selections.
   2.   **Create a Network:** Form a private email list or private social media group so participants can confidentially share ideas, questions and experiences between meetings.
   3.   **Procure Workbook(s):** Each participant needs a personal copy of *The Paleovation Workbook*. These can either be attained individually prior to the first meeting or they can be procured by the group leader and distributed at the first meeting (to purchase books in bulk at a discounted rate, contact BulkOrder@Paleovation.com).
   4.   **Review the Book Structure:** Note the program rules, book layout and the general long-term goals.
       ➢   The information is broken into manageable pieces with daily W*hy* (Paleo-Wise) and *How* sections
       ➢   Paleo lifestyle, shopping and further reading tips are interspersed through the text and include recipes, food and nutritional supplement resources, online articles and book recommendations
       ➢   Paleo staple cooking assignments provide foundational foods often used in other Paleo recipes that may be difficult to find or expensive to purchase
       ➢   Resource Section extras:
           •   **Summary Guides** – Problems with Modern Foods, Paleo Reference Guide, Fats Guide
           •   **Charts** – additional copies of forms such as Kitchen Cleanout and Stock-up Lists
           •   **Key Graphics** – magnified images for better comprehension
           •   **Recipes** – suggested foundation recipes
           •   **Nutritional Supplements** – information, options and resources
   5.   **www.Paleovation.com:** Our website has additional information to introduce the Paleo Protocol.
       a.   **Paleo Synopsis** – *Free Paleo Synopsis and Guidelines* is a 10-page overview of the Paleo Diet
       b.   **Baby Steps Page** – ideas for a gradual approach to Paleo eating
       c.   **Recommended Reading** – compilation of links to articles recommended in the book

⚓ Meeting #1 – Preparing for Success

Note: Schedule the first meeting *prior* to starting the Strict Paleo Protocol. Meeting #1 is designed to establish group rapport and clarify program specifications before participants begin Day 1 of the Strict Paleo Protocol.

A. Group Leader Preparation Checklist

☐ **Book Introduction** – Acquaint yourself with book layout. Scan the Intro, Prep A-G and Resource sections.

☐ **Discussion Topics (below)** – Browse the subject matter. Jot down ideas to share in the agenda margins.

    a. Sticky flag / dog-ear pages referenced in the topics (activity in Prep A, excuses in Prep D, etc).

    b. Write down any additional ideas, questions and concerns particularly relevant to your group: Examples include establishing a support network, staying compliant, modifying an exercise routine, collecting recipe ideas, locating groceries, incorporating nutritional supplements, etc.

☐ **Optional Enrichment (below)** – Preview the options and arrange logistics for activity selections.

☐ **Locate Assorted Paleo Cookbooks / Online Recipes** – Bring these to Meeting #1 (suggestions are listed in the book Introduction and Prep B). Libraries often have selections. Alternative: share this activity and request that participants bring a Paleo cookbook and/or copies of some savory Paleo recipes.

☐ **"Show & Tell" Homework Assignment** – Complete this on your own ahead of time to provide an example for the group. It's possible to overlap with items in the Enrichment Label-Reading activity.

☐ **Communicate with Participants** (email or otherwise) before Meeting #1 – Content may include:

    a. Those under medical management need to coordinate care with their healthcare providers during the transition to the Paleo Diet. Suggestions can be found in these articles:

          ⌁ <u>Whole30</u> Talk to your Doc: What to Do if your Doctor Says "No"

          ⌁ <u>Whole30</u> Talk to your Doc: Prescription Medications

    b. Clarify when/how each participant acquires their copy of *The Paleovation Workbook*. Optional: If members already have a copy, they may read through the Prep sections before the first meeting.

    c. If books are not attained prior to Meeting #1, plan to distribute them at the first meeting. In the meantime, direct the group to the website ⌁ <u>Paleovation</u> for general information:

          ⌁ The *Free Paleo Synopsis and Guidelines* will outline specifics of the Paleo Protocol

          ⌁ <u>Paleovation</u> Baby Steps provides starting points to instill new healthy habits

    d. Alert members that the first meeting lays out the rules of the program. They will begin eating the Strict Paleo Protocol between the 1st and 4th day following Meeting #1.

    e. Encourage participants to compile any questions or concerns they may have for discussion.

☐ **Anything else to bring?** Pens, slips of paper for sharing results, additional topics list, waiver forms, etc:

B. Meeting Agenda [Participants have not yet started the 28-day challenge]

This is the opportunity to meet others in the group, share questions and concerns, discuss personal goals for the program and enjoy the company of like-minded individuals. The facilitator has two main goals: help the group understand the Paleo Protocol and build an open and sharing environment. The Paleo transition period is challenging; therefore, these two factors build the groundwork for group success.

Meeting #1: Discussion Topics	
Objectives	**Subject Matter and Dialogue Cues**
Set the Tone	Encourage participants to be as candid as they wish during these meetings. Emphasize that privacy is respected, and all personal information shared within the group sessions *and* online support network remains confidential.
Introductions – to each other and to Paleo-eating	1. Optional: introductions can include why each participant has decided to join this program; use the Prep A chart "Symptoms of Chronic Inflammation" to spark ideas 2. Pass around Paleo cookbooks and point out recipes that catch the eye
Book Format	Explain features of the workbook layout including the prep sections, fast fare, daily pages, *why* and *how* info, resource section, recommended articles, supplements, etc.

Objectives	Subject Matter and Dialogue Cues (Meeting #1 Continued)
Discuss Start Date	Group members can begin as they are ready – they do not all need to be on the exact same day. Plan to finish all preparation sections and start the 28-day program within 4 days after Meeting #1 - this ensures participants will at least be on Day 4 by Meeting #2.
Clarify Program Rules	1. Define Paleo foods – for guidance, use Clean Out (Prep A) and Stock-Up (Prep B) charts as well as the Paleo Pyramid and Reference Guide in the Resource Section 2. Discuss the "Practice Removing Not-for-Now Foods" chart in Prep A and complete the blank chart together [Optional: Prep B has a similar activity for extra practice] 3. Identify any group-specific rules in addition to the basic *Paleovation* program: Examples can include additional supplements, signing the facility's insurance waiver, taking a daily walk, no potatoes, keeping a food or exercise journal, etc
Group Motivation	Have participants review the text in Prep D, Section II, regarding mental excuses. Discuss personal concerns regarding commitment to the program and how group support helps overcome those. Brainstorm additional strategies as necessary.
Answer Questions	• Let participants review the list of questions they prepared before arrival. Some topics will already be addressed within the rules discussion. Use any remaining questions for discussion purposes. • If any questions are not answered satisfactorily during Meeting #1, have *each* group member record them – they can search for answers in Paleo-Wise reading sections and recommended articles before Meeting #2.
Cooking Assignment #1 Bone Broth	Participants can begin preparation for Cooking Assignment #1 (Prep E). Review the directions and direct members to bone suggestions listed in Prep E and online here: <u>NourishedKitchen Bone Broth: How to Make it and Why It's Good</u>

Optional Enrichment Activities: These activities can be completed or discussed during Meeting #1
- Complete the Pre-Paleo Check-In Form in Prep C: score and share thoughts (not required to share scores; however, anonymously shared scores can be averaged into a 'group starting score' if interested)
- Read food labels to identify non-Paleo foods: discuss the example in the Kitchen Clean Out form in Prep A and/or bring in sample grocery items for the group members to decide which ones are Paleo safe
- Take a group photo and/or headshots: the pictures are used to mark progress over the next 4 weeks
- Survey group interest on a food-related documentary discussion (selections listed at the end of Day 5): choose a video to watch at home before Meeting #2 or watch one together following Meeting #2's discussion (and extend Meeting #2' length; a volunteer can arrange projection and sound requirements)
- Assess interest in casually meeting for coffee/lunch once per week during the *Paleovation* program
- Survey interest in a weekly Paleo recipe exchange, each member brings in copies for the group

Homework Assignment for Meeting #2: Show & Tell
This is an either/or assignment. Each participant selects one of the following to bring to Meeting #2:
1. Bring in 1-3 Paleo foods or packages as examples of how to stock the kitchen. Share the purchase price, local store(s) where it is available, whether you sampled it yet, etc.
2. Print a copy of a recommend reading article noted in the Prep sections or Days 1-4. Be prepared to share a brief synopsis and pass around the article if necessary.

Adjourning Thoughts
- ✓ Use the social media/email list for questions and answers, sharing recipes, posting articles, posting pictures of Paleo meals, identifying local sales on Paleo foods, etc.
- ✓ Meeting #2's topics cover Prep Sections C-G and Days 1-4. Please keep up with the daily reading.
- ✓ Take notes directly in the *Paleovation* text; consider highlighters, sticky flags or dog-eared pages.
- ✓ Next week's discussion revolves around sugar withdrawal and potential low-carb flu. To be prepared, each individual should pay close attention to low-carb flu symptoms and relief strategies.
- ✓ Keep a running list of questions and concerns to discuss at Meeting #2.

⅄ Meeting #2 – Getting through the Low-Carb Flu

Background and Basics: Participants are on Days 4-7 of the program. This meeting covers topics from Prep C through Day 4. Low-carb flu is very likely affecting them – do not be surprised by a less lively discussion.

A. Group Leader Preparation Checklist:

☐ **Content Research** – Read *The Paleovation Workbook* through Day 4.
   a. Compile a list of low-carb flu symptoms and relief strategies
   b. Take notes on the information and activities you personally want to highlight at Meeting #2

☐ **Discussion Topics** – Browse the subject matter. Jot down ideas to share in the agenda margins.
   a. Review all information referenced, including future book topics that appear after Day 4
   b. Sticky flag / dog-ear pages referenced in the topics for quick access during the meeting
   c. [Optional]: Enlarge a copy of the Sugar UN-Merry-go-Round (Resource Section) for a visual aide
   d. Compile ideas for complementary topics or concerns relevant to your group
   e. Preview Cooking Assignment #2 (mayo): Complete ahead of time to share your experience

☐ **Optional Enrichment** – Preview the options and arrange logistics for activity selections.

☐ **"Eating Out" Homework Assignment** – Complete this on your own ahead of time. Use your personal example(s) to introduce dining out solutions to the group.

☐ **Group Communication** – Check in with the group via email or social media during the week:
   a. Encourage members to use the online group support as necessary for motivation, questions, etc
   b. Remind the group of their Show & Tell Homework a day or two before Meeting #2
   c. Coordinate and remind participants of any optional enrichment activities selected at Meeting #1 (watch selected documentary, specifics for lunch/coffee meet-ups, recipe exchange, etc)

☐ **Anything else?** Pens, signup sheets, recipe copies, supplementary topics, unanswered question list, etc.

B. Meeting Agenda [Participants are on Day 4-7]

The main objective of this meeting is to support the initial transition to the Paleo Protocol. Some individuals may have symptoms of the low-carb flu and need reminders about how to support themselves during the withdrawal period. Others will need assistance finding appropriate groceries and meals.

Meeting #2: Discussion Topics	
Objectives	**Subject Matter and Dialogue Cues**
Share Experiences	1. Let participants share their experience so far. Use the "Day 2 Review" questions to stimulate discussion (the last activity of Day 2). 2. Suggested experiences to highlight: foundation meal selections, bone broth (both making it and incorporating it), low-carb flu symptoms, favorite meals/recipes so far, best Paleo-eating strategy up to now, ease of using the Veggie + Protein + Fat template, interesting grocery purchases or local deals. 3. Show & Tell Homework: Allow each member to share either the Paleo foods they purchased or give a brief synopsis of the recommended article they printed.
Understanding Low-Carb Flu	Review Prep E, Section II on the low-carb flu together. Ask participants to share their current symptoms and any relief strategies they've used or plan on using.
Sugar UN-Merry-go-Round Graphic (Prep C, Resources)	This is a perpetual cycle of sugar/starch intake, insulin response, sugar crash and cravings generation. Discuss the implications of not paying attention to sugar/starch consumption. Describe the key to breaking the cycle and why Paleo is a solution.
Answer Questions	Paleo-Wise sections covered sugar, grains, insulin/leptin, fats and fat-burning. 1. Begin with unanswered questions from the end of Meeting #1. Discuss answers found in the text, recommended reading articles or from personal experience. 2. Guide discussion with the questions participants encountered during the week. 3. Record any remaining questions to see if answers emerge by the next meeting.

Objectives	Subject Matter and Dialogue Cues (Meeting #2 Continued)
Group motivation	**Crutches** – Review the potential crutches discussed on Day 3 and discuss pros/cons, personal preferences, if they are necessary with the support of this group, etc. **Assistance** – Allow each member to raise personal concerns (staying compliant, finding groceries, withdrawal support, etc). The group can strategize an appropriate solution.
Cooking assignment #2 Paleo mayo	Review the assignment directions in Day 4. Survey the group's experience. A. Has anyone made homemade mayonnaise before? Share technique used, recipe used and tips. B. Have any members purchased a commercial Paleo mayo? Share thoughts.
Cooking assignment #3 veggie as a grain	Preview assignment directions in Day 7. Which participants have already incorporated some of these suggestions? Share experiences, recipe sources, results, tips, etc.

Optional Enrichment: These activities can be completed or discussed during Meeting #2
- Share the "Good Health Results" (Prep C, Section IV) each participant hopes to realize.
- Connect low-carb flu to the chronic inflammation and inflammatory behavior charts in Prep A. How are symptoms reinforcing that the body is detoxing from western foods vs reacting to influx of Paleo foods?
- Discuss ideas to help embrace healthy dietary fat: How did our great-grandparents cook with traditional fats? Is food tastier with the fat? What fats are easiest to include?
- Watch/review the optional food-related documentary (listed at the end of Day 5): Share thoughts on initial reactions, arguments presented that reinforce Paleo eating principles, takeaway points, etc.
- Asses interest in an additional documentary to include in next week's discussion or meeting.
- Survey interest in sharing a "Paleo bar" meal at the end of Meeting #3: suggestions listed on the last page of Day 10 – Family-Friendly Dinners. Select a style; brainstorm a list of the base foods and potential toppings. Each participant signs up to bring specific foods and/or supplies such as plates, napkins, silverware, etc.

Homework Assignment: Eating Out
Group leader shares his/her own experience to introduce this project. Each participant selects one of the following to complete before Meeting #3:
1. Create a restaurant strategy for a local eatery including what you would normally order, how you can change that order to make it Paleo, how you will voice your food preferences to the server, etc.
2. Actually go to a restaurant to eat and report back on the overall experience.
3. Visit a Paleo blog/website and print off their dining out strategies to pass around at Meeting #3.

Adjourning Thoughts
- ✓ Take a moment after the meeting to read any printed article(s) brought in by others.
- ✓ Use the social media or email groups for clarification, sharing meal photos, tips and tricks, etc
- ✓ Take notes directly in the *Paleovation* text; consider highlighters, sticky flags or dog-eared pages.
- ✓ Next week focuses on Paleo foods and resources found locally as well as personalized Paleo habits
  - o Pay attention to Paleo-eating strategies (to establish a Paleo Groove, Day 10) that work for you. Share your best approaches next week or via the email list or social media group.
  - o Create a list of Paleo items you've found useful. Include brands, stores and companies you like, especially highlighting information for locally-produced vegetables, meats, eggs, etc.
- ✓ Meeting #3's topics cover information on Days 5-10. Please keep up with the daily reading.
- ✓ If you find a useful recommended reading article, print a copy to share with the group.
- ✓ Keep a running list of questions and concerns to discuss at Meeting #3.

⚑ Meeting #3 – Establishing Paleo Habits

Background and Basics: Participants are on Days 11-14. Members are still rather new to Paleo eating and may need help solidifying their approach. Some individuals are starting to feel the physical improvements and benefits. This meeting covers topics from Days 5-10. **Note:** The stress topics (Days 11 and 12) will be discussed in detail at Meeting #4, this gives all members a chance to read and reflect on both Cortisol topics.

A. Group Leader Preparation Checklist:

☐ **Content Research** – Read *The Paleovation Workbook* through Day 10.
   a. Compile a list of strategies to establish Paleo eating habits
   b. Take notes on the information and activities you personally want to highlight at Meeting #3

☐ **Discussion Topics** – Browse the subject matter. Jot down ideas to share in the agenda margins.
   a. Review all information referenced in the outline, especially sections that appear after Day 10
   b. Sticky flag / dog-ear pages referenced in the topics for quick access during the meeting
   c. Compile ideas for any additional topics or concerns relevant to your group
   d. Preview Cooking Assignment #4 (jerky or granola): Complete ahead to share your experience

☐ **Optional Enrichment** – Preview the options and arrange logistics for activity selections.

☐ **"Lifestyle Support" Homework Assignment** (next page) – Complete this on your own ahead of time. Use your personal example(s) to introduce the idea of supporting other pillars of health.

☐ **Group Communication** – Check in with the group via email or social media during the week:
   a. Encourage members to use the online group support as necessary for motivation, questions, etc
   b. Remind the group to complete Eating Out Homework and lists of interesting local Paleo foods
   c. Coordinate and remind participants of optional enrichment activities selected at previous meetings (watch documentary, specifics for meet-ups, recipe exchange, potluck, volunteers, etc)

☐ **Anything else?** Pens, signup sheets, recipe copies, supplementary topic list, unanswered questions, etc.

B. Meeting Agenda [Participants are on Day 11-14]

Participants are still quite new to the Strict Paleo Protocol. This week's discussion focuses on meal-building strategies plus local resources to support the Paleo transition. By this time, some individuals will notice positive changes (even if just a lessening of low-carb flu); sharing these experiences strengthens group morale.

Meeting #3: Discussion Topics	
Objectives	**Subject Matter and Dialogue Cues**
Share Experiences	1. Overall health: How is everyone feeling? Are low-carb flu symptoms dissipating? Are you noticing positive changes (Day 9, Section IV)? 2. Results of Cooking Assignments #2: Paleo mayo, how did it go? 3. Specific Paleo-eating strategies: successful Paleo substitutions (Day 6), Day 7's initial questions, understanding meat labels and consuming enough protein (Day 7), digestive strategies (Day 8), Paleo Groove questions (Day 10)
Customizing the *Veggie + Protein + Fat* Template	Let participants share what is working for their meal-building – each individual will have varying needs. To stimulate discussion, review the following together: ▪ SAD-Paleo-Ketogenic teeter-totter graphic and protein chart (Day 6) ▪ Carbohydrate tweaking (Day 10, Section III) ▪ Abundant vegetable suggestions (Day 13)
Answer Questions	Paleo-Wise topics covered proteins, dairy, legumes and movement. Answers can be found in the text, recommended articles or from personal experience. Note: Stress topics will be discussed at Meeting #4; focus on topics from Days 5-10. 1. Review questions from the end of Meeting #2. 2. Let participants share the questions they encountered since the last meeting. 3. Record unanswered questions to see if answers emerge by meeting #4.

Objectives	Subject Matter and Dialogue Cues (Meeting #3 Continued)
Movement Discussion	Share thoughts on sedentary behaviors (Day 9) or chronic cardio exercise (Day 10). Are any participants revamping their exercise plans? What will they do differently?
Group Motivation	**Restaurant Strategies** – Discuss strategies and experiences from the last week's Eating Out homework and/or pass around printed dining out tips from websites. **Local Info** – Encourage each other to share information on local grocers, sale items, meat farmers, farmer's market products and potential restaurant meals. **Paleo Entertaining Ideas (Day 10)** – Why do these approaches work? What makes these ideas valuable beyond the *Paleovation* program? Which ideas appeal to the group members? Brainstorm additional recipes that fit into each category.
Cooking Assignment #4 Jerky or Granola	Review the assignment directions in Day 11. Ask the group for any personal experiences in making jerky or granola. Share tips, tricks, recipes, results, etc.

Optional Enrichment: These activities can be completed or discussed during Meeting #3
- Share results of the Rising Test (Day 9) and/or personal strategies to reduce sedentary behaviors.
- Review the non-dairy calcium foods (Day 7). Identify specific foods each participant is including. Discuss why less total calcium is necessary when following a Paleo Diet.
- Discuss misleading food labels. Use information from the Marketing Magic boxes (Prep C, Prep E, Day 6, Day 22) and animal product terms (Days 5 and 7) to illustrate why labels are difficult to interpret. Brainstorm solutions to locate quality food products.
- Watch/review the optional food-related documentary selected at Meeting #2 (Day 5): Share thoughts on initial reactions, arguments presented that reinforce Paleo eating principles, takeaway points, etc.
- Survey interest levels of ending Meeting #4 with a guided meditation and/or breathing exercise; a volunteer can locate an appropriate activity (CD/DVD, app, online site/channel or library resource; Day 18 has breathing exercise info; also arrange for a speaker system, player, projector, wi-fi access, etc).
- Assign each participant a shake-it-up recipe (Day 13) and/or unsweetened beverage (Day 16). Bring in samples at the next meeting. Split up supplies such as plates, napkins, cups, silverware, etc.

Homework Assignment: Lifestyle Support
Diet is one pillar of health, but sleep, stress, movement, connections to others are equally important. Each participant selects one of the following to complete before Meeting #4, the group leader shares his/her homework results to introduce the project:
1. Complete the non-sedentary plan (Day 9) and movement plan (Day 19), tailoring to your personal needs.
2. Remove any remaining crutches and adhere to the Strict Paleo Protocol for the rest of the program.
3. Write 5-10 *new* actions you are taking to actively manage stress and sleep (Days 12 and 13).

Adjourning Thoughts
- ✓ Take a moment after the meeting to read the printed off articles brought in by others.
- ✓ Use the social media or email groups for motivation, clarification, sharing meal photos, tips & tricks, etc.
- ✓ Meeting #4's topics cover information in Days 11-18. Please keep up with the daily reading.
- ✓ Pay attention to stress reduction and sleep support strategies, report on techniques that work for you (and if you have a pair of blue-light blocking glasses *bring them to the next meeting* for Show & Tell).
- ✓ Compile questions, concerns and any useful recommended articles to discuss at Meeting #4.

⚐ Meeting #4 – Stress Management and Sleep Importance

Background and Basics: Participants are on Days 18-22 of the program. They currently are tapering off the low-carb flu and beginning to experience real health improvements. This is the perfect time to expand the focus on whole lifestyle support, not just dietary support. This meeting covers topics from Days 11-18.

A. Group Leader Preparation Checklist:

- ☐ **Content Research** – Read *The Paleovation Workbook* through Day 18.
  - a. Compile a list of stress management and sleep support techniques
  - b. Take notes on the information and activities you personally want to highlight at Meeting #4
- ☐ **Discussion Topics** – Browse the subject matter. Jot down ideas to share in the agenda margins.
  - a. Review all information referenced in the outline; there may be questions about reintroducing fruits upon reaching Day 22 so also scan Days 21 and 22 for basic background information
  - b. Sticky flag / dog-ear pages referenced in the topics for quick access during the meeting
  - c. [Optional]: Make a blown-up copy of the Cortisol Tube for a visual aide
  - d. Compile ideas for supplementary topics or concerns relevant to your group
  - e. Preview Cooking Assignment #5 (roast a chicken): Complete ahead to share your experience
- ☐ **Optional Enrichment** – Preview the options and arrange logistics for activity selections.
- ☐ **"Reading Ahead" Homework Assignment** – Preview the text in Days 22-27. Take note of any topics you want the group to focus on during their reading. For instance, how the reintro rules and long-term strategies are interspersed throughout; ideas especially relevant for your group (variety of long-term approaches, determining individual carbohydrate tolerance, establishing a healthy baseline); etc.
- ☐ **[Optional]: Meeting #6's Homework** – if Meeting #5 will be the final meeting, it is possible incorporate the Kitchen Gadget homework. The group leader brings in a favorite gadget to introduce the project.
- ☐ **Group Communication** – Check in with the group via email or social media during the week:
  - a. Encourage members to use the online group support as necessary for motivation, questions, etc
  - b. Remind the group of their Lifestyle Support Homework a day or two before meeting #4
  - c. Coordinate and remind participants of any optional enrichment activities selected (lunch/coffee, potluck signups, recipe exchange, wear comfortable clothing for meditation, volunteers, etc)
- ☐ **Anything else to bring?** Pens, list of complementary topics, unanswered questions list, scissors, etc.

B. Meeting Agenda [Participants are on Day 18-21]

By this point, participants will understand that establishing good health is not achieved by diet alone. A well-balanced, wholesome lifestyle includes a nutritious diet but also sensible exercise, stress reduction and sleep support. This meeting is an opportunity to discuss the importance of these additional pillars of optimal health.

Meeting #4: Discussion Topics	
Objectives	**Subject Matter and Dialogue Cues**
Share Experiences	1. Have each individual discuss positive changes they are observing. Compare their current benefits against their notations in Day 9, Section IV and Day 13, Section III. What other positive health benefits are emerging? 2. What grain substitutes were made for Cooking Assignment #3? Results? Will participants make these recipes again? Is there another they would like to try? 3. Discuss Halfway Hooray (Day 15, Section II). Congratulations to the group! Did anyone incorporate a non-food reward? Other reward possibilities? 4. Discuss homework: adjusting movement plan, crutches or sleep/stress support.
Tweaking the Paleo Protocol	Day 14 addresses common modifications to tweak the Paleo protocol for personal needs. Share individual experiences with the too-much and too-little chart topics.
Cortisol Tube	**Chronic Cortisol Tube** – Remove the copy from the Resource Section, roll and tape into place. Pass around for those who did not do this at home.

Objectives	Subject Matter and Dialogue Cues (Meeting #4 Continued)
Sleep and Stress Support	**Stress:** Discuss the critical points of stress elevation and stress reduction: 1. Excessive cortisol overrides hormonal signaling throughout the body. Discuss these implications as a group: raises blood sugar levels, prevents fat burning, interrupts sleep cycles, affects heart and breathing rates, etc. 2. Discuss keys for calming the cortisol response. The stress reducing techniques on Day 12 can prompt discussion on what works for each individual. **Sleep:** The sleep topic on Day 13 lays out different approaches to enhance sleep. What techniques have participants tried? Did anyone bring blue-light glasses?
Answer Questions	Paleo-Wise sections covered cortisol, stress, sleep, fiber, bone health, cholesterol* and heart disease*. Answers can be found in the text, via personal experience or in additional reading recommendations. 1. Review questions from the end of Meeting #3. 2. Use the members' questions on new topics to guide the group discussion. 3. Record remaining questions to see if answers emerge by the next meeting. *Please note, some facilitators are not as familiar with the nonstandard viewpoints presented in these topics. It is possible to have a casual conversation to recap the information presented, but an answer of "I don't know" is completely acceptable.
Group Motivation	Cooking assignments include Paleo staple recipes for hard-to-find or expensive foods. Are participants motivated to try another vegetable-as-a-grain recipe? Cooking assignment #4: Survey participants to see which recipe (jerky or granola) they will make by their Day 19. Has anyone already finished? The program allows more fruit on Day 22 – is the group excited? What fruits are the participants missing? Is anyone concerned about fruit creating sweet cravings? The **Healthy Baseline Chart** in the Resources is a fundamental piece for food group reintroductions and construction of long-term strategies. Review this chart together and note all the facets of health that are affected by dietary choices.
Cooking Assignment #5 Roast a Chicken	Review the assignment directions on Day 15. Survey the group to see who has experience roasting a whole chicken. Share tips, tricks, recipes, results, etc.

Optional Enrichment: These activities can be completed or discussed during Meeting #4.
- Turn part of this meeting into a *walking meeting* or a *stand-up-and-stretch discussion*
- Share thoughts on connections to self, others, nature and spirituality (Day 12)
- Discuss personal stress manifestation symptoms (Day 11, Section II) and how it's helpful to recognize these in order to dissipate overall stress levels
- Practice a guided meditation or breathing exercise together (Day 18 has belly breathing suggestions)

Homework Assignment: Reading Ahead – The Reintroduction Guidelines
Read sections on reintroduction guidelines and long-term strategies up through Day 27 before next week's meeting. This means some members need to read ahead to be fully prepared for the discussion.
[**Optional:** If next week is the final gathering, it's possible to assign Meeting #5's Kitchen Gadget Homework]

Adjourning Thoughts
- ✓ Take a moment after the meeting to read the articles brought in by others.
- ✓ Next week's discussion will be about reintroductions and long-term strategies, specifically note:
  - ○ Healthy Baseline Chart in the Resource Section
  - ○ Markers of health (Day 25)
  - ○ Carb tolerance topics and flowsheet (Days 23 and24)
  - ○ Long-term lifestyle strategies that appeal to you
- ✓ Meeting #5 covers topics in Days 19-27. Keep up with the daily reading and *read ahead if necessary*.
- ✓ Keep a running list of questions, concerns or articles to share and discuss at Meeting #5.
- ✓ Cholesterol and Heart Disease are mentally challenging topics (Days 17 and 18), reread if desired.

Meeting #5 – Long-Term Strategies and Guidelines

Background and Basics: Participants are on Days 25-28 of the program. For some groups this will be the final meeting – formulating long-term strategies is the main focus. This meeting covers topics from Days 19-27.

A. Group Leader Preparation Checklist:

☐ **Content Research** – Read *The Paleovation Workbook* through Day 27.
    a. Compile a list of low-carb flu symptoms and relief strategies
    b. Take notes on the information and activities you personally want to highlight at Meeting #5

☐ **Discussion Topics** – Browse the subject matter. Jot down ideas to share in the agenda margins.
    a. Review all information referenced in the outline, especially sections that appear after Day 27
    b. Sticky flag / dog-ear pages referenced in the topics for quick access during the meeting
    c. Compile ideas for supplemental topics or concerns relevant to your group
    d. If this will be the group's final meeting, review the agenda for Meeting #6 to incorporate any additional topics and ideas into Meeting #5

☐ **Optional Enrichment** – Preview the options and arrange logistics for activity selections.

☐ **[Optional Homework for Meeting #6]**: Kitchen Gadget Homework– Bring in one of your own gadgets to provide an example of tools that make Paleo eating easier.

☐ **Group Communication** – Check in with the group via email or social media during the week:
    a. Encourage members to use the online group support as necessary for motivation, questions, etc
    b. Remind the group of their homework assignment(s) a day or two before Meeting #5
    c. Coordinate and remind participants of any optional enrichment activities selected at previous meetings (lunch/coffee meet-ups, recipe exchange, "after" photos, etc)

☐ **Anything else?** Pens, slips of paper to share results, additional topics list, unanswered question list, etc.

B. Meeting Agenda [Participants are on Day 25-28]

Today's goals are to solidify the food reintroduction process and help participants develop long-term strategies to support and maintain life-long health. If this is the last meeting, *congratulate the group on a job well done!*

Meeting #5: Discussion Topics	
Objectives	**Subject Matter and Dialogue Cues**
Share Experiences	1. Discuss the Healthy Baseline Chart. Draw attention to the importance of monitoring multiple aspects of health to maintain long-term success. Do members like the chart? Did any member experience additional improvement over the week? What other areas of body awareness are important to health? 2. Review results of cooking assignments #4 and #5: how did the recipes turn out, share experience of cooking a whole chicken, what will they make again, etc 3. [Optional: Kitchen Gadget Homework if assigned at Meeting #4]
Bye to Conventional Wisdom	Day 19 discusses which conventional wisdom points have not served the general population well. To maintain life-long health, it is useful to denote which conventional wisdom health strategies do not nurture optimal well-being.

Reintroduction Guidelines	Day 25 emphasizes the individual must be ready for food reintroduction – some people take more time than others to reset their health.
	  A. The Markers of Health (Day 25) break down optimal health into a few categories. Let participants discuss how they feel about their current markers and readiness.
	  B. Continued Complications Table (Day 25) identifies areas where more improvement can develop. Is anyone borderline on extending the protocol for 2 more weeks?
	Day 26 outlines the reintroduction methods. Use the Healthy Baseline Chart and Food Reintroduction Diary (Resource Section) to illustrate how to compare and contrast health factors during food reintroduction trials. Are participants clear on the process?

Objectives	Subject Matter and Dialogue Cues (Meeting #5 Continued)
Answer Questions	Paleo-Wise sections covered environmental toxins, gut health, fructose, organ meats and controversial foods such as coffee, GMOs and exogenous ketone supplements. 1. Review questions from the end of Meeting #4. 2. Discuss any new questions that emerged during the past week. Brainstorm additional information resources for participants to use in the future.
Group Motivation	Complete Post-Paleo Check Out (Day 28) and score. Potential to share how many points gained, best improvement categories so far, benefits that remain slow to improve, surprising results or categories marked with the extra 'blown away' point, etc. Days 22-27 highlight numerous maintenance mode strategies including food tolerance, other ancestral diet paradigms, the author's long-term approaches, carb cravings, etc. How will the ground rules (Day 23) be useful for each participant? What specific strategies appeal to each member and why? Permanent dietary and lifestyle transformation requires conscientious choices and proper understanding of how facets of health are intertwined. Discuss how each participant will monitor their pillars of health: diet, movement, stress, sleep, connecting to self/others/nature/spirituality and creating a healthy environment. Strategies to regain control after straying too far outside the Strict Paleo Protocol will be necessary for each member at some point. Discuss suggestions in Day 24.

Optional Enrichment: These activities can be included during Meeting #5 or saved for optional Meeting #6*

- Walk through an example of the Carb Tolerance Flowchart (Day 24 or in the Resource Section); optional: to enlarge a copy as a visual aide
- Ask the members to describe ways they've fallen off a healthy diet in the past; as a group, form a comprehensive plan to address that situation in the future (examples in Day 27)
- Discuss how personal health strategies will change once this group discontinues meeting
- Compile the group average on the Post-Paleo Check Out for comparison with original score, if taken
- Each participant anonymously writes down their best health benefit so far and gives to group leader – the group then guesses who wrote them
- * Revisit optional photos taken during the 1st meeting and take follow up photos and headshots; use the before/after photo comparison questions on Day 28 for discussion
- * Plan a reunion in 1-2 months to discuss how reintroductions and long-term strategies are working

Homework Assignment: Reintroduction Discussion [Optional Meeting #6: Kitchen Gadget Homework]
Report back on the first reintroduction including what was eaten, how it tasted, if the body had any reaction, strategies to narrow down tolerance and what was learned to assist in future reintroductions.

> **If this is the final meeting:** Use the support email list or social media group to share your personal reintroduction experience.

> **[If planning the optional Meeting #6]:** Be prepared to share your reintroduction experience at the next meeting. Additionally, bring in favorite kitchen gadget(s) that make Paleo eating easier (or a description of them). How often did you use it? What recipes did you make with it? How did it save you time/money?

Adjourning Thoughts
- ✓ Congratulate your group and highlight the positive changes seen in each member.
- ✓ Take a moment after the meeting to read the article print offs brought in by others.
- ✓ Encourage continued communication via email or social media for recipe sharing, local food products or restaurant strategies, planning a get together, meditation or exercise meet ups, local events, etc.
- * [Optional] Meeting #6's topics include a more in-depth coverage of "advanced" Paleo methods: fermented foods, intermittent fasting, Paleo treats, tweaking the Paleo Protocol, resource articles, etc. Review pertinent sections noted in Meeting #6's agenda.
- * [Optional] Meeting #6 can include specific topic requests from the members. Survey participants to determine which subjects to revisit (use the Paleo-Wise Wrap-Up chart in Day 24).

⚓ Meeting #6 – Discuss Reintroduction Trials

Background & Basics: Participants have completed the 28-days of Strict Paleo Protocol portion of the program and have already reintroduced their first non-Paleo food. This meeting covers topics from Day 28, Resource Sections and initial reintroduction experiences (browse discussion list below for other topics to re-read).

A. Group Leader Preparation Checklist:

☐ **Content Research** – Read *The Paleovation Workbook* through Day 28 and all the Resource Section topics. Take notes on the information and activities you personally want to highlight at Meeting #6.

☐ **Discussion Topics** – Browse the subject matter. Jot down ideas to share in the agenda margins.
   a. Review all information in the agenda, including topics the group members want to revisit
   b. Sticky flag / dog-ear pages referenced in the topics for quick access during the meeting
   c. Compile ideas for complementary topics or concerns relevant to your group

☐ **Group Communication** – Check in with the group via email or social media during the week:
   a. Encourage members to use the online group support as necessary for motivation, questions, etc
   b. Remind the group of their Kitchen Gadget Homework a day or two before Meeting #6
   c. Coordinate and remind participants of any optional enrichment activities previously selected (specifics for lunch/coffee meet-ups, recipe exchange, "after" photos, etc)

☐ **Anything else?** Pens, additional topics, unanswered questions list, etc.

___

B. Meeting Agenda:
This final meeting is the opportunity to walk through and analyze food reintroductions and revisit previous topics for additional clarification. *Congratulate your group on a job well done!*

Meeting #6: Discussion Topics	
Objectives	**Subject Matter and Dialogue Cues**
Share Experiences	1. Share current reintroduction experiences including reinstated foods, reactions, ease of using the Healthy Baseline Chart, unexpected tolerance/reaction, etc. 2. Pass around or describe favorite kitchen gadgets. Each participant can share why this tool is useful for them, the recipes they were able to make with it, stores where it is available, etc.
Answer Questions	Topics may include fermented foods, prebiotics and probiotics for gut health (Day 21), incorporating organ meats (Day 23), intermittent fasting (Day 27), treats (Day 28), autoimmune protocol and nutritional supplements (Resource Section). 1. Review questions from the end of Meeting #5. 2. Discuss any new questions that emerged during the past week. Brainstorm additional information resources for participants to use in the future.
Group Motivation	Tweaking Paleo is an ongoing lifestyle experiment. Options are outlined in Days 14 and 25 as well as the AIP (autoimmune protocol) guidelines in the Resource Section. Which suggestions has the group already put into practice? Which ideas are appropriate to use long-term?

Optional Enrichment: These activities can be completed during Meeting #6
- Revisit optional photos taken during the 1st meeting and take follow up photos and headshots; use the before/after photo comparison questions on Day 28 for discussion
- Plan a reunion in 1-2 months to discuss how reintroductions and long-term strategies are working

Adjourning Thoughts
✓ Take a moment after the meeting to read the article print offs brought in by others
✓ Use the support email list or social media group to share your continued reintroduction experience.
✓ Encourage continued communication via email or social media for recipe sharing, local food products or restaurant strategies, planning a get together, meditation or exercise meet ups, local events, etc.

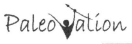 **KITCHEN CLEAN-OUT: FOODS TO ELIMINATE**

These foods must be avoided during your first Paleo month: No *Exceptions*!

Refined Grains

- ☐ Bread
- ☐ Cereal
- ☐ Tortillas
- ☐ Granola
- ☐ Protein bars
- ☐ Popcorn
- ☐ Crackers
- ☐ Pretzels
- ☐ Cookies
- ☐ Granola bars
- ☐ Pita bread
- ☐ Oatmeal
- ☐ Croissants
- ☐ Muffins
- ☐ Pancake mix
- ☐ Bagels
- ☐ Grits
- ☐ Pasta
- ☐ Rice
- ☐ Starch/Flour
- ☐ Corn chips
- ☐ Tortilla chips
- ☐ Muffin mix
- ☐ Couscous

Whole Grains and Pseudo-Grains

- ☐ Wheat
- ☐ Quinoa
- ☐ Bran
- ☐ Rye
- ☐ Corn
- ☐ Spelt
- ☐ Germ
- ☐ Rice
- ☐ Amaranth
- ☐ Wheat berries
- ☐ Buckwheat
- ☐ Chia
- ☐ Barley
- ☐ Bulgur
- ☐ Groats
- ☐ Oats
- ☐ Millet
- ☐ Teff

Potatoes - Everyone should eliminate processed versions of potatoes for the program. If interested in losing weight, we recommend eliminating *all* potatoes until you have reached your goal weight.

- ☐ White
- ☐ Red
- ☐ Gold
- ☐ Fingerling
- ☐ Chips/Fries
- ☐ Other Processed

Legumes

- ☐ Black beans
- ☐ Refried beans
- ☐ Peanut butter
- ☐ Lima beans
- ☐ Edamame
- ☐ Soybeans
- ☐ Mung beans
- ☐ Kidney beans
- ☐ Soy lecithin
- ☐ Chickpeas
- ☐ Navy beans
- ☐ Pinto beans
- ☐ Tofu
- ☐ Soy sauce
- ☐ Peanuts
- ☐ Lentils
- ☐ Peas
- ☐ Tamari
- ☐ White beans
- ☐ Miso
- ☐ Tempeh
- ☐ Hummus

High-Sugar Fruits (all fruit except those labeled in the low-sugar fruits section in Prep B)

- ☐ Fresh
- ☐ Canned
- ☐ Frozen
- ☐ Dried
- ☐ Juice
- ☐ Jam/Jelly

Dairy Products

- ☐ Cow milk
- ☐ Goat milk
- ☐ Sheep milk
- ☐ Cottage cheese
- ☐ Yogurt
- ☐ Whey Protein
- ☐ Coffee creamer
- ☐ Whipped cream
- ☐ Cream
- ☐ Sour cream
- ☐ Powdered milk
- ☐ Conventional butter (grass-fed is okay)
- ☐ Half † half
- ☐ Ice cream
- ☐ Cheeses
- ☐ Kefir

Beverages

- ☐ Alcohol
- ☐ Sweet teas
- ☐ Soda
- ☐ Diet soda
- ☐ Juice
- ☐ Soft drinks
- ☐ Presweetened coffee drinks
- ☐ Energy/sports drinks
- ☐ Shake or smoothie mixes

Sweeteners

- ☐ Sugar
- ☐ Corn syrup
- ☐ Sweet'N Low®
- ☐ Brown sugar
- ☐ Honey
- ☐ Agave nectar
- ☐ Maple syrup
- ☐ Coconut sugar
- ☐ Nutrasweet®
- ☐ Molasses
- ☐ Sugar alcohols
- ☐ Splenda®
- ☐ Dates
- ☐ Equal®

Fats and Oils

- ☐ Canola oil
- ☐ Soybean oil
- ☐ Coffee creamer
- ☐ Safflower oil
- ☐ Margarine
- ☐ Whipped topping
- ☐ Grapeseed oil
- ☐ Vegetable oil
- ☐ Shortening
- ☐ Sunflower oil
- ☐ Butter spreads
- ☐ Corn oil
- ☐ Crisco

Questionable Foods – Examine Ingredients

READ LABELS! The following items may be perfectly acceptable *if they have clean ingredients*. However, these products typically contain non-Paleo additives, so you must read EVERY LABEL. If the following ingredients are present, remove the item from your kitchen.

Chemicals and Additives to Avoid:

MSG, carrageenan, food colorings, sodium benzoate, soy ingredients, casein/whey, corn-derived additives, wheat-derived ingredients, grains, dairy, sweeteners, industrialized oils, sulfites and anything you can't pronounce or don't recognize. Check ☝ Pinterest.com/Paleovation Sneaky Food Additives

---

Reading the Ingredients Label: Just because a product is organic or gluten-free does not mean it is anti-inflammatory. In this example Sauce #2 is the clear winner.

Marinara Sauce 1: Organic Tomato Puree (Water, Tomato Paste), Organic Diced Tomatoes in Juice, Organic **Soybean** Oil, Organic **Sugar**, Organic Extra Virgin Olive Oil, Organic Onions, Sea Salt, Organic Garlic, Organic **Romano Cheese** (Organic Cultured Part Skim **Milk**, Salt, Enzymes), Organic Basil, Organic Black Pepper

Marinara Sauce 2: Imported Italian Plum Tomatoes, Extra Virgin Olive Oil, Onions, Garlic, Basil, Salt

---

PANTRY

- ☐ Gluten-free goods (often contain other grains)
- ☐ Canned goods like fish, sauce and vegetables
- ☐ Boxed/canned broth or stock
- ☐ Bottled items such as marinara sauce
- ☐ Premade or boxed meals/mixes
- ☐

- ☐ Nut butters (legumes, sugar, veg oil)
- ☐ Nuts roasted in seed oils
- ☐ Soups / soup mix
- ☐ Boxed drinks and drink mixes
- ☐ Sauce mixes
- ☐

FRIDGE/FREEZER

- ☐ Salad dressing
- ☐ Ketchup
- ☐ Mustard
- ☐ Teriyaki sauce
- ☐ Hot sauce
- ☐ Olives
- ☐ Other condiments
- ☐

- ☐ Marinades
- ☐ Nut milks
- ☐ Barbecue sauce
- ☐ Salsa
- ☐ Mayonnaise
- ☐ Pickles
- ☐ Pre-made meals
- ☐

SPICE CUPBOARD

- ☐ Table salt (dextrose and anti-caking ingredients)
- ☐ Bouillon cubes
- ☐ Soft drink mixes
- ☐ Vanilla extract (contains alcohol)

- ☐ Seasoning mix packs (taco, onion soup mix)
- ☐ Baking powder (contains corn starch)
- ☐ Purchased seasoning salts
- ☐

OTHER

- ☐ Prepared tea and coffee drink mixes (watch for sugars)
- ☐ Kombucha (no added sugar)
- ☐ Dried tea (some have soy or wheat)
- ☐

Autoimmune Protocol (AIP) Resources

> *I did as much research as I could and I took ownership of this illness,*
> *because if you don't take care of your body, where are you going to live? ~Karen Duffy*

Discover Relief with Dietary Change

Dietary change is an instrumental first step in renewing health...and the nourishing Paleo Diet has the power to soothe autoimmune symptoms. Many people with autoimmune conditions have been able to rekindle their health and rebuild their bodies healthier and stronger just by changing the foods they eat.

Success stories are abundantly shared in the online autoimmune community. Feel free to search "Paleo + [your condition] success stories" to read input from others. "Success" varies from person to person – lowering pain intensity is one person's success while to another, major flare-ups can be minimized with diet alone.

Although it's impossible to know exactly where you will fall on this spectrum, know that dietary change is the perfect place to begin the healing process. As always, talk with your medical providers. Let them know you intend to eliminate inflammatory foods for one month to observe your body's reaction.

AIP Resource Topics:

1. Autoimmune Protocol (AIP) Defined
2. The AIP Community
3. AIP Implementation
4. AIP Expectations for Healing
5. Food Reintroductions after Completing an AIP Elimination

> *All autoimmune diseases are characterized by an overactive immune system, which leads to chronic inflammation and tissue destruction. In fact, the main feature that differentiates one autoimmune disease from another, is simply the part of the body (the type of tissue) that is under attack by the immune system. For example, rheumatoid arthritis is the result of the immune system attacking the joints, whereas multiple sclerosis is caused by the immune system attacking the myelin sheath surrounding nerves. ~Sara Gottfried MD*

Section I: Autoimmune Protocol (AIP) Defined

The AIP is a step beyond Paleo, just like Paleo is a step beyond gluten-free. Due to the connection between autoimmune disease and leaky gut, the AIP identifies additional foods which irritate the immune system and/or gut lining. The following foods contain common triggers for autoimmune flare-ups: eggs, nightshade vegetables, nuts, seeds, nightshade- and seed-based spices, coffee, cocoa and the usual non-Paleo foods (grains, legumes, dairy, industrial seed oils, additives).

The AIP is designed to simultaneously remove all the likely food culprits while incorporating even more gut-soothing foods. Without the interference of these irritants, the body is given its very best chance to heal. These items do not need to be avoided forever, but they are eliminated until the individual feels better. At that point, tolerance to these typical triggers is tested via controlled reintroduction.

> **Case for the Full AIP Elimination:** Because removing one item at a time may not reveal the same personal insights or health benefits, consider implementing the full AIP at some point in the future. It is perfectly acceptable to begin with the standard Strict Paleo Protocol and work your way into AIP.

Focus on Healing Foods

Respect that this is a fresh start. Many individuals never realize that common, everyday foods significantly interfere with the gut lining and overall health. But once we know better, we can do better...the AIP provides nutrients the body needs in the forms it prefers.

> *Let food be thy medicine and medicine be thy food. ~Hippocrates*

To begin, focus on consuming more healing foods than harming foods, listed in the next table.

AIP Food Categorization	
Healing	**Harming**
<ul><li>**Abundant Vegetables** focus on deep colors, leafy greens and those which contain sulfur such as cruciferous*, onions and mushrooms</li><li>**Sea Vegetables** (*excluding* immune-stimulating algae like chlorella and spirulina)</li><li>**Organ Meats and Other Offal**</li><li>**Fish and Shellfish** especially wild-caught</li><li>**Quality Meats** especially free-range, wild-caught, grass-fed and pasture-raised</li><li>**Quality Fats** high-quality lard, tallow, duck fat and olive, avocado, coconut and palm oils</li><li>**Low-Sugar Fruit** enjoy 10-20g of fructose daily</li><li>**Probiotic Foods** fermented vegetables, kefir (from wate or coconut milk), homemade coconut milk yogurt, kombucha, supplements</li><li>**Glycine-Rich Foods** any foods with connective tissue including joints, skin, organ meats, collagen/gelatin and bone broth</li><li>**Bone Broth** straight from a mug, as a soup base or added into recipes or leftovers</li><li>**Well-Cooked Foods** are easier to digest: soups, stews, slow-cooked meats, crock pot meals</li><li>**Herbs and Teas** especially ginger and turmeric for anti-inflammatory benefits</li><li>**Trace Minerals** use Himalayan pink salt, Celtic sea salt or add a trace mineral supplement</li></ul>	<ul><li>**Non-Paleo foods**: all grains, dairy, *all* legumes (*including* green beans and snow/snap peas), industrial seed oils</li><li>**Eggs**</li><li>**Nuts**</li><li>**Seeds** including seed-based spices[†]</li><li>**Nightshades**: potatoes, tomatoes, bell peppers, eggplant, tomatillos, chili peppers, goji berries and nightshade-based spices[†]</li><li>**Coffee**</li><li>**Cocoa**</li><li>**Fructose:** use low-sugar fruits</li><li>**Alcohol**</li><li>**Caffeine**</li><li>**Potential "Gluten Cross-Reactive" Foods**: all grains, quinoa, hemp, teff, tapioca, potato, soy, dairy products *including ghee*, chocolate, yeast, sesame, eggs, coffee</li><li>**NSAIDS[‡]** certain painkillers such as aspirin, ibuprofen, some prescriptions</li><li>**Additives** such as emulsifiers, preservatives, colorings and natural or artificial sweeteners</li><li>**Food Allergens/Sensitivities**, do not consume any foods that create discomfort for you even if they are AIP-friendly (such as coconut or shellfish)</li></ul>

* **C**ruciferous vegetables include broccoli, cabbage, cauliflower, Brussels sprouts, kale, turnips, arugula, mustard greens, watercress, etc (tip: cooked or fermented versions may be easier to digest than raw).

[†] See *AIP Spice Guide* on the next page.

[‡] Do not stop pain medication if you are still in pain. Your medical providers must supervise all medication adjustments to fine-tune your body needs (direct links available from ⏎ Paleovation).

⏎ PhoenixHelix Where Medication Fits on a Healing Diet

⏎ PhoenixHelix When Painkillers Are Good for You

The take home point about AIP is that if you have an autoimmune issue, you most likely have a poorly functioning digestive tract. Because your gut is not in the best shape, byproducts of all of the things passing through your intestines are leaking through your gut barrier into your blood stream, causing your immune system to respond. This concept is fundamental to understanding why the AIP works in decreasing inflammation and immune system stimulation. ~Megan McGrane, PA, writer for UltimatePaleoGuide.com

As you compile your thoughts about the healing versus harming foods, remember that this is a temporary protocol to enhance healing. Numerous resources exist to help embrace this dietary tool to reestablish health.

⏎ ThePaleoMom 20 Keys to Success on the Autoimmune Protocol

⏎ ThePaleoMom AIP Mindset: Getting Beyond Feeling Deprived

⏎ ThePaleoMom AIP Mindset: Cooking is Not a Burden

⏎ ThePaleoMom AIP Mindset: Putting Myself First

⏎ ThePaleoMom AIP Mindset: Optimism, Hope and Healing

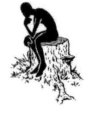

Autoimmune Seasoning

The AIP-restricted nightshade- and seed-based spices are grayed in the following table:

AIP Seasoning Guide		
Spices	**Herbs**	**Spice Blending†**
Allspice	Basil*	
Anise	Chamomile*	*Italian Herbs* – Oregano, basil, rosemary,
Bay Leaf	Chervil	thyme, marjoram
Black Pepper*	Chives*	
Caraway	Cilantro*	*Italian Sausage/Pizza* – salt, pepper,
Cardamom*	Dill weed	fennel/anise, + Italian herbs
Cayenne Pepper*	Dill seed	
Celery Seed	Lavender	*Chili Seasoning* – chili powder, cumin, garlic,
Chili Peppers	Lemon Balm	oregano, onion, paprika
Cinnamon*	Lemongrass	
Clove*	Marjoram	*Curry Powder (purchased)* – turmeric,
Cocoa Powder	Mint	coriander, cumin, ginger, nutmeg, cinnamon,
Coriander	Oregano	garlic, clove, pepper
Cumin	Parsley*	
Fennel	Rosemary*	*Herbes de Provence* – thyme, rosemary, basil,
Garlic Powder*	Sage	oregano, dill, tarragon, fennel
Garlic*	Savory	
Ginger*	Tarragon	*Mexican* – paprika, salt, onion, garlic, cumin,
Horseradish	Thyme	oregano, pepper, cocoa
Lemon Zest		
Mace		*Asian 5-Spice* – ginger, nutmeg, cinnamon,
Mustard		anise, clove, pepper
Nutmeg*		
Onion Powder		*Lemon Pepper* – pepper, lemon zest, salt
Paprika		
Poppy seed		*Garlic & Herb* – garlic, basil, parsley, oregano
Saffron		
Shallots		
Star anise		
Turmeric*		
Vanilla Bean (not extract)		

   * Anti-inflammatory properties, especially turmeric and ginger

     <u>Interesting note</u>: *Anise* is from a seed (non-AIP) while *star anise* is from a berry (AIP-friendly)

   † For spice blending recipes check ⌐ WellnessMama 14 Homemade Spice Blends

Flavorful Food

Notice how *nearly half* the spices and *all* the green herbs are safe! Even the spice blends will taste amazing without the nightshade/seed spices. Use citrus zest to brighten a dish, mix your own seasoning blends, add a spicy kick with ginger or horseradish and focus on including flavors you enjoy.

> **"Herbamare" Herbed Sea Salt by A. Vogel:** This AIP-friendly sea salt and herb blend is widely available

Again, this is not a *forever and ever* ban on nightshade- and seed-based spices. It's only until the body is ready to test individual sensitivities. Daunting? Yes. Do-able? Yes. It's all part of committing to better health. Remember, there is help available:

   ⌐ PhoenixHelix Nightshade-Free Survival Guide

   ⌐ ThePaleoMom Spices on the Autoimmune Protocol

Section II: The AIP Community
When Doubt Sets In

Looking over the AIP restricted foods list generates many questions: Am I really supposed to make meatloaf without eggs or breadcrumbs? Is it possible to make marinara without tomato? Can I make taco filling without the tomato and chili powder? What about salsa...or chili...or BBQ sauce? Is there anything left to eat?

Rather than feel discouraged or alone, realize there are many people who already feel better by following the AIP – you can be next. The AIP community is tightly knit...extensive information is available to help educate about your body and embrace the changes it takes to implement the AIP.

The AIP community adapts favorite recipes like Nomato Sauce, Notato Salad, Egg-Free Mayo, AIP Tacos, sauces, condiments and even tips on finding AIP-friendly prepared foods. These various tidbits are always presented with the wisdom and personal experiences of others who restored health through dietary change:

AIP Information (direct links availbale from ◌ Paleovation)	
Author with Autoimmune: Website	**Notable Material**
Sarah Ballantyne: ◌ ThePaleoMom	• Online overview of the AIP: ◌ ThePaleoMom AIP Protocol • Detailed autoimmune information: ▭ *The Paleo Approach* • Cookbooks: ▭ *The Paleo Approach Cookbook* and co-authored ▭ *The Healing Kitchen* with Alaena Haber
Terry Wahls, MD: ◌ TerryWahls	▭ *The Wahls Protocol* ⊛ TEDx talks by Terry Wahls, MD 🎧 Popular guest on many podcasts • The nonprofit Wahls Foundation supports clinical trials to study the effect of lifestyle change on chronic disease and educates the public about integrative treatment
Eileen Laird: ◌ PhoenixHelix	◌ PhoenixHelix AIP Recipe Roundtables ◌ PhoenixHelix Inspirational Stories • Podcast, AIP eBooks ◌▭ including *A Simple Guide to the Paleo Autoimmune Protocol*

Mickey Trescott and Angie Alt: ◌ AutoimmuneWellness	• Coauthors of ▭ *The Autoimmune Wellness Handbook: A DIY Guide to Living Well with Chronic Illness*
	◌ AutoimmuneWellness AIP Stories of Recovery Series
	• Programs for purchase: ◌ RealPlans menu plans based on sensitivities, ◌ AIPBatchcook for full make-ahead AIP menus
	• Cookbooks:
	  1. Alt: ▭ *The Alternative Autoimmune Cookbook*
	  2. Trescott: ▭ *The Autoimmune Paleo Cookbook*

Rachael Bryant: ◌ Meatified	• Cookbook: ▭ *Nourish: The Paleo Healing Cookbook* ◌ Meatified Autoimmune Paleo Resources
Bre'anna Emmitt: ◌ HeWontKnowItsPaleo	• Cookbook: ▭ *He Won't Know It's Paleo*
Christine Feindel: ◌ ACleanPlate	◌ ACleanPlate Resources • Various AIP eBooks available ◌▭ ACleanPlate

Good to Know: As more individuals use the AIP elimination diet to control their autoimmune conditions, new blogs, books, cookbooks and premade products will make their way into the market. There is no way to create a comprehensive list – keep researching.

Here is an *excellent* online compilation of *All-Things-AIP* including coaches and meet-up groups:
  ◌ ThePaleoMom AIP Community

Section III: AIP Implementation

Many individuals with known autoimmune conditions find basic relief of symptoms by following Paleo 'out-of-the-box;' however it is likely additional sensitivities exist. It's a personal choice whether to begin with Strict Paleo, slightly modify Strict Paleo (we recommend an egg-free version) or even jump straight into the AIP...some individuals are highly motivated because they've never before had a tool of this magnitude!

Tips for Getting Started

1. **Eat to Nourish:** In the beginning, focus on using food as a healing nutrient-delivery system...eat more healing foods than harming. Don't worry, you will eventually build an AIP repertoire.
2. **Meal Building:** Create meals using the Vegetable + Protein + Fat template (described in Day 1). Even if it doesn't look like a normal meal (maybe it's jerky, carrot slaw and some cucumber slices dipped in coconut butter), the body needs these nutrients and doesn't mind how they get in.
3. **Breakfast:** Because AIP is egg-free, traditional breakfast ideas are difficult to recreate. Instead, think of breakfast as an earlier version of lunch and rely on combinations you enjoy such as seasoned ground meat with sautéed sweet potatoes, meatballs and steamed broccoli, soups and stews or even salad.
4. **Educate Yourself:** Research online AIP articles; read an AIP book or ebook.
5. **Create a Support Network:** The AIP can be intimidating. Establish a strong, supportive foundation.
   a. Educate friends/family so they understand this next step in regaining your health
   b. Motivate yourself by reading AIP testimonials
   c. Use online forums to research and ask AIP-specific questions
   d. Join Facebook groups: AIP Support, Autoimmune Paleo Recipes, AIP for You and Me, etc
   e. Accept your efforts, even if you have a setback you are still heading in the right direction
6. **Eat Abundant Vegetables:** More than you think...Sarah Ballantyne recommends 8-14 cups per day and Wahls Protocol is 9+ cups (3 cups dark greens, 3 cups sulfur-rich and 3 cups brightly-colored). Do not be afraid – 3 cups of spinach cooks down to ~1/2 cup serving.

Finding Appropriate Recipes

Online AIP recipes (#AIP) are abundant but often accidentally include a non-AIP ingredient such as black pepper or mustard. Even on AIP-designated blogs, if the author has successfully reintroduced a few AIP items, those ingredients may start appearing in their recipes.

1. It is safest to use AIP print cookbooks for recipes; see previous table for recommendations.
2. The best online options
   ⤳ PhoenixHelix AIP Recipe Roundtables
   ⤳ Pinterest.com/Eileen1365 PhoenixHelix Pinterest
3. The ⤳ AIPBatchcook program adheres to sugar-free AIP recipes and is available for purchase.
4. Start slowly. Use simple meals as a foundation and gradually build an AIP recipe rotation. Follow the *Turn Back Time* recommendation to select 5 AIP Foundation Recipes that batch-cook or freeze well.

Budgeting

1. Purchase the best quality foods within your budget. Even with conventional meats and produce, the AIP easily surpasses the standard American diet (dietary benefits also stem from what you're *not* eating).
   ⤳ ThePaleoMom Can I Still Do Paleo if I Can't Afford Grass-Fed Beef?
2. Inexpensive nutritional powerhouses: homemade bone broth, organ meats, some shellfish like mussels.
3. Inexpensive anti-inflammatory foods: fresh or ground turmeric and ginger, gelatin or collagen (the price tag looks hefty, but a can lasts a long time).

Shopping

1. Use the downloadable ⤳ Whole30 Shopping List AIP
2. Some online stores like ⤳ GrasslandBeef US Wellness Meats include AIP filtering on their product lists
3. AIP Starter Kits are available ⤳ BarefootProvisions The Paleo Mom's AIP Survival Pack
4. Purchase AIP or Wahls Protocol meals at ⤳ PetesPaleo, ⤳ PreMadePaleo and ⤳ PaleoOnTheGo

Five Healing Foods
These restorative foods should have a place in your diet every week, or better – every day:

Top Five Restorative Foods	
Bone Broth (Prep F)	Bone broth is easily digested and provides unique amino acids often absent in western diets. Make your own or buy a high quality product. Consume at least one mug per day. <u>Tip</u>: A small percentage of the population is sensitive to histamines in food (<1%). If this describes you, a shorter-cooked broth (stock) may be more beneficial than a longer-cooked, traditional bone broth. ⌁ <u>PaleoLeap</u> All About Histamines ⌁ <u>AutoimmuneWellness</u> Could Histamine Intolerance Be Impacting Your Autoimmune Healing
Gelatin and Collagen (Days 6 and 16)	These proteins are anti-inflammatory, soothing for the digestive tract and healing for the entire body. Consume them via bone broth or by supplement. We recommend high quality brands such as Great Lakes or Vital Proteins. Gelatin dissolves in hot liquids and gels as it cools. Collagen powder readily blends into any food and does not gel.
Turmeric and Ginger	These roots offer anti-inflammatory, immune-boosting and digestive-enhancing properties. Use fresh or dried – in foods, teas or capsules*. ⌁ <u>PrimallyInspired</u> Turmeric Tea Liver Detox (omit pepper for full AIP, and honey during the program) ⌁ <u>WeedEmAndReap</u> The Best Natural Anti-Inflammatory
Liver and Other Offal (Day 23)	Organ meats are nutritional powerhouses containing all the nutrients necessary to support organ function. This technique is useful if you do not care for the taste (as a precaution, *cook the liver* before freezing): ⌁ <u>PrimallyInspired</u> Frozen Raw Liver Pills Alternatively, you can purchase a high quality desiccated liver product – Dr. Ron's and Vital Proteins are popular brands.
Omega-3's: EPA & DHA (Day 3)	Select fatty fish such as sardines or mackerel, or invest in a high quality EPA/DHA supplement*†.

*Caution: Work with your medical provider for drug interactions, especially blood thinners.

†Nutritional supplement information and recommendations in the Resource Section.

Other Often-Overlooked Factors
Healing from an autoimmune disorder isn't only about diet. It is also about creating and sustaining an entire atmosphere to promote healing. Each individual has his/her own challenges.

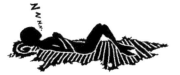

1. **Loving the Self:** A positive outlook and self-nurturing environment are both necessary for the body to heal. Autoimmune isn't a battle, it's about working with your body and learning to understand your unique challenges. The journey is very much about acceptance, gratitude and refusing to judge the self.
2. **Peaceful Sleep:** Sleep is a crucial component for all healing. For those who struggle with restless sleep, these dietary and lifestyle changes will help you rest more soundly. In the meantime, give yourself permission to use naps as appropriate. More sleep recommendations on Day 13.
3. **Stress Reduction:** Stress is counterproductive to healing, and functioning with daily autoimmune symptoms creates its own unique stressors. Do your best to calmly approach dietary change and not fret over the little details. The good news is, by eliminating non-Paleo and non-AIP foods, you reduce stress on the digestive system, which in turn reduces overall stress load. More de-stressing tips on Day 12.
4. **Patience with a Positive Attitude:** You will heal in the manner *you* are supposed to heal, not like anyone else. Do not rely on strict timelines or comparisons between others with similar circumstances. There may be highs, lows and plateaus, but they all mark progress in your healing experience.

5. **Gentle movement:** Talk a daily walk, be part of nature, use calming stretches.
6. **Vitamin D or sunshine:** If you do not spend time in the sun, you need a D3 supplement – more information is in the Resource Section. Discuss medication contraindications and appropriate dosage with your medical providers.

AIP Goal: Over time, you'll understand how to nourish your body to feel your best. At that point, healthy eating will become habit and won't feel like work anymore.

Section IV: AIP Expectations for Healing

Many individuals report that the AIP has given them their lives back, but the process of undoing damage and restoring health takes time. One month of the AIP will set the stage to reestablish your health.

Depending upon the state of your autoimmune condition(s) and current medical protocol, you may find your body needs a longer commitment to the AIP before it is ready for other food reintroductions. It is common to regain abilities and energy over a course of 6-24 months.

How the Body Responds to AIP

1. Expect an initial slump as the body adjusts to the changes (more about Low-Carb Flu in Prep E).
2. After the first month, you may notice less systemic inflammation (joints may move easier, gradually less pain through the body, reduced brain fog, less bloating, better blood pressure).
3. Over time, digestion will heal (especially when incorporating the top 5 restorative foods). Nutrient absorption and energy levels also improve.
4. Gradually you will become more comfortable in your own skin, but not necessarily healed or 'cured.' However, you will gain knowledge of your personal triggers and begin to understand how to move *with* your condition rather than against it.

Realistic Expectations and Reasons to Celebrate

This post appeared on the Phoenix Helix Facebook page on Aug 12, 2015. It is written by Eileen Laird (Phoenix Helix founder) who uses lifestyle interventions to support her rheumatoid arthritis symptoms:

I am not cured. I've never met anyone with autoimmune disease who was cured. Nor am I 100% symptom-free. Complete remission is rare with autoimmunity. I have improved my symptoms by 95% through the autoimmune paleo diet and lifestyle, and where I started (excruciating pain and disability) to where I am today (a full and beautiful life) is night and day. But it's not perfection.

In addition to diet and supplements, I take 1 Aleve tablet twice daily to manage my remaining inflammation. For someone with a severe form of RA, that's amazing, and I'm grateful. It's the only medication I take. I've been honest about this on my blog, but sometimes people miss these details. I'm sharing this today, because I want you to know that if you haven't achieved perfect healing you aren't alone.

Some people need more medication than I do. Some people need less. Some people regain all of their abilities. Some people regain some. I interview a lot of people for my blog and podcast, and I believe every step forward is cause for celebration: any ability you reclaim, and [SIC] pain you relieve, any energy you regain. That's reversing autoimmune disease. It's not about perfection. It's about living your best possible life.

Other Articles on AIP Expectations

- AIPLifestyle You Don't Have to Be an Autoimmune Warrior
- ThePaleoMom How Long Is this Going to Take?
- ThePaleoMom How Do I Know when it's Working?
- PhoenixHelix Top 5 Mistakes People Make on the Paleo AIP

AIP Advantage: Once you know your triggers, it's quite easy to *want* to avoid them because it is not worth feeling rotten. You deserve to know what foods hold you back from your true potential.

Staying on Track

The following template is valuable in adhering to the AIP. Make copies of the plan until you settle into an AIP routine (explanation on using the chart on Day 1). An extra tear-out form is located at the end of this section.

My AIP Paleo Meals			
Meal	**Veggies**	**Protein**	**Healthy Fats**
Breakfast	Green Yellow/Orange Red Blue/Purple/Black White/Tan		
Lunch	Green Yellow/Orange Red Blue/Purple/Black White/Tan		
Dinner	Green Yellow/Orange Red Blue/Purple/Black White/Tan		
Snack	Green Yellow/Orange Red Blue/Purple/Black White/Tan		

Daily Vegetable Allotment	Daily Healing Foods
Record the number of cups you consumed in each category (if a vegetable overlaps, only count it toward one category):	Checkmark each of the top 5 restorative foods you consumed today:

Daily Vegetable Allotment	Daily Healing Foods
Dark-green vegetables such as kale, mustard greens, chard, collards, spinach	Bone broth
Sulfur-rich such as onions, garlic, leeks, chives, mushrooms and brassica family (broccoli, arugula cauliflower, Brussels sprouts, kale, cabbage)	Collagen or gelatin Ginger or turmeric Organ meats or supplement
Deeply-colored like carrots, purple or golden beets, winter squash, pumpkin, olives, herbs	Fatty fish or EPA/DHA
Total of 8-14 cups of vegetables Y N	

Notes (completeness of nutrients / variety, foods you enjoyed, items to include in tomorrow's rotation, etc):

_____

To develop your AIP repertoire, pay attention to the foods you enjoy and wish to include in a more permanent recipe rotation. Highlight, circle, strike through or otherwise rate the AIP meals to plan future meals you enjoy.

Section V: Food Reintroductions after Completing the AIP

The AIP is designed as a temporary, healing diet but there is no one-size-fits-all timeline. Autoimmune disease is not straightforward and healing time differs. For some individuals, additional time on the therapeutic diet is welcomed and/or necessary.

> *Healing is a matter of time, but it is sometimes also a matter of opportunity.* ~Hippocrates

It's okay to continue the AIP for 3, 6 or even 12 months to extend the opportunity for further health benefits. Once an individual gains significant improvement in the Markers of Optimal Health (described on Day 25), the body has sufficiently healed and is ready to test for personal food sensitivities.

1. Take your time when it comes to food reintroductions; carefully separate each group into its distinct foods.
    * For example, yogurt may not induce a negative response whereas soft cheeses do.
2. Reintroduction is the opportunity to determine which foods help you thrive!
3. Leaky gut continues to heal on the AIP and Paleo Protocols. Some foods that cause sensitivities today may not be as troublesome in the future.

> *You deserve to know what foods trigger your flare ups.*

AIP Reintroduction Anomalies

The general Reintroduction Guidelines (Days 25 and 26) lay out the basic rules, but due to the nature of autoimmune disease, there are modifications:

1. Select a single food to reintroduce each cycle (versus multiple items from a related group).
2. Instead of three full servings across the day, take 15 minutes to monitor reactions to the first bite. If no negative response occurs, eat a few more bites and assess for 2-3 hours. If still symptom-free, eat a small serving. Return to the AIP over the observation period (minimum of 3 additional days).
3. If there is a negative reaction, *take the appropriate time to return to a healthy baseline before starting the next reintroduction.* This may increase the waiting period to a 7-day cycle or longer.
4. Some AIP-restricted foods are better to separate into components during reintroduction – for example, plain egg yolks are much better tolerated than either egg whites or whole eggs.
    a. Egg yolk versus egg white (soy-free, pasture-raised eggs are better tolerated than conventional)
    b. Ripe, raw tomatoes versus cooked
    c. Sweet, bell peppers versus hot, chili peppers
    d. Hard cheeses versus soft cheeses
5. Seriously consider never reintroducing gluten. Individuals with autoimmune conditions tend to be highly sensitive to gluten – a single exposure can disrupt health for weeks, if not months.
6. Use AIP-specific guidance during food reintroductions:
    * ThePaleoMom Reintroduction Quick Start-Guide: A New Free Download
    * PhoenixHelix Reintroducing Foods on the Paleo AIP
    * Consult Eileen Laird's ebook, 📖 *The Paleo AIP Reintroduction Guide*
    * Explore online AIP support groups or AIP-specific books for additional assistance

Closing Thoughts

The AIP holds incredible potential to heal the gut lining and reestablish health over time. Though it's not necessarily a cure, it is the biggest self-supporting health tool available to those with autoimmune conditions.

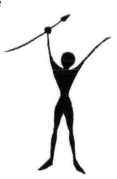

> *In order to change, we need to be sick and tired of being sick and tired.* ~Anonymous

You may or may not be interested in implementing the AIP right now, but always remember this information is available and is right here waiting for you when you're ready.

~ This page intentionally left blank ~

⚡ My AIP Paleo Meals: Day _____			
Meal	**Veggies**	**Protein**	**Healthy Fats**
Breakfast	Green		
	Yellow/Orange		
	Red		
	Blue/Purple/Black		
	White/Tan		
Lunch	Green		
	Yellow/Orange		
	Red		
	Blue/Purple/Black		
	White/Tan		
Dinner	Green		
	Yellow/Orange		
	Red		
	Blue/Purple/Black		
	White/Tan		
Snack	Green		
	Yellow/Orange		
	Red		
	Blue/Purple/Black		
	White/Tan		

Daily Vegetable Allotment	**Daily Healing Foods**
Record the number of cups you consumed in each category (if a vegetable overlaps, only count it toward one category):	Checkmark each of the top 5 restorative foods you consumed today:

	Daily Vegetable Allotment		Daily Healing Foods
	Dark-green vegetables such as kale, mustard greens, chard, collards, spinach		Bone broth
	Sulfur-rich such as onions, garlic, leeks, chives, mushrooms and brassica family (broccoli, arugula cauliflower, Brussels sprouts, kale, cabbage)		Collagen or gelatin
			Ginger or turmeric
			Organ meats or supplement
	Deeply-colored like carrots, purple or golden beets, winter squash, pumpkin, olives, herbs		Fatty fish or EPA/DHA
	Total of 8-14 cups of vegetables, Y/N		

To develop your AIP repertoire, highlight, circle, strike through or otherwise rate the AIP meals to plan future meals you enjoy. Additional notes (completeness of nutrients / variety, flavor combinations you enjoyed, items to include in tomorrow's rotation, etc):

_____

_____

Basic Paleo Meal Template

My Paleo Meals	Date: _____		
Meal	**Veggies**	**Protein**	**Healthy Fats**
Breakfast	Green Yellow/Orange Red Blue/Purple/Black White/Tan		
Lunch	Green Yellow/Orange Red Blue/Purple/Black White/Tan		
Dinner	Green Yellow/Orange Red Blue/Purple/Black White/Tan		
Snack	Green Yellow/Orange Red Blue/Purple/Black White/Tan		

Meal Building

Remember this is not about cutting calories, it's about building nourishing and satisfying meals – portion sizes are to your satisfaction.

Checkmark the meal-building principles you are following well. Circle or highlight the areas for improvement.

- ☐ Eating lots of veggies
- ☐ Eating a colorful range of veggies
- ☐ Eating protein at every meal
- ☐ Eating a wide variety of proteins
- ☐ Eating healthy fats at every meal
- ☐ Adding traditional fats to a naturally lean meal

What is your plan to address any shortcomings and/or build well-balanced Paleo meals tomorrow?

_____

What was your favorite food from today? _____

Quick Paleo Reference Guide

Paleo-Approved Foods

- **Unlimited Vegetables** (organic preferred) – Although classified as a root vegetable, white potatoes are high in starch. If weight loss is a goal, limit consumption until weight tapers. (<u>Note</u>: potato chips and french fries *don't qualify* as whole foods – Tarzan didn't eat them!).

- **Protein from Animal Sources** – Note that *farm-raised* fish and *feedlot* beef/pork/poultry are fed an inflammatory diet high in grains and/or legumes (usually corn and soy) and should be avoided when possible. Lean conventional meats are acceptable if budget is a concern, but realize that the nutritional quality is diminished. In the following list, fats from these natural sources are *anti-inflammatory* – embrace them!
  - Grass-fed beef, bison, lamb, goat
  - Pasture-raised pork
  - Wild caught fish and seafood
  - Pasture-raised, free-range poultry
  - Eggs (from pasture-raised sources)
  - Wild game

- **Healthy Fats/Oils** – Coconut and coconut oil, olives and extra virgin olive oil, avocados, butter/ghee (from grass-fed sources). Note: clarified butter / ghee removes potentially irritating milk proteins.

- **Fruit** occasionally – Focusing on low sugar fruits like berries, green apples, grapefruit, etc. (remember, fruit was not available year-round until recently and has been bred to be increasingly sweeter).

- **Nuts and Seeds** – Those with highest anti-inflammatory properties listed first: macadamias, hazelnuts, cashews, almonds, pecans, pistachios; corresponding nut butters (but not peanuts – they're a legume).

- **Spices** – All spices. FYI, the following have been shown to have high anti-inflammatory properties: turmeric, ginger, garlic, basil, cayenne, cinnamon.

- **Drinks** – Water, coconut water, herbal tea, sparkling water, kombucha (with no sugar added to final product); black tea and coffee if you must (NO fruit juice - it's nearly all sugar, even the 100% varieties).

- **Salad Dressing** – Extra virgin olive oil, vinegar, lemon juice, salsa, guacamole, pureed berries, spices.

- **Treats** occasionally – Dark chocolate 85+% or a periodic Paleo dessert.

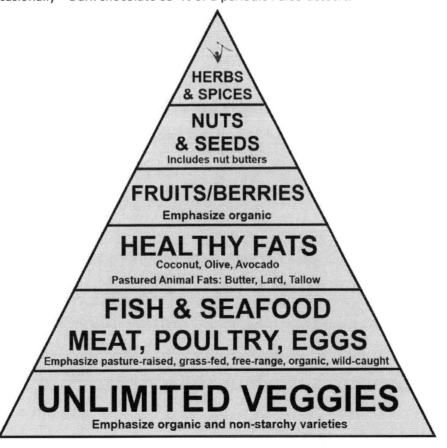

325

~ This page intentionally left blank ~

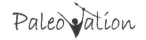 **KITCHEN STOCK-UP: FOODS TO PURCHASE**

Start assembling your Paleo kitchen. Use the following guide to purchase items you want, need and *will actually use* in the next month. Just because they're on the list doesn't mean you have to buy them. An extra tear-out copy is located in the Resource Section. Read labels carefully – common non-Paleo additives are noted.

VEGETABLES

Fresh, frozen, dehydrated and organic are preferred. Nearly all veggies are a thumbs up! Remember, no corn (it's a grain) or legumes (except snow peas, sugar snap peas and green beans – the ones you eat raw in the pod). If weight-loss is a goal, no white, yellow, or red potatoes. Veggie Guide is located on Day 1.

PROTEINS

Emphasize quality sourcing when possible: grass-fed, pastured / pasture-raised, free-range and wild-caught.
- ➤ **Meats** – (Careful! Processed meats often contain sugar and preservatives – select products with less than 1g of carbohydrate per serving, 0g is best) Beef, pork, veal, buffalo, lamb, venison, goat, wild game, bacon, jerky, ground, sausage, soup bones, grass-fed (pastured) hot dogs, organ meats
- ➤ **Poultry / Eggs** – (Read labels, poultry lunch meats often contain carrageenan) Chicken, turkey, duck, goose, Cornish hens, game birds, eggs from well-raised birds (pasture-raised)
- ➤ **Seafood** – Salmon (sockeye red salmon is always wild-caught), cod, perch, whitefish, snapper, halibut, tilapia, herring, grouper, trout, catfish, tuna, lobster, shrimp, mussels, clams, scallops, oysters, calamari, sardines, anchovies, caviar, other shellfish/seafood

NUTS and SEEDS

Dry roasted, in the shell or raw. Macadamias, cashews, hazelnuts, almonds, pecans, pistachios, pumpkin seeds, walnuts, pine nuts, sunflower seeds, sesame seeds, nut butters (no peanut products – legume).

PANTRY

- ☐ Canned fish in 100% olive oil or water (watch for soy, even if packed "in water")
- ☐ Canned vegetables like pumpkin, tomatoes
- ☐ Tomato paste
- ☐ Canned coconut milk
- ☐ Dried seaweed
- ☐ Vinegars (avoid malt, sulfites and sweetened)
- ☐ Coconut butter
- ☐ Broth or Stock (Most have sugar, Imagine® or Costco® organic is okay)
- ☐ Raw or dry roasted nuts and seeds
- ☐ Nut/seed butter (not peanut)
- ☐ Nut flours/meal
- ☐ Arrowroot or tapioca starch/flour (occasional use)
- ☐ Unsweetened applesauce (occasional use in cooking, not as a low-sugar fruit serving)

OILS/FATS

- ☐ Extra virgin coconut oil
- ☐ Extra virgin olive oil (dark bottle and bold taste)
- ☐ Pastured animal fats – lard, duck fat, tallow
- ☐ Drippings from pastured bacon or meats
- ☐ Avocados and avocado oil
- ☐ Olives
- ☐ Grass-fed butter or ghee
- ☐ Unsweetened coconut flakes
- ☐ Walnut, macadamia nut or toasted sesame oils (small amounts occasionally, keep refrigerated)

LOW SUGAR FRUITS

- ☐ Strawberries
- ☐ Raspberries
- ☐ Blackberries
- ☐ Blueberries
- ☐ Lemon
- ☐ Lime
- ☐ Grapefruit
- ☐ Green apples
- ☐ Unripe banana
- ☐ Fresh figs
- ☐ Unsweetened applesauce (occasional use)

SPICE CUPBOARD

- ☐ Salt – Himalayan, Celtic, Real Salt® or sea salt
- ☐ Pepper
- ☐ Sugar-free and additive-free spice mixes
- ☐ Dried herbs
- ☐ Cinnamon
- ☐ Bouillon – Rapunzel® is okay (low-sugar)
- ☐ Onion powder
- ☐ Garlic powder
- ☐ Seaweed flakes
- ☐ Dried mushrooms

FRIDGE

- ☐ Fresh cut veggies, ready to eat
- ☐ Eggs - preferably raised on a pasture
- ☐ Sugar-free mayo like Primal Kitchen® Mayo or Chosen Foods® Avocado Mayo (minimal sugar)
- ☐ 100% olive oil dressings – Tessamae's®, Whole Foods 365® Herbes de Provence, Bolthouse® has one
- ☐ Guacamole – most prepackaged are fine
- ☐ Nut milk, unsweetened (avoid carrageenan, soy lecithin) Silk® or Whole Foods 365® organic are okay
- ☐ Dill pickles (often contain coloring), Vlassic Market® pickles, Bubbies® are okay
- ☐ Fresh herbs (dill, parsley, rosemary, thyme, basil, oregano, chive, etc)
- ☐ Garlic, horseradish or ginger root
- ☐ Sauerkraut (buy refrigerated to preserve healthy bacteria, read label carefully for active, live cultures)
- ☐ Kimchee (watch out for MSG)
- ☐ Fish Sauce like Red Boat® brand
- ☐ Hot sauce (watch for colorings), Cholula® is okay
- ☐ Coconut aminos to replace soy sauce
- ☐ Ketchup by Tessamae's® has a little bit of dates for sweetener (use sparingly)
- ☐ Mustard (most are okay)

FREEZER

- ☐ Frozen burgers (chicken, grass-fed beef, turkey, bison, salmon) for quick protein
- ☐ Other frozen meats (whole chicken, ground beef)
- ☐ Veggies w/no additives
- ☐ Cauliflower rice
- ☐ Puréed veggies to add to soups and sauces
- ☐ Frozen berries
- ☐ Guacamole – purchased guacamole servings can be frozen and put in lunch bags
- ☐ Sausage, easy to make your own and freeze (raw or pre-cooked)
- ☐ Homemade freezer meal
- ☐ Herb purées or minced herbs
- ☐ Soup bones

OTHER

- ☐ Herbal tea
- ☐ Root teas (ginger, turmeric)
- ☐ Other teas
- ☐ Coffee, preferably organic
- ☐ Coconut water (occasional)
- ☐ Kombucha, no sugar added to final product
- ☐ Sparkling water
- ☐ Dark chocolate, soy-free 85%+, (occasional treat)

ᐱ Suggested Foundation Recipes

Note: Additional tips for "batch-cooking" are detailed in Prep E, Section VI

--------------------------------PALEO TURKEY CHILI--------------------------------

Makes 6 servings.

- 3 tablespoons coconut oil, divided
- 1 1/2 pounds ground turkey
- 1 packet organic taco seasoning mix*
- 1 tsp ground coriander
- 1 tsp dried oregano
- 1 tsp red pepper flakes (optional)
- 1 tsp salt
- 1 tsp black pepper
- 2 T tomato paste
- 2 cups beef broth (bone broth!)

- 1 (7 ounce) jar salsa
- 1 (14.5 ounce) can crushed tomatoes
- 1 (7 ounce) can chopped green chili peppers
- 1 medium onion, finely chopped
- 1 green bell pepper, diced
- 3 medium zucchini, halved lengthwise and sliced
- 1 bunch green onions, chopped
- 1 cup guacamole

Directions:

1. Brown turkey in 1 tablespoon of oil in a large stock pot over medium-high heat. Add seasonings and tomato paste. Reduce heat to medium and continue cooking until turkey is well browned.
2. Add broth and simmer about 5 minutes.
3. Add salsa, tomatoes, and green chilies; continue cooking at a moderate simmer for ten minutes.
4. Thin with water if necessary.
5. While chili is simmering, sauté onion and green pepper in 1 tablespoon of oil in a large skillet. Add onion and bell pepper to the chili pot; continue cooking at a very low simmer.
6. In the same skillet, sauté zucchini with the last tablespoon of oil for 2-3 minutes. Add zucchini to the chili, reduce heat and continue cooking 15 minutes more. Adjust the consistency with water as needed.
7. Ladle chili into serving bowls. Top with guacamole, green onion and fresh cilantro if you have it.
   * Spices in place of taco seasoning mix: 1 Tbsp chili powder, 1 ½ tsp ground cumin, 1 tsp garlic powder, 1 tsp onion powder, ½ tsp oregano, ½ tsp paprika, ¼ tsp salt, ¼ tsp cayenne (optional)

--------------------------------FISH CAKES/CASSEROLE--------------------------------

Makes 1 dozen pan-fried cakes, 1 dozen muffins or one loaf pan.

- 10-14 oz canned fish (Read labels to avoid soy. Use tuna, salmon, sardines, mackerel, baby shrimp, etc)
- 2 Tbsp olive, avocado or coconut oil plus extra to grease pans
- 2 eggs, beaten
- 4 cups leftover cooked veggies cut into bite-sized pieces (broccoli, sweet potato, green beans)
- 3 Tbsp green or sweet onion, minced
- ½ tsp lemon zest or juice (zest is the colored outer peel, use a fine grater)
- 2 Tbsp fresh cilantro/parsley, minced (or 1 tsp dried herbs like dill)
- Salt, pepper and/or hot pepper sauce to taste

Directions:

1. Gently mix all ingredients so mixture is still chunky.
2. To pan fry: heat pan to medium-high, add butter, olive or avocado oil, scoop ¼ cup portions onto hot skillet and fry 3-5 minutes per side.
3. For muffins: preheat oven to 350°F, grease muffin tin or use silicon/parchment cup liners, scoop ¼ cup in each muffin cup and bake 20-25 min until eggs is set.
4. For loaf: preheat oven to 350°F, grease loaf pan and bake for 45-50 min until egg is set.

Tip: Leftovers are delicious warm or cold (super easy for a snack or packed lunch). The muffins freeze very well…bake first, then cool and freeze. Quintuple (5x) the recipe to make two 9x13 cake pans (takes 35-40 min to bake), once cool you can even freeze in the pan.

----------------------------SEASONED HAMBURGERS----------------------------

Makes four ¼-pound burgers or three ⅓-pound burgers. Easy to double or triple recipe.

- 1 lb grass-fed ground beef (or mixture of any ground meats)
- 2 cloves garlic, minced
- 2 Tbsp avocado oil (alternatively use olive oil or another Paleo-friendly fat)
- 1 tsp salt (Celtic or Himalayan)
- 1 tsp fresh ground black pepper
- ½ tsp dried basil leaves (or 1 Tbsp fresh chopped)

Directions:
1. Preheat outdoor grill (or optionally, fry in skillet over medium heat).
2. Mix all ingredients and divide into ¼ lb portions and flatten into patties (try a hamburger press to make patties denser and uniform).
3. Grill about 3-5 min on each side or to desired doneness.
4. Serve with lettuce, tomato, pickles, a pat of grass-fed butter and/or guacamole.

Note: Make an ice burg lettuce "bun" – take the whole head of lettuce and cut a semi-circle off either side to form the top and bottom of the bun. This holds together better than a lettuce "wrap" formed from single leaves.

Tip: For a large batch, prepare all into patties, cooking some for immediate use and reserving some for leftovers. Freeze the rest raw on a cookie sheet lined with parchment paper. Once frozen, stack the patties between squares of parchment paper to prevent sticking and freeze in a plastic bag. Cook directly from frozen.

----------------------------COCONUT CURRY----------------------------

Makes 4 servings.

- 1 lb meat of choice cut into bite-sized pieces – chicken, shrimp, pork, beef, mixed seafood, lamb
- 2 Tbsp grass-fed butter or coconut oil
- ½ - 1 onion, chopped
- 2 Tbsp curry powder (most are Paleo-friendly; sweet curry powder is available if for those sensitive to spicy foods)
- ½ - ¾ can of coconut milk
- Variety of bite-size vegetables like carrots, sweet potato, cauliflower, broccoli, green beans, celery, tomato, zucchini, chopped greens
- Salt to taste
- Optional garnish: toasted coconut flakes, chopped green onion, chopped cilantro

Directions:
1. Heat large skillet or stock pot to medium-high and add oil.
2. Sauté onion for 2 min.
3. Add meat and sprinkle on curry powder, mixing to coat evenly. Cook 5 min.
4. Continue cooking the meat and add any hard veggies, cook for 5 min.
5. Add the softer vegetables and coconut milk, reduce heat and simmer for 15-20 min stirring occasionally.
6. Serve with cauliflower rice or in a bowl as a soup.

Tip: You can have two pots cooking simultaneously on the stove top, one for now and one to cool and freeze. If you prefer firmer vegetables, do not cook the softer vegetables for the frozen meal. Instead, chop them up, freeze them raw and add them to the curry when reheating.

-------------------------------TUNA LETTUCE WRAPS-------------------------------

Makes 1-2 servings.

- Can of tuna (read label to avoid soy)
- 1-2 Tbsp olive oil
- Salt and pepper to taste or Paleo All-Purpose Seasoning Salt (see below)
- Fresh veggies cut into strips (carrots, bell peppers, cucumber, celery, kohlrabi, slaw mix)
- Fats like avocado, olives, guacamole, Paleo mayo (Day 4 has directions for Paleo mayonnaise)
- Leaves from romaine or butter lettuce, cabbage sometimes works (smaller heads are better)

Directions:

Mix tuna with oil and seasonings. Open the lettuce leaf and spread in the tuna, some veggies and some fats. Roll up or fold in half, whatever works for your leaf. Optional to secure with toothpick.

-------------------------------ROASTED CHICKEN-------------------------------

Makes 5-7 servings.

- 4-5 lb free range or organic chicken, consider roasting two chickens
- 2 Tbsp grass fed butter or olive oil
- Seasonings of choice: onion powder, garlic powder, parsley, thyme, rosemary, lemon

Directions:

Day 15 has detailed instructions on how to roast a whole chicken as part of Cooking Assignment #4.

-------------------------------ROASTED VEGETABLES-------------------------------

Makes as many servings as you wish to prepare. More detailed instructions in Prep E, Section VI.

- Variety of vegetables cut into evenly sized pieces (onion, carrot, sweet potato, bell pepper, broccoli, cauliflower, green beans, cabbage, beets, turnips, zucchini)
- Olive oil, coconut oil or avocado oil
- Salt and pepper, or Paleo All-Purpose Seasoning Salt (recipe on next page)

Directions:

Preheat oven to 350°F and place vegetables on a cookie sheet. Coat with oil, sprinkle on seasonings and toss to evenly spread. Roast depending on hardness of vegetables...zucchini takes 15-20 minutes, cubed beets take 45-55 min (whole beets up to 90 min). Use a spatula to turn over or stir approximately half-way through roasting for even cooking. Do not be afraid if the vegetables start to brown – they're not burning, they're caramelizing and the flavor is amazing!

-------------------------------CAULIFLOWER RICE -------------------------------

Makes 4-6 servings.

- 1 medium head cauliflower
- Coconut or olive oil
- Seasonings of choice (if desired): sea salt, pepper, garlic, ginger, curry, herbs

Directions:

Grate the cauliflower by hand or run through a food processor using the shredder blade. Heat oil in skillet. Sauté cauliflower for 10 min, adding seasonings if desired. Optional to bake in a 350°F oven for 20 min.

---------------------------------**GUACAMOLE**------------------------------

Makes 2 servings.

- 1 ripe avocado (has a bit of give when you gently squeeze it)
- 1 tsp lime or lemon juice
- Paleo All-Purpose Seasoning Salt to taste
- Optional: chopped onion, chopped jalapeno, hot sauce or salsa

Directions:

Slice avocado in half, spoon out the flesh into a bowl. Mash with a fork, add the rest of the ingredients and mix. Optional: place all ingredients in a food processor and process until smooth.

-----------------------------**PALEO ALL-PURPOSE SEASONING SALT**------------------------------

Makes about 1 cup, stores well.

- ¼ cup salt (sea salt, pink Himalayan, Real Salt®)
- ¼ cup garlic powder
- ¼ cup onion powder
- 2 Tbsp black pepper, ground
- 2 Tbsp paprika
- 2 Tbsp parsley or thyme, dried and ground
- Optional – 1 Tbsp red pepper flakes/chili powder

Directions:

If you have leafy dried herbs, use a mortar/pestle or coffee grinder to pulverize into a powder. Mix all ingredients and store in a glass container or shaker jar. Keeps for months. Use on everything: beef roast, chicken, steamed veggies, marinades, eggs, salad, burgers...

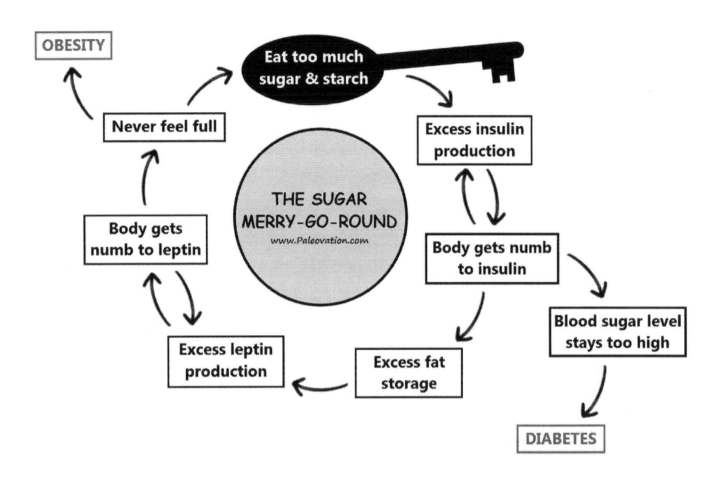

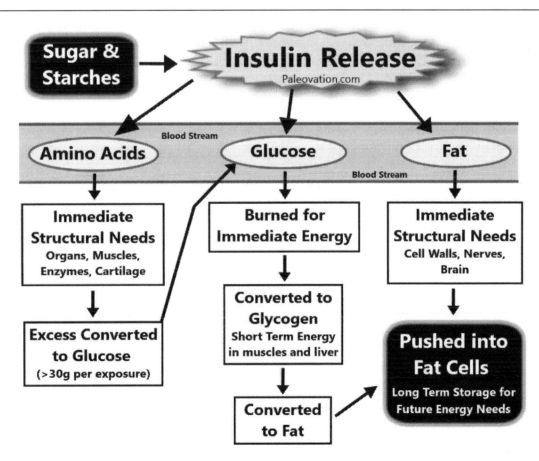

~ This page intentionally left blank ~

~ This page intentionally left blank ~

Science Behind Paleo Cheat Sheet
Problems with the Standard American Diet (even a "healthy" version)

Grains – Inflammatory
- Grains (even whole grains) are starches and break down to pure glucose during digestion
- Grains contain anti-nutrients which bind minerals making them unavailable to the body
- Grains contain certain difficult-to-digest proteins (such as gluten) which cause digestive inflammation and create holes in the intestinal lining, allowing foreign matter to pass directly into the bloodstream

Vegetable Oils (canola, soybean, corn, safflower, sunflower, grapeseed, etc) – Inflammatory and toxic
- Highly susceptible to rancidity with exposure to light and heat
- Highly processed with chemicals, stabilizers and deodorizers, and could never be made at home in a traditional manner (using a pressing or grinding technique)
- Trans fats are inherently created during industrial processing (deodorizing or hydrogenation) and again when heated for cooking; the body uses these damaged fats to build (damaged) cellular membranes
- Comprised mostly of omega-6 oils; though some omega-6 fats are necessary for a healthy diet, this skews the omega-6 to omega-3 ratio which ancestrally was 1:1 or 2:1 and now exceeds 30:1
- When oxidized (rancid) they can cause plaque build-up in the arteries

Legumes – Inflammatory without proper preparation (soaking, fermenting, boiling, sprouting)
- Legumes contain anti-nutrients which bind minerals making them unavailable to the body
- Legumes are high in starch which breaks down to pure glucose in digestion
- Soy contains phytoestrogens which interfere with the body's own hormonal messaging system
- Peanuts often contain aflatoxin, produced by certain molds which is toxic to humans

Dairy – Hormonal influx
- Insulinogenic: dairy product consumption can raise insulin levels leading to insulin resistance (diabetes)
- Contain hormonal and growth signaling messages for a newborn animal but not necessary in adults

Added Sugars and Chemicals – Inflammatory and toxic
- Added sugars contribute to blood sugar spikes and insulin resistance
- Sugar goes by many names and is hidden in nearly all processed foods – sauces, condiments, salad dressings, crackers, yogurt, etc.
- Excitotoxins such as MSG or aspartame cause brain cells to repeatedly fire until they become damaged
- Even FDA-approved GRAS ("Generally Regarded as Safe") additives are known triggers for ill health effects and are often banned in other countries

Other Diet Problems – Omissions and over-consumptions
- Avoidance of cholesterol – Cholesterol is a necessary building block, including the brain, so the body produces most of its own cholesterol. Dietary cholesterol only contributes up to ~5% of blood levels, and though we don't need to consume lots of cholesterol, there's no reason to avoid it.
- Low in protective saturated fats – Natural saturated fats from animals raised on a pasture are stable and contain fat-soluble vitamins necessary for a healthy body.
- Low in traditionally-cooked foods – Eating food cooked on the bone provides more nutrients than boneless/skinless cuts. Time-honored bone broth is incredibly nutritious and healing for the digestive tract. Organ meats are valued in traditional cultures, though are typically avoided in the western diet.
- High in fruits – Originally fruit was only available seasonally and was less sweet. With modern farming practices and availability, many tend to over-consume. Berries and green apples are low sugar fruits.
- Low in vegetables – Vegetables provide a majority of the water, fiber, minerals, vitamins and precursors for the body to produce building blocks for proper functioning and healing. Most people consume just a handful of veggies, but abundant vegetables with a wide variety of deep colors are best.

~ This page intentionally left blank ~

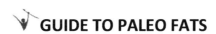 GUIDE TO PALEO FATS

Eliminate the fear that "eating fat makes us fat." Simply incorporate a variety of natural fats and avoid chemically-manufactured fats to replenish our bodies with the nutrients needed to thrive.

Paleo-Approved Fats		
Naturally Saturated	**Monounsaturated**	**Polyunsaturated (Omega 3, 6)**
• Coconut and coconut oil • Palm oil • Grass-fed Butter • Pasture-raised animal fats (lard, tallow, duck fat, etc)	• Olives and olive oil • Avocados and avocado oil • Select nuts, especially macadamias, hazelnuts and cashews (followed by almonds, pecans and pistachios)	3- Wild-caught fatty fish 3- Free range or omega-3 eggs 3- CLA found in pasture-raised red meat and dairy products 3- Fish oil supplements 6- Flax, chia, hemp and walnuts

Healthy Habits for Paleo Fats	
Usage	**Details**
Fats for cooking	Use naturally saturated fats, olive oil or avocado oil
Safest processing	Choose extra virgin, virgin or organic (expeller-pressed is a distant second)
Minimalize oxidation of fragile Paleo-friendly PUFA oils	These oils include walnut oil, flaxseed oil, fish oil ✓ Select oils in dark glass or metal bottles ✓ Refrigerate nut oils and flaxseed oils ✓ Purchase in small amounts and do not store for long periods ✓ Do not heat or cook with these oils
Consume EPA & DHA	Liberally eat sardines, herring, salmon, mackerel, etc; supplement with fish oil*

*Speak to your doctor regarding dosage if you are taking blood thinners or have a bleeding disorder

Unhealthy Products	
Foods to Avoid	**Details**
Industrialized Fats	✓ Read labels to avoid hydrogenated, interesterified, mono/diglycerides ✓ All omega-6 PUFA oils such as canola, soybean, corn, vegetable, safflower, sunflower, cottonseed, etc (the deodorization process creates trans fat) ✓ All processed or restaurant foods where PUFA oils are exposed to heat: *Ask for food to be cooked in butter; buy products with safe cooking fats
Avoid processed "low-fat" products	✓ Low-fat often means high sugar/starch ✓ Healthy fats are removed and replaced with sugars, chemicals, emulsifiers, etc

~ This page intentionally left blank ~

~ This page intentionally left blank ~

Fridge Efficiency Chart

Paleo Vation

Leftovers to Eat

Grocery List

Meal Ideas
+Ingredients to Save

Fresh Foods
Use Immediately

~This page intentionally left blank~

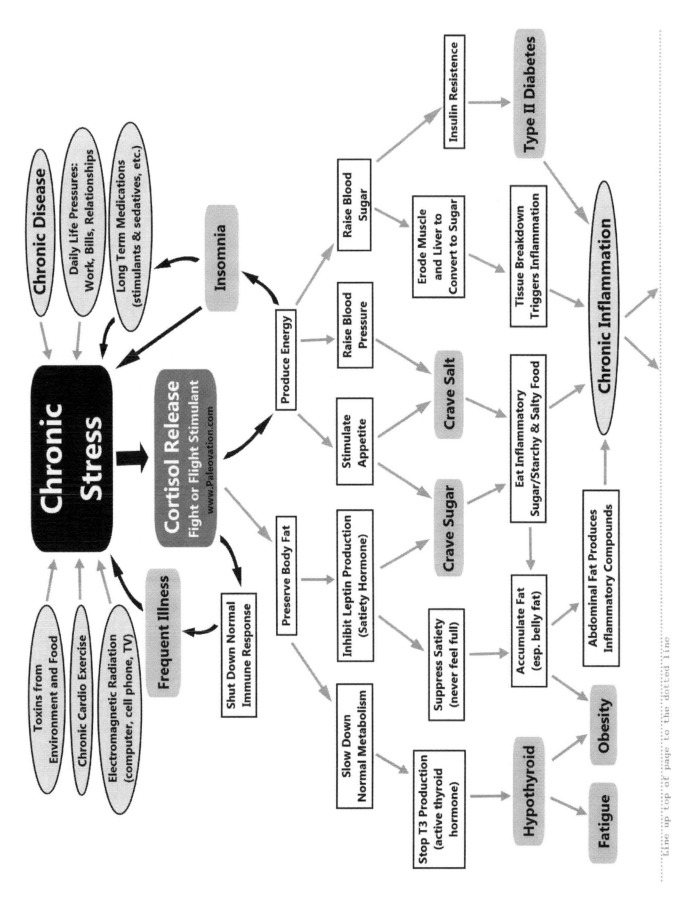

~This page intentionally left blank~

~This page intentionally left blank~

Carb Tolerance Flowchart

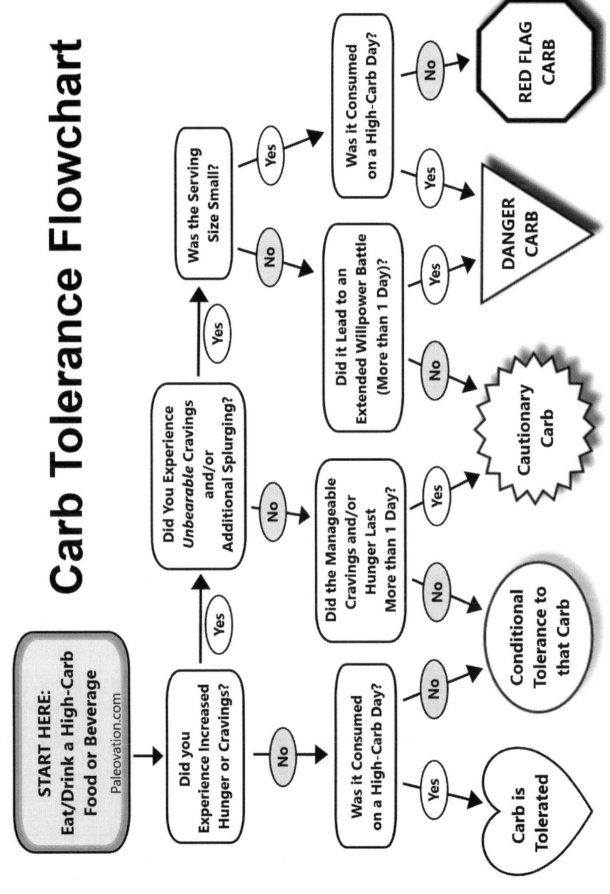

START HERE: Eat/Drink a High-Carb Food or Beverage
Paleovation.com

Did you Experience Increased Hunger or Cravings?

— **Yes** → Did You Experience *Unbearable* Cravings and/or Additional Splurging?

— **No** → Was it Consumed on a High-Carb Day?

Did You Experience *Unbearable* Cravings and/or Additional Splurging?

— **Yes** → Was the Serving Size Small?

— **No** → Did the Manageable Cravings and/or Hunger Last More than 1 Day?

Was the Serving Size Small?

— **Yes** → Was it Consumed on a High-Carb Day?

— **No** → Did it Lead to an Extended Willpower Battle (More than 1 Day)?

Was it Consumed on a High-Carb Day?

— **No** → RED FLAG CARB

— **Yes** → DANGER CARB

Did it Lead to an Extended Willpower Battle (More than 1 Day)?

— **Yes** → DANGER CARB

— **No** → Cautionary Carb

Did the Manageable Cravings and/or Hunger Last More than 1 Day?

— **Yes** → Cautionary Carb

— **No** → Conditional Tolerance to that Carb

Was it Consumed on a High-Carb Day?

— **No** → Conditional Tolerance to that Carb

— **Yes** → Carb is Tolerated

Healthy Baseline Chart

Before you are ready for reintroduction, a "Paleo healthy" needs to be established. During the last week of the program, record the quality of your health as a reference point for future comparison. When you are ready to reintroduce non-Paleo foods, it will be easy to compare your body's response to this baseline. Comment in the notes if extenuating circumstances potentially interfered, such as high pollen count, high stress, etc.

The following body functions are typically affected during reintroduction.

Rate your symptoms from 0 – 3 (0 = no symptoms, 1 = mild, 2= moderate, 3 = severe):

Structure/ Function	Common Symptoms and Ratings	Day 22	Day 23	Day 24	Day 25	Day 26	Day 27	Day 28
Digestion	0 = smooth, efficient digestion and elimination 3 = bloating, stool changes, painful gas, cramps	0 1 2 3	0 1 2 3	0 1 2 3	0 1 2 3	0 1 2 3	0 1 2 3	0 1 2 3
Stomach	0 = comfortable stomach function 3 = heartburn, nausea, 'butterflies'	0 1 2 3	0 1 2 3	0 1 2 3	0 1 2 3	0 1 2 3	0 1 2 3	0 1 2 3
Skin	0 = clear, glowing, supple skin 3 = blemishes, rashes, itching, hives, canker sores	0 1 2 3	0 1 2 3	0 1 2 3	0 1 2 3	0 1 2 3	0 1 2 3	0 1 2 3
Muscles & Joints	0 = good range of motion, strong, pain-free movement 3 = joint/muscle pain, muscle cramps, restricted motion	0 1 2 3	0 1 2 3	0 1 2 3	0 1 2 3	0 1 2 3	0 1 2 3	0 1 2 3
Circulation	0 = normal blood pressure, regular heart rate 3 = abnormal pulse, chest pain, finger/ankle/eye swelling	0 1 2 3	0 1 2 3	0 1 2 3	0 1 2 3	0 1 2 3	0 1 2 3	0 1 2 3
Brain	0 = normal cognition, good memory, ability to focus 3 = foggy, headache, poor concentration, poor memory	0 1 2 3	0 1 2 3	0 1 2 3	0 1 2 3	0 1 2 3	0 1 2 3	0 1 2 3
Mood	0 = even tempered, feeling positive and calm 3 = anxious, depressed, irritable, short temper, angry	0 1 2 3	0 1 2 3	0 1 2 3	0 1 2 3	0 1 2 3	0 1 2 3	0 1 2 3
Sleep	0 = sound sleep, wake up refreshed 3 = insomnia, restlessness, groggy in morning	0 1 2 3	0 1 2 3	0 1 2 3	0 1 2 3	0 1 2 3	0 1 2 3	0 1 2 3
Energy Level	0 = steady, even energy through the day 3 = lethargy, hyper/buzzing, unstable, need to nap	0 1 2 3	0 1 2 3	0 1 2 3	0 1 2 3	0 1 2 3	0 1 2 3	0 1 2 3
Appetite	0 = healthy appetite for meals, no cravings in between 3 = driving hunger, lack of appetite, cravings	0 1 2 3	0 1 2 3	0 1 2 3	0 1 2 3	0 1 2 3	0 1 2 3	0 1 2 3
Sinuses	0 = smooth, clear breathing 3 = stuffed up / congested, runny nose, snoring	0 1 2 3	0 1 2 3	0 1 2 3	0 1 2 3	0 1 2 3	0 1 2 3	0 1 2 3
Immunity	0 = free from symptoms, good overall health 3 = swollen glands, cold/flu symptoms, allergy symptoms	0 1 2 3	0 1 2 3	0 1 2 3	0 1 2 3	0 1 2 3	0 1 2 3	0 1 2 3

Additional Notes:

⚑ Reintroduction Diary for _____

[Food or food group being reintroduced]

Carefully record everything you eat/drink during the entire 4-day reintroduction cycle:
- **Day 1:** Reintroduce the item/group 3-4 times through the day
- **Days 2, 3 and 4:** Return to strict Paleo-eating for observations*

	Day 1	*Day 2	*Day 3	*Day 4
Breakfast				
Lunch				
Dinner				
Snacks				
Beverages				

Rate your response to the reintroduced food on a scale of 0-3 (0 = no symptoms, 1=mild, 2=moderate, 3=severe)

Common Symptoms During Reintroduction	Day 1	Day 2	Day 3	Day 4
Digestive: bloating, stool changes, painful gas, cramps	0 1 2 3	0 1 2 3	0 1 2 3	0 1 2 3
Stomach: heartburn, nausea, 'butterflies'	0 1 2 3	0 1 2 3	0 1 2 3	0 1 2 3
Skin: blemishes, rashes, itching, hives, canker sores	0 1 2 3	0 1 2 3	0 1 2 3	0 1 2 3
Muscle/Joints: joint/muscle pain, cramps, poor motion	0 1 2 3	0 1 2 3	0 1 2 3	0 1 2 3
Circulation: rapid pulse, face flush, finger/ankle/eye swelling	0 1 2 3	0 1 2 3	0 1 2 3	0 1 2 3
Brain: foggy, headache, poor concentration, poor memory	0 1 2 3	0 1 2 3	0 1 2 3	0 1 2 3
Mood: anxious, depressed, irritable, short temper, angry	0 1 2 3	0 1 2 3	0 1 2 3	0 1 2 3
Sleep: insomnia, restlessness, groggy in morning	0 1 2 3	0 1 2 3	0 1 2 3	0 1 2 3
Energy: lethargy, hyper/buzzing, unstable, need to nap	0 1 2 3	0 1 2 3	0 1 2 3	0 1 2 3
Appetite: driving hunger, lack of appetite, cravings	0 1 2 3	0 1 2 3	0 1 2 3	0 1 2 3
Sinuses: stuffed up / congested, runny nose, snoring	0 1 2 3	0 1 2 3	0 1 2 3	0 1 2 3
Immune: swollen glands, cold/flu symptoms, allergy	0 1 2 3	0 1 2 3	0 1 2 3	0 1 2 3

Additional observations (note anything peculiar):

Day 1: _____

Day 2: _____

Day 3: _____

Day 4: _____

Compare these past 3-4 days to your Healthy Baseline Chart to gauge your response to this food.

Definite reaction to this food includes these symptoms: _____

Possible reactions include: _____

Tolerance level to this food: Low   Medium   High

⬇ **Reintroduction Diary for** _____
[Food or food group being reintroduced]

Carefully record everything you eat/drink during the entire 4-day reintroduction cycle:
- **Day 1:** Reintroduce the item/group 3-4 times through the day
- **Days 2, 3 and 4:** Return to strict Paleo-eating for observations*

	Day 1	*Day 2	*Day 3	*Day 4
Breakfast				
Lunch				
Dinner				
Snacks				
Beverages				

Rate your response to the reintroduced food on a scale of 0-3 (0 = no symptoms, 1=mild, 2=moderate, 3=severe)

Common Symptoms During Reintroduction	Day 1	Day 2	Day 3	Day 4
Digestive: bloating, stool changes, painful gas, cramps	0 1 2 3	0 1 2 3	0 1 2 3	0 1 2 3
Stomach: heartburn, nausea, 'butterflies'	0 1 2 3	0 1 2 3	0 1 2 3	0 1 2 3
Skin: blemishes, rashes, itching, hives, canker sores	0 1 2 3	0 1 2 3	0 1 2 3	0 1 2 3
Muscle/Joints: joint/muscle pain, cramps, poor motion	0 1 2 3	0 1 2 3	0 1 2 3	0 1 2 3
Circulation: rapid pulse, face flush, finger/ankle/eye swelling	0 1 2 3	0 1 2 3	0 1 2 3	0 1 2 3
Brain: foggy, headache, poor concentration, poor memory	0 1 2 3	0 1 2 3	0 1 2 3	0 1 2 3
Mood: anxious, depressed, irritable, short temper, angry	0 1 2 3	0 1 2 3	0 1 2 3	0 1 2 3
Sleep: insomnia, restlessness, groggy in morning	0 1 2 3	0 1 2 3	0 1 2 3	0 1 2 3
Energy: lethargy, hyper/buzzing, unstable, need to nap	0 1 2 3	0 1 2 3	0 1 2 3	0 1 2 3
Appetite: driving hunger, lack of appetite, cravings	0 1 2 3	0 1 2 3	0 1 2 3	0 1 2 3
Sinuses: stuffed up / congested, runny nose, snoring	0 1 2 3	0 1 2 3	0 1 2 3	0 1 2 3
Immune: swollen glands, cold/flu symptoms, allergy	0 1 2 3	0 1 2 3	0 1 2 3	0 1 2 3

Additional observations (note anything peculiar):
Day 1: _____
Day 2: _____
Day 3: _____
Day 4: _____

Compare these past 3-4 days to your Healthy Baseline Chart to gauge your response to this food.

Definite reaction to this food includes these symptoms: _____
Possible reactions include: _____

Tolerance level to this food:	Low	Medium	High

⚡ Reintroduction Diary for _____

[Food or food group being reintroduced]

Carefully record everything you eat/drink during the entire 4-day reintroduction cycle:
- **Day 1:** Reintroduce the item/group 3-4 times through the day
- **Days 2, 3 and 4:** Return to strict Paleo-eating for observations*

	Day 1	*Day 2	*Day 3	*Day 4
Breakfast				
Lunch				
Dinner				
Snacks				
Beverages				

Rate your response to the reintroduced food on a scale of 0-3 (0 = no symptoms, 1=mild, 2=moderate, 3=severe)

Common Symptoms During Reintroduction	Day 1	Day 2	Day 3	Day 4
Digestive: bloating, stool changes, painful gas, cramps	0 1 2 3	0 1 2 3	0 1 2 3	0 1 2 3
Stomach: heartburn, nausea, 'butterflies'	0 1 2 3	0 1 2 3	0 1 2 3	0 1 2 3
Skin: blemishes, rashes, itching, hives, canker sores	0 1 2 3	0 1 2 3	0 1 2 3	0 1 2 3
Muscle/Joints: joint/muscle pain, cramps, poor motion	0 1 2 3	0 1 2 3	0 1 2 3	0 1 2 3
Circulation: rapid pulse, face flush, finger/ankle/eye swelling	0 1 2 3	0 1 2 3	0 1 2 3	0 1 2 3
Brain: foggy, headache, poor concentration, poor memory	0 1 2 3	0 1 2 3	0 1 2 3	0 1 2 3
Mood: anxious, depressed, irritable, short temper, angry	0 1 2 3	0 1 2 3	0 1 2 3	0 1 2 3
Sleep: insomnia, restlessness, groggy in morning	0 1 2 3	0 1 2 3	0 1 2 3	0 1 2 3
Energy: lethargy, hyper/buzzing, unstable, need to nap	0 1 2 3	0 1 2 3	0 1 2 3	0 1 2 3
Appetite: driving hunger, lack of appetite, cravings	0 1 2 3	0 1 2 3	0 1 2 3	0 1 2 3
Sinuses: stuffed up / congested, runny nose, snoring	0 1 2 3	0 1 2 3	0 1 2 3	0 1 2 3
Immune: swollen glands, cold/flu symptoms, allergy	0 1 2 3	0 1 2 3	0 1 2 3	0 1 2 3

Additional observations (note anything peculiar):

Day 1: _____

Day 2: _____

Day 3: _____

Day 4: _____

Compare these past 3-4 days to your Healthy Baseline Chart to gauge your response to this food.

Definite reaction to this food includes these symptoms: _____

Possible reactions include: _____

Tolerance level to this food:	Low	Medium	High

⌄ Reintroduction Diary for _____

[Food or food group being reintroduced]

Carefully record everything you eat/drink during the entire 4-day reintroduction cycle:

- **Day 1:** Reintroduce the item/group 3-4 times through the day
- **Days 2, 3 and 4:** Return to strict Paleo-eating for observations*

	Day 1	***Day 2**	***Day 3**	***Day 4**
Breakfast				
Lunch				
Dinner				
Snacks				
Beverages				

Rate your response to the reintroduced food on a scale of 0-3 (0 = no symptoms, 1=mild, 2=moderate, 3=severe)

Common Symptoms During Reintroduction	**Day 1**	**Day 2**	**Day 3**	**Day 4**
Digestive: bloating, stool changes, painful gas, cramps	0 1 2 3	0 1 2 3	0 1 2 3	0 1 2 3
Stomach: heartburn, nausea, 'butterflies'	0 1 2 3	0 1 2 3	0 1 2 3	0 1 2 3
Skin: blemishes, rashes, itching, hives, canker sores	0 1 2 3	0 1 2 3	0 1 2 3	0 1 2 3
Muscle/Joints: joint/muscle pain, cramps, poor motion	0 1 2 3	0 1 2 3	0 1 2 3	0 1 2 3
Circulation: rapid pulse, face flush, finger/ankle/eye swelling	0 1 2 3	0 1 2 3	0 1 2 3	0 1 2 3
Brain: foggy, headache, poor concentration, poor memory	0 1 2 3	0 1 2 3	0 1 2 3	0 1 2 3
Mood: anxious, depressed, irritable, short temper, angry	0 1 2 3	0 1 2 3	0 1 2 3	0 1 2 3
Sleep: insomnia, restlessness, groggy in morning	0 1 2 3	0 1 2 3	0 1 2 3	0 1 2 3
Energy: lethargy, hyper/buzzing, unstable, need to nap	0 1 2 3	0 1 2 3	0 1 2 3	0 1 2 3
Appetite: driving hunger, lack of appetite, cravings	0 1 2 3	0 1 2 3	0 1 2 3	0 1 2 3
Sinuses: stuffed up / congested, runny nose, snoring	0 1 2 3	0 1 2 3	0 1 2 3	0 1 2 3
Immune: swollen glands, cold/flu symptoms, allergy	0 1 2 3	0 1 2 3	0 1 2 3	0 1 2 3

Additional observations (note anything peculiar):

Day 1: _____

Day 2: _____

Day 3: _____

Day 4: _____

Compare these past 3-4 days to your Healthy Baseline Chart to gauge your response to this food.

Definite reaction to this food includes these symptoms: _____

Possible reactions include: _____

Tolerance level to this food: Low   Medium   High

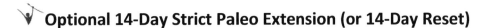 Optional 14-Day Strict Paleo Extension (or 14-Day Reset)

Carefully build your meals over the next 14 days to extend the program and encourage further healing. There will be a Post-Extension Check-Out form at the end of the additional two weeks.

Suggestions for Your Extension:

1. For portion-size recommendations, review Day 2, Section II: Building a Paleo Meal.
2. If interested, the AIP Guidelines in the Resource Section include a more extensive Meal Template detailing types of vegetables eaten through the day plus additional suggestions for anti-inflammatory and gut-healing foods such as bone broth, turmeric, EPA/DHA, etc.
3. Additional tactics to boost the benefits of the Strict Paleo Protocol are offered on Day 25, Section II: Tweaking Your Paleo Protocol.
4. The Supplement Guide in the Resource Section describes specific nutrients that are difficult to attain from food alone. If you are still not feeling well, consider adding a few recommended vitamins, minerals or anti-inflammatory supplements to your routine.

My Paleo Meals: Extension Day 1			
Meal	**Veggies**	**Protein**	**Healthy Fats**
Breakfast	Green Yellow/Orange Red Blue/Purple/Black White/Tan		
Lunch	Green Yellow/Orange Red Blue/Purple/Black White/Tan		
Dinner	Green Yellow/Orange Red Blue/Purple/Black White/Tan		

Evaluate your day. Check the Paleo principles you followed well (add any missed food categories tomorrow):

☐ Lots of veggies   ☐ Colorful range of veggies   ☐ Wide variety of proteins   ☐ Traditional fats

My Paleo Meals: Extension Day 2			
Meal	**Veggies**	**Protein**	**Healthy Fats**
Breakfast	Green Yellow/Orange Red Blue/Purple/Black White/Tan		
Lunch	Green Yellow/Orange Red Blue/Purple/Black White/Tan		
Dinner	Green Yellow/Orange Red Blue/Purple/Black White/Tan		

My Paleo Meals: Extension Day 3			
Meal	**Veggies**	**Protein**	**Healthy Fats**
Breakfast	Green Yellow/Orange Red Blue/Purple/Black White/Tan		
Lunch	Green Yellow/Orange Red Blue/Purple/Black White/Tan		
Dinner	Green Yellow/Orange Red Blue/Purple/Black White/Tan		

My Paleo Meals: Extension Day 4			
Meal	**Veggies**	**Protein**	**Healthy Fats**
Breakfast	Green Yellow/Orange Red Blue/Purple/Black White/Tan		
Lunch	Green Yellow/Orange Red Blue/Purple/Black White/Tan		
Dinner	Green Yellow/Orange Red Blue/Purple/Black White/Tan		

My Paleo Meals: Extension Day 5			
Meal	**Veggies**	**Protein**	**Healthy Fats**
Breakfast	Green Yellow/Orange Red Blue/Purple/Black White/Tan		
Lunch	Green Yellow/Orange Red Blue/Purple/Black White/Tan		
Dinner	Green Yellow/Orange Red Blue/Purple/Black White/Tan		

My Paleo Meals: Extension Day 6			
Meal	**Veggies**	**Protein**	**Healthy Fats**
Breakfast	Green Yellow/Orange Red Blue/Purple/Black White/Tan		
Lunch	Green Yellow/Orange Red Blue/Purple/Black White/Tan		
Dinner	Green Yellow/Orange Red Blue/Purple/Black White/Tan		

My Paleo Meals: Extension Day 7			
Meal	**Veggies**	**Protein**	**Healthy Fats**
Breakfast	Green Yellow/Orange Red Blue/Purple/Black White/Tan		
Lunch	Green Yellow/Orange Red Blue/Purple/Black White/Tan		
Dinner	Green Yellow/Orange Red Blue/Purple/Black White/Tan		

My Paleo Meals: Extension Day 8			
Meal	**Veggies**	**Protein**	**Healthy Fats**
Breakfast	Green Yellow/Orange Red Blue/Purple/Black White/Tan		
Lunch	Green Yellow/Orange Red Blue/Purple/Black White/Tan		
Dinner	Green Yellow/Orange Red Blue/Purple/Black White/Tan		

My Paleo Meals: Extension Day 9			
Meal	**Veggies**	**Protein**	**Healthy Fats**
Breakfast	Green Yellow/Orange Red Blue/Purple/Black White/Tan		
Lunch	Green Yellow/Orange Red Blue/Purple/Black White/Tan		
Dinner	Green Yellow/Orange Red Blue/Purple/Black White/Tan		

My Paleo Meals: Extension Day 10			
Meal	**Veggies**	**Protein**	**Healthy Fats**
Breakfast	Green Yellow/Orange Red Blue/Purple/Black White/Tan		
Lunch	Green Yellow/Orange Red Blue/Purple/Black White/Tan		
Dinner	Green Yellow/Orange Red Blue/Purple/Black White/Tan		

My Paleo Meals: Extension Day 11			
Meal	**Veggies**	**Protein**	**Healthy Fats**
Breakfast	Green Yellow/Orange Red Blue/Purple/Black White/Tan		
Lunch	Green Yellow/Orange Red Blue/Purple/Black White/Tan		
Dinner	Green Yellow/Orange Red Blue/Purple/Black White/Tan		

My Paleo Meals: Extension Day 12			
Meal	**Veggies**	**Protein**	**Healthy Fats**
Breakfast	Green Yellow/Orange Red Blue/Purple/Black White/Tan		
Lunch	Green Yellow/Orange Red Blue/Purple/Black White/Tan		
Dinner	Green Yellow/Orange Red Blue/Purple/Black White/Tan		

My Paleo Meals: Extension Day 13			
Meal	**Veggies**	**Protein**	**Healthy Fats**
Breakfast	Green Yellow/Orange Red Blue/Purple/Black White/Tan		
Lunch	Green Yellow/Orange Red Blue/Purple/Black White/Tan		
Dinner	Green Yellow/Orange Red Blue/Purple/Black White/Tan		

My Paleo Meals: Extension Day 14			
Meal	**Veggies**	**Protein**	**Healthy Fats**
Breakfast	Green Yellow/Orange Red Blue/Purple/Black White/Tan		
Lunch	Green Yellow/Orange Red Blue/Purple/Black White/Tan		
Dinner	Green Yellow/Orange Red Blue/Purple/Black White/Tan		

Markers of Health Quiz

At the end of Extension Day 14, note how many of these markers of health apply to you:

Markers for Optimal Health	
☐ Excitement about your body's potential	☐ Clear skin
☐ Over the hump of the low-carb flu	☐ Stable energy levels
☐ Sound sleep	☐ Enjoying being active
☐ Noticeable relief of aches/pains	☐ Improved exercise recovery
☐ Increased range of motion	☐ Healthier food relationship (ex: no stress-eating)
☐ Comfortable stool consistency & frequency	☐ Mind/Body/Spirit feel balanced
☐ Improved digestion	☐ Improved ability to cope with stress
☐ Headache relief	☐ Better libido
☐ Hunger/cravings controlled	☐ Improved concentration and focus
☐ Better hormonal balance	☐ Mood stabilization
☐ Increased brain function	☐ Fat-adapted status

Compare your results with your responses from Day 25 to quantify your progress:
Have you achieved a better health profile? Do you feel you could make more gains than you already have?
Explain:

_____

_____

Fill out the Post-Extension Check-Out form on the next page to help with decision-making about the next step to support your total health.

Post-Extension Check-Out Form   Date: _____

Please record any specific observations or clarifications in the notes below.	Strongly Disagree -2	Disagree -1	Neutral 0	Agree +1	Strongly Agree +2	Blown Away +3
I have even energy levels throughout the day.	☐	☐	☐	☐	☐	☐
I fall asleep easily and sleep soundly.	☐	☐	☐	☐	☐	☐
I rarely have food cravings.	☐	☐	☐	☐	☐	☐
I'm satisfied with both my hunger levels and my response to hunger.	☐	☐	☐	☐	☐	☐
My joints and tendons are comfortable and work smoothly.	☐	☐	☐	☐	☐	☐
I am satisfied with my range of motion (flexibility) throughout my body.	☐	☐	☐	☐	☐	☐
I have relatively few aches or pains (including neck, back, headache, joint, muscle, etc).	☐	☐	☐	☐	☐	☐
I am satisfied with my athletic performance and body's response to physical activity.	☐	☐	☐	☐	☐	☐
My body heals quickly from overuse or injury.	☐	☐	☐	☐	☐	☐
My immune system functions properly (rarely catch a cold, recover from illness well, etc).	☐	☐	☐	☐	☐	☐
My skin, complexion, hair, nails, teeth and gums are all healthy and strong.	☐	☐	☐	☐	☐	☐
My moods are stable and easy to control.	☐	☐	☐	☐	☐	☐
I am satisfied with my mental clarity and ability to focus.	☐	☐	☐	☐	☐	☐
In general, I am able to calmly respond to stressful situations.	☐	☐	☐	☐	☐	☐
My digestion functions properly (no stomach cramps, heartburn, bloating, painful gas, etc).	☐	☐	☐	☐	☐	☐
My elimination function is normal and comfortable (no diarrhea, constipation, etc).	☐	☐	☐	☐	☐	☐

*This category is provided for improvements that truly were above and beyond expectations

Notes:

Post-Extension Check-Out Form

Score your form below. A "Strongly Agree" response is +2 points, a "Strongly Disagree" is -2, and Neutral is zero. The "blown away" category scores +3!

Extension Day 14: Post-Extension Check-Out Score: _____

Go back to compare your responses:

Prep C: Pre-Paleo Check-In Score: _____

Day 28: Post-Paleo Check-Out Score: _____

How do you feel about your progress at this point?

_____

Where have you made your biggest health gains?

_____

Are there any issues that are slow to improve or not improving at all?

_____

Are you satisfied with your progress?   Yes   No   Not sure

Potential Autoimmune Condition

Including this 2-week extension, which of these symptoms persist after 42 Days on the Strict Paleo Protocol?

Continued Health Complications		
Fatigue	Inability to lose weight	Memory issues
Muscle weakness	Yeast infections	Allergies
Low immune system	Bowel issues	Rashes
Swollen glands	Anxiety/depression	PMS
Poor sleep	Migraines	Thyroid problems
Low blood sugar	Absence of any of the optimal health markers listed above	

After reviewing this list of continued complications, do you wish to continue tweaking the diet to find better health?   Yes   No   Explain:

_____

The more issues persisting after this length of time following strict Paleo, the higher the chance you may feel better following the stricter Autoimmune Protocol (AIP)*. If you are unsure about your next step, read about the Autoimmune Protocol (AIP). Details and additional resources are listed in the AIP Guidelines located in the Resource Section.

Further Reading:
- ThePaleoMom The Autoimmune Protocol
- ThePaleoMom You May Have an Autoimmune Disease but Don't Know It

Healthy Baseline: We want you to feel exceptional before you reintroduce any foods...this is the only way you can compare potential reactions to how good you *know you feel* without those foods.

Are you ready to begin reintroductions? Explain:

_____

_____

⍦ Nutritional Supplements

A Case for Adding Supplements
When pursuing optimal health, quality diet is the first priority; nutritional supplements are second. Ideally, eating nutrient-dense Paleo foods alone would eliminate the need for nutritional supplements. Though diet is clearly a starting place, realistically, it's difficult to eat exclusively Paleo and our food supply is imperfect. It's challenging to regularly consume all necessary nutrients in sufficient amounts for a variety of reasons:
1. **Limited Food / Nutrient Variety**
   a. **Seasonal** – Some nutrients are only attainable during limited times of the year: Vitamin D from sun exposure is at risk for deficiency during cool seasons or if sunscreen is regularly used
   b. **Regional** – Certain key nutrients are limited by region:
      i. **Iodine** – Found in sea greens, sea salt and coastal areas but deficient in inland regions
      ii. **EPA/DHA** – Best source is small fatty fish but difficult to find locally in arid climates
      iii. **Selenium and Magnesium** – Over-farmed areas have depleted soil and inadequate amounts
   c. **Habits**
      i. **Unfamiliarity** – Foods with exceptional nutrients are either avoided or not consumed in sufficient quantities: sardines, fermented foods, organ meats, seaweed or bitter greens
      ii. **Limited Food Variety** – Most regular meal rotations include only a handful of vegetables and 2-3 meat/protein sources
      iii. **Processed Convenience Foods** – High processed food intake restricts nutrient quality and quantity
2. **Compromised Quality**
   a. **Poor Agricultural and Animal Husbandry Standards:** Non-organic produce or CAFO animal products fail to maximize nutrient content and are tainted with antibiotic, hormone and chemical residues
   b. **Interference from Other Foods:**
      i. Phytates in grains and legumes interfere with mineral absorption
      ii. Lectins in grains and legumes damage gut lining and contribute to toxin exposure
   c. **Commercial Agricultural Practices**
      i. **Depleted Soil:** Reduces trace minerals and microorganism activity
      ii. **Limited Fertilizers:** Only replace several minerals; trace minerals are depleted
      iii. **Contamination:** Pesticide, herbicide and fungicide toxin residues
      iv. **Irradiation:** This process increases produce shelf life but reduces vitamins and enzymes
   d. **Industrial Processing**
      i. Preservatives, colorings, flavor enhancers, etc interfere with nutrient availability
      ii. Heating, spray-drying or flash cooking damages fragile nutrients (EPA/DHA or vitamin C)
      iii. Toxin residues from bleaching, separating, extracting, flavoring, etc

Supplement Regimens
Depending on state of health, history of illness, genetics, current stress levels, etc, supplementation can be a valid method to fill in nutritional gaps either temporarily or as long-term support (itemized in the next tables).
1. **Temporary** – Taking specific supplements for a particular therapeutic purpose for a fixed period of time
2. **Therapeutic** – To support long-standing, chronic health problems; may be temporary or long term
3. **Maintenance** – Some nutrients are universally difficult to attain from diet alone; almost everyone would benefit from supplementing these on a regular or semi-regular basis

Consider Professional Assistance
The following table presents general supplementation guidelines for a few commonly deficient key nutrients; however nutritional needs vary (see Supplement Chart for details). Although supplementation can be self-administered and managed, those with complicated health conditions will benefit from assistance with selection, quantity and duration of supplements. Consider consulting a knowledgeable healthcare provider who can screen medication contraindications, monitor personal progress and recommend adjustments to your plan.

Maintenance Supplements[†] – Nutrients Universally Difficult to Attain from Diet Alone			
Nutrient[‡]	**Source**	**Function**	**How Much**
Vitamin D3* (Read more about vitamin D3 in Bone Health on Day 16 and Cholesterol on Day 17)	✓ Sunlight ✓ Vitamin D3 is compromised with low sun exposure or regular sunscreen use ✓ There are no foods that can possibly provide the entire required amount	• Proper bone formation • Calcium absorption • Neuromuscular health • Anti-viral • Anti-inflammatory	4000-5000 IU/day, or enough to maintain blood levels of 25-OHD* in the range of 40-60 mg/mL **Note:** The FDA approves 2000 IU daily as a base dose
Magnesium	✓ Vegetables, fruits, grazing animal products – due to modern agricultural soil depletion, these foods tend not to contain sufficient quantities of magnesium	• Bone formation - more than half of the body's magnesium is in the bones • Muscle relaxer • Natural laxative • Encourages restful sleep • Cofactor in over 300 enzyme reactions	Best bioavailability tends to be forms ending in *'ate'* for (ex: citrate, aspartate, malate); 400mg/day
EPA/DHA (Read more about EPA/DHA on Day 3) *Note:* Flax only contains ALA which does not convert well to EPA/DHA	✓ Oily fish ✓ Fats from grass-fed or wild animals ✓ Shellfish ✓ Egg yolks ✓ Seaweed	• Anti-inflammatory • Protects against heart disease, joint pain • Supports immune system • *Major* component of brain health • Mild laxative	1000-3000mg (1-3g) daily
Probiotic + **Prebiotics** + **Soil-Based Organisms (SBOs)** (Read more on Gut Health on Day 21)	**Probiotic:** Fermented foods (sauerkraut, kefir, yogurt, kimchi, kombucha), products labeled *raw, unpasteurized* or *'contains live cultures'* as heat kills the beneficial organisms **Prebiotic:** Resistant starch **SBOs:** Healthy soils	• Help digest food • Synthesize and activate B vitamins and vitamin K2 • Breakdown complex lipids and cholesterol • Strengthen immune system • Improve cholesterol ratios • Displace harmful gut flora	✓ **Probiotics:** Variety of *Lactobacillus & Bifidobacterium* strains – usually refrigerated are best, 10-50 billion ✓ **SBOs:** *Prescript Assist* or *MegaSpore:* follow product label
Iodine **Caution:** Those with autoimmune thyroid issues must consult a healthcare professional and co-supplement with selenium	✓ Celtic sea salt (Himalayan pink salt has a trace) ✓ Shellfish ✓ Ocean fish ✓ Seaweed (dulse, kelp, nori, kombu, wakame) – amount varies by product	• Thyroid support which regulates metabolism, body temperature, weight gain/loss, energy levels • Protective for breast tissue • Protective against radioactive iodine exposure	Varies: 225mcg-12mg (*yes* a very large range) depending the expert opinion consulted and personal health status. Often better to take with selenium. Start at lower doses and gradually increase.

† These statements have not been evaluated by the Food & Drug Administration. These products are not intended to diagnose, treat, cure or prevent any disease.

‡ Some supplements may cause initial digestive upset as the body acclimates to the influx of nutrients. If any unusual symptoms develop, discontinue, then try reinstating at a lower dosage and gradually increase.

* Vitamin D level can be tested with the *25-hydroxyvitamin D* (also abbreviated as 25(OH)D or 25-OHD). Levels tend to fluctuate seasonally with sunshine exposure.

Temporary Supplements[†] – May need short term while transitioning to Paleo			
Nutrient[‡]	**Source**	**Function**	**How Much**
Digestive Enzymes Genetics or health conditions can prevent sufficient production of particular enzymes **Enzyme Categories:** **Amylase** – carbohydrates **Protease** – proteins **Lipase** – fats	**Mouth** - carbohydrate digestion begins with saliva **Stomach** – protein digestion begins here **Pancreas** – releases enzymes that digest starches, fats and protein **Small Intestine** – digestion and absorption of sugars, amino acids and fatty acids **Raw Foods** – cooking destroys enzymes	Breaks down foods into the smallest possible size for better absorption and best nutrient extraction.	Follow packaging for starting dose. Generally okay to increase dosage (one extra pill per sitting) until a 'burning sensation' registers (drink water then to dilute). Highest dose is then one pill less than the number that caused the warmth.
Carb Craving Product (such as: *Pure Encapsulations* CarbCrave)	A variety of amino acids, vitamins and trace minerals necessary for healthy carbohydrate metabolism	Supports neurotransmitters that control mood and appetite. Used short-term to ease into fat-burning mode.	Follow product directions. **Caution:** often interferes with SSRI prescriptions.
Liver and Detoxification Support (such as: *Pure Encapsulations* Detox Pure Pack)	A variety of trace minerals, amino acids and antioxidant micronutrients which support the liver (ex: broccoli, milk thistle, silymarin, curcumin, artichoke, glutathione, NAC, chlorella, taurine, etc)	Assist the liver by providing nutrients necessary for effective detoxification pathways.	Follow product directions.

† These statements have not been evaluated by the Food & Drug Administration. These products are not intended to diagnose, treat, cure or prevent any disease.

‡ Some supplements may cause initial digestive upset as the body acclimates to the influx of nutrients. If any unusual symptoms develop, discontinue, then try reinstating at a lower dosage and gradually increase.

Additional Hard-to-Attain Nutrients

Other choices for supplementation include vitamin K2, methyl-B12, trace minerals, desiccated liver, selenium, turmeric and collagen/gelatin. Though a well-rounded diet of high quality produce, animal products and real salt provides these nutrients, some prefer to supplement for 'insurance' or an occasional nutrition boost.

Choose Quality! (You Get What You Pay For)

The US government does not regulate supplement production, so manufacturers rely on third-party inspections to establish purity and quality. Good manufacturing practices (GMP) are evaluated and include verification of ingredients, cleanliness of the facilities and testing of final products. The GMP are *voluntary guidelines* issued by the FDA to ensure the label accurately reflects the contents of the bottle. Quality companies will use third-party verification to certify their products. Look for these labels:

- NSF International – also certifies GMP
- United States Pharmacopeia (USP)
- Consumer Labs

Choose the highest quality you can afford from a reputable source or healthcare professional. Also scan labels for artificial colors, flavorings or added sugar.

🖰 PureRXO.com/Paleovation

This partner site offers many brands of quality, pharmaceutical-grade products. Nearly all the above recommendations can be found at the online store. Select 'My Picks' for our preferred products.

~ This page intentionally left blank ~

⅄ **Optional Nutritional Supplement Chart**

This chart is included for those who wish to supplement nutrients. The listed supplements are difficult to attain via diet alone and are offered as suggestions. Please read Nutritional Supplements in the Resource Section for more specific information. To personalize this chart for your deficiencies, work with a healthcare practitioner[†].

<u>Caution</u>: *Check contraindications to current prescriptions, over-the-counter medications or other supplements.*

✓	Supplement	Daily Dosage	Comments	Provider Notes
☐	**Vitamin D3**	2000 IU, test blood levels for higher dose	Maintain 25-OHD blood test at 40-60ng/mL	
☐	**Magnesium**	400 mg	Other sources: Epsom Salt bath, EASE magnesium oil	
☐	**EPA / DHA**	1000-3000 mg (1-3g)	ALA form from flax does not provide EPA/DHA	
☐	**Probiotic**	10-50 billion CFU (colony forming units)		
☐	**Soil-Based Organisms (SBOs)**	*	Brands: Prescript Assist or MegaSpore	
☐	**Iodine*** (consider taking with selenium)	Large range: 225mcg – 12mg, supervision needed for high doses	Start small and work up to dose; *autoimmune thyroid must consult a professional*	
☐	**Digestive Enzymes** Until digestion mends	*	Take before meals, reduce dosage if burning sensation	
☐	**Vitamin K2**	180mcg	MK-4 and MK-7 forms	
☐	**Vitamin B12**	1-3 mg (1000-3000mcg)	Choose Methyl-B12 or methylcobalamin form	
☐	**Multi-Trace Minerals** Many in this category	*	Ex: chromium, manganese, selenium, boron, zinc, copper	
☐	**Desiccated Liver**	*	Vital Proteins, Radiant Life or Dr. Ron's are quality brands	
☐	**Turmeric (curcumin) and/or Ginger**	*	Available in capsules, tablets, powdered, fresh, extracts, tea	
☐				
☐				
☐				
☐				
☐				
☐				

[†] **Healthcare Professionals:** Personalize for your client

*Follow product label.

~ This page intentionally left blank ~

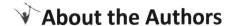 About the Authors

Kelly C. Andrews, DC

Kelly has been a staff chiropractor at Group Health Cooperative of South Central Wisconsin since 1992. She received her bachelor's degree in biochemistry and nutrition from the University of Wisconsin in 1984 and her doctor of chiropractic degree from Palmer Chiropractic University in 1987. She is a Certified Nutritional Counselor in the state of Wisconsin.

Rachel D. Carlson, BS, RYT

Rachel received her bachelor's degree in mathematics and secondary education from the University of Wisconsin in 1998 and completed her 200RYT yoga teacher training at Jiva Yoga Center in 2017. She has taught a wide variety of subjects in both the public and private sectors (math, dietary change, music, swim, cooking, organizational skills). She is a registered yoga teacher with Yoga Alliance.

Paleovation, LLC

A chance meeting – that was all it took for Kelly and Rachel to discover that, not only are they both passionate about nutrition, diet and maximizing health naturally, but also about sharing their success by supporting others.

Kelly's experience in healthcare, nutrition and exercise combined with Rachel's background in education, cooking and yoga is the perfect combination to educate and assist others with adopting a healthy diet and lifestyle. Their initial venture involved developing a class to guide participants through the first month of Paleo. *The Paleovation Workbook* is a natural progression of their efforts – and the Group Manual in the Resource Section is based on their class structure.

The term, "Paleovation," was coined to represent the merging between the anti-inflammatory Paleo Diet and the ovation one deserves for implementing healthful, revitalizing food choices and releasing old dietary habits.

Paleovation® is a registered trademark.

~ This page intentionally left blank ~

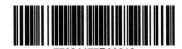

Made in the USA
Lexington, KY
30 December 2017